STUDIES IN INFLUENZA AND PNEUMONIA

E. C. Rosenow
Mayo Foundation

An 11-part series

As originally published in the

Journal of the American Medical Association, 1919
Volumes 72 (31-4, 1604-9) and 73 (396-401)
and the
Journal of Infectious Diseases, 1920
Volume 26 (469-622)

***

APPENDIX A

E. C. Rosenow, *Minnesota Med.*, June 1929, 12, 366-368

APPENDIX B

E.C. Rosenow, *A.M.A. Arch. Otolaryng.* 58: 609-622, Nov. 1953

***

FOREWORD
Pandemic Centennial
By S. H. Shakman

AFTERWORD
Influenza, Encephalitis, Implications
By S. H. Shakman

INSTITUTE OF SCIENCE
InstituteOfScience.com / I-o-S.org

©Copyright S. H. Shakman 2014, 2018

All rights reserved. No part of the Foreword of this book (or related materials posted on the world-wide-web under the auspices of the INSTITUTE OF SCIENCE via www.instituteofscience.com or associated sites) may be integrated into any database, public or private, or reproduced or transmitted in any form by any means - except by a reviewer who may quote brief passages in a review - without written permission of the publisher. For information please contact:

INSTITUTE OF SCIENCE
1217 Wilshire Blvd., #3234
Santa Monica, CA 90403

InstituteOfScience.com / I-o-S.org
mail@InstituteOfScience.com / mail@I-o-S.org
phone: 1-424-248-5635

Published by the INSTITUTE OF SCIENCE

First Printed 2014; reprinted February 16, 2018, with a revised Foreword.

Warning and Disclaimer: Although every possible effort has been made to assure the accuracy and correctness of information herein, the publisher hereby: apologizes and disclaims liability for any errors which have escaped editing; and disclaims any and all medical or legal liability in the event the contents of this book are utilized as a direct source of any dental or medical advice. The reader is encouraged to access original works discussed herein to assure accuracy of information, particularly on such critical matters as vaccine preparation, etc., and to refer any medical questions concerning discussions herein and related medical treatment to appropriate professionals. A proper professional assessment of all of a person's medical conditions must always be taken into account prior to development of a treatment plan. In this regard, as differing professional opinions abound, a "second opinion" (or more) is highly recommended.

Printed in the United States of America

CONTENTS

FOREWORD – Pandemic Centennial by S. H. Shakman.................……. i-xii

Studies in Influenza and Pneumonia by E.C. Rosenow MD

Jour. Am. Med. Assn. 1919, Vol. 72-73
  I. "Prophylactic inoculation against respiratory infections
  during the present pandemic of influenza. Preliminary report."
  (Vol. 72) ………………………………..……………… [31-4]* …… 1-7

  II. "The experimental production of symptoms and lesions
  simulating those of influenza with streptococci isolated during the
  present pandemic." (Vol. 72) ………………..………… [1604-1607] …… 8-15

  III. "The occurrence of a pandemic strain of streptococcus during
  the pandemic of influenza.". (Vol. 72) ……....……… [1608-1609]…… 16-18

  IV. "Further results of prophylactic inoculation." (With B.F. Sturdivant),
  (Vol. 73) …………………………………….………….. [396-401]…… 19-29

Jour. Infect. Dis. 1920, Vol.26 ……………..……… [469-622+11 plates] … (30-194)
  V. "Observations on the bacteriology and certain clinical features of
  influenza and influenzal pneumonia." ………....………. [469-91] …….. 30-52

  VI. The leukocytic reaction in influenza and influenzal pneumonia."
  ……………………………………………………….... [492-503] …… 53-64

  VII. "A study of the effects following the injection of bacteria found in
  influenza in normal throats, in simple nasopharyngitis, and in lobar
  pneumonia." ……………………………………………. [504-556] ….. 65-117
      Plates ... [pages not numbered in original article – 556a-556k] …. 118-128

  VIII. "Experiments on the etiology of "gastrointestinal" influenza."
  ……………………………………………………..………. [557-566] ….. 129-138

  IX. "Changes in the green-producing streptococcus induced by
  successive animal passage and their significance in epidemic
  influenza." ……………………………………......………… [567-596] ……. 139-168

  X. "The immunologic properties of the green-producing streptococci
  from influenza. …………………………………………….. [597-613] ….. 169-185

  XI. Therapeutic effects of a monovalent antistreptococcus serum in
  influenza and influenzal pneumonia." ………………… [614-622] ….. 186-194

  * [WHITE numbers on BLACK background denote original article page numbers]

APPENDIX A: Rosenow, E.C., "Observations on the Cause and
Prevention of Influenza and Influenzal Pneumonia" *Minnesota Med.* **12**, 1929
.... [366-368] 195-197

APPENDIX B: Rosenow, E.C., "Diagnostic cutaneous reactions,
specific prevention and treatment in epidemic respiratory infections",
A.M.A. Arch. Otolaryng. **58,** Nov. 1953 .... [609-622] 198-211

AFTERWORD – Influenza, Encephalitis, Implications by S.H. Shakman ... 212-223

* [WHITE numbers on BLACK background denote original article page numbers]

****

FOREWORD

PANDEMIC CENTENNIAL

S. H. Shakman
InstituteOfScience.com

The Influenza Pandemic of 1918-1919 rivals only the Bubonic Plague of 1347-1351 as among the greatest global disasters in recorded history. This Pandemic killed an estimated 20-50 million persons world-wide, including some 675,000 Americans. In comparison, three U.S. influenza pandemics since 1919 have caused far fewer deaths, i.e., 68,900 in 1957-8, 33,800 in 1968-9, and 8,870-18,300 in 2009-10. [flu.gov/pandemic/history/]

Unfortunately this downward trend in deaths can't wholly be attributed to advancements in therapy and vaccines, but rather, at least partly, to luck. The particularly-deadly strain of influenzal-pneumonia that struck in 1918-19 seemingly has not re-emerged since. But it could. Notwithstanding presumed advances in vaccine technology, e.g., development of trivalent and quadrivalent vaccines (three or four strains resp.), vaccines have proved to be merely just about 50 to 60 percent effective most years. [cnbc.com/2015/10/19/the-16-billion-business-of-flu.html]

Thus, it is not surprising that the medical community and government(s) approach annual influenza "season(s)" with heightened caution. According to the CDC, while flu activity can occur throughout the year, it tends to start in October and peak between December and March. [cdc.gov/] (The opposite pattern is observed in the Southern Hemisphere, which gives respective hemispheres a "heads-up" as to the possible identities of upcoming flu threats.)

More than a half-year in advance of each impending flu season, authorities around the world mobilize the necessary resources to attempt to identify probable or possible strains of the presumed-causative influenza microbe for inclusion in the ultimate vaccine(s) to be used. Manufacturing and testing vaccines begins, with the ironic hope that these efforts may in the end prove unnecessary if the flu fizzles out on its own.

The costs of these annual exercises are not trivial. For example, the U.S. market for flu vaccine had been estimated at $1.6 billion in 2015, within a worldwide market of $4 billion. In addition there may be special efforts directed at special situations; e.g., in 2009 U.S. had indicated it would spend $1 billion to start the process of making an H1N1 influenza vaccine, beyond amounts being spent on the conventional flu program.

And while the attention in any flu season has been understandably directed to potential victims of influenza itself, special attention is also directed toward those who may be susceptible to associated, potentially deadly, strains of influenzal pneumonia. The 2009 Pandemic turned out to be not the killer that had been feared; however, it had nonetheless fostered discussion of particular concerns regarding pneumonia:

"Preliminary results presented to the CDC vaccine committee in June by Dr. Matthew R. Moore, a CDC medical epidemiologist, indicated that about 40% of swine-flu-related pneumonia had an unknown cause -- and that about 30% were caused by *S. pneumoniae*. This suggests that at least a third of flu-related pneumonia deaths could be prevented by vaccination." [T.H. Baugh III, *Los Angeles Times*, August 4, 2009]

This suggestion sparked the recollection that E.C. Rosenow, through the Mayo Foundation, had reported a much larger reduction in deaths during the 1918-1919 pandemic with a vaccine he had developed at that time. The mortality rate in a group inoculated three times with Rosenow's vaccine was less than 1/4 (1.00/4.45) that of un-inoculated persons. Thus, Rosenow's vaccine might have prevented *three-fourths of pneumonia deaths* (in persons receiving his vaccine, versus those not) linked to the 1918-1919 Influenza Pandemic (see last column in Table i, below.) – *much better than the mere one-third* anticipated for the modern pneumonia vaccine!

This was the initial impetus for compiling and re-publishing E. C. Rosenow's comprehensive series of Pandemic articles. Notwithstanding that these 1919-1920 articles are available through most medical libraries, publication in a much more easily accessible combined book form seemed appropriate. As the world keeps a watchful lookout for whatever scourge may strike next, Rosenow's work may be as germane as ever.

E.C. Rosenow, MD, had joined the Mayo Foundation at its inception in 1915, after having worked closely for more than a decade with AMA Presidents Frank Billings and Charles Mayo, among a cadre of the finest medical minds of the era. He went on to serve as head of the Division of Experimental Bacteriology at the Mayo Foundation for nearly three decades (1915-1944). Thus he was well established at Mayo when the pandemic of 1918-9 occurred. He was Mayo's primary investigator during the crisis and was uniquely positioned to conduct exhaustive, definitive studies, including extensive vaccine trials.

Rosenow's work on the 1918-1919 pandemic had built on his prior work on pneumonia dating from 1903, including early reports on immunization (JAMA 59:795-796, 1912, and Science Mag., 1908) and treatment with autolysed pneumococci (JAMA 59:2203-2240, 1913, with L. Hektoen.) Prior to 1919, he had already published over 30 articles in medical journals with titles referring to "pneumonia" and/or "pneumococci".

The state of medicine prior to the pandemic of 1918-9:

There were two particularly-relevant **distinct** medical histories coming into the 1918 pandemic:
(a) The "influenza bacillus" or "Pfeiffer's bacillus" hypothesis, carried over from the Pandemic of 1889-92; and
(b) A separate pneumonia vaccine experience in the early 1900s, following on the prior works of Sir Almroth Wright, Leishmann, Rosenow and others.

(a) *The "influenza bacillus", or "Pfeiffer's bacillus", hypothesis*, carried over from the Pandemic of 1889-92, was the widely-considered claim by Richard Pfeiffer to have found the cause of that pandemic in the so called "Influenza Bacillus" (aka *Hemophilus influenzae*). Despite considerable and widespread doubt concerning the role of Pfeiffer's bacillus by the time the 1918-1919 pandemic struck, the lack of a proven alternative kept Pfeiffer's bacillus prominently in consideration. Thus it became somewhat of a requisite for inclusion in seemingly most initially-proposed vaccines by various organizations such as the New York Department of Public Health and the Public Health Service.

And even a century later, it is nonetheles surprising that some portion of the general medical population is still subject to this apparently persisting wrongful impression, i.e., that *Hemophilus influenzae* caused the 1918 Pandemic.

> "The etiology of influenza was unknown at the time of the 1918 pandemic. Many contemporaneous investigators erroneously believed that bacteria, in particular Bacillus influenzae (Pfeiffer's bacillus, now known as Haemophilus influenzae) was the cause of influenza" [YW Chien, KP Klugman ,DM Morens, *JID* 2010:202, 1639]
>
> -------
>
> "... the notion that B. influenzae was the true cause of influenza persisted up to the time of the ... pandemic in 1918 ... when Rockefeller scientists Peter Kosciusko Olitsky [of Sabin-polio fame] (1886–1964) and Frederick L Gates (1886–1933) [*J Am Med Assoc* 1920;74:1497–1499] provided strong evidence against a causal association, documenting that the infective influenza agent survived passage through filters that excluded B. influenzae" [JK Taubenberger etal, *Antivir Ther* 2007; 12(4 Pt B): 581–591]
>
> -------
>
> "Bacterium pneumosintes appeared as a minute bacilloid body of regular morphology, measuring 0.15 to 0.3 micron in the long axis. Usually solitary, the bacteria were often found in diplo form, and occasionally in short chains of three or four members. ... When grown on media containing nutrient broth, and especially in the presence of dextrose, Bacterium pneumosintes has developed larger bacillary forms up to 1 micron in length. The identity of these microorganisms with the original strains has been proved by serological reactions and by their reversion to the minute forms on transfer to the original medium." [PK Olitsky, FL Gates, *J Exp Med* 1922 October 31; 36(5): 501–519]

(b) *The pneumonia vaccine experience*: Meanwhile, a large and distinct other body of work addressing the pandemic at its outset was the pneumonia vaccine experience, following from the prior and coincident works of Sir Almroth Wright, Lister, Leishmann, E.C. Rosenow and others. Pneumonia- directed vaccines were widely used during the Pandemic, e.g., by U.S. and British armed forces, by

> -- Wright, A. E.; Morgan, W. P., et al., Lancet X: 1-10 (Jan. 3) 1914..
> -- Lister, F. S.: South African Institute for Medical Research, W. E. Horton and Company, Ltd., 1917, pp. 1-30.
> -- Cecil, R. L., and Austin, J. H.: J. Exper. M. 28:19-41 (July 18) 1918.

Rosenow and the Mayo Foundation, and many others. They made a lot of sense: While it was generally agreed that the cause of pandemic influenza had not been established, at least there was indeed a well-documented and successful history of immunization against pneumonia.

Not only do Rosenow's earlier pneumonia articles provide a fitting background for his 1918-1919 work on the Pandemic, and his associated work well beyond, but his continuing impact and importance have been prominently recognized well into the 21st Century. For example, among Rosenow's early pneumonia articles is his 1904 study of pneumonia and pneumococcus, which was reprinted and lavishly praised in a 2004 *J Infect Dis* article by Morton N. Swartz: "The large body of evidence presented in a logical sequence, the use of appropriate controls, and the clear and thorough explication of results in this article published a century ago in the first issue of the Journal set a suitable standard for future investigators." (Swartz, M.N., *J Infect Dis*, 2004: 189, 1, 128-164, "Commentary: Rosenow EC. Studies in Pneumonia and Pneumococcus Infection". *J Infect Dis 1904; 1:280-312*).

And a 2010 article in this same journal (Chien, Y,W., K.P. Klugman, D.M. Morens, *J Infect Dis* 2010, **202**, 11, "Efficacy of Whole-Cell Killed Bacterial Vaccines in Preventing Pneumonia and Death during the 1918 Influenza Pandemic") illustrates the continuing importance of Rosenow's pandemic work. Notably, one of the co-authors of Chien 2010, David M. Morens, is Senior Scientific Advisor to Anthony Fauci of the National Institutes of Health (NIH), with whom Morens has also co-authored other Pandemic-related articles. And co-author, Keith P. Klugman, heads up pneumonia research for the Bill and Melinda Gates Foundation. As such this article may easily be considered to represent an, if not **the**, authoritative NIH view.

As correctly listed by Chien 2010, half-million Rosenow-via-Mayo survey responses attest to substantial reductions (4.21-4.45:1) in pneumonia and death incidence rates resp. (see Table i). Moreover, while unintended, they also reduced influenza rates (2.96).

Indeed, most of the 220,000 anti-pneumonia vaccines listed in Chien 2010 had been provided by Rosenow – his 143,760 plus ¾ of Cadham's civilian 52,999 doses. (*See the postscript clarification of the Chien data on page x.)

> "In considering prophylactic inoculations in this epidemic of influenza, we put aside the debated question as to the cause of the initial symptoms and considered primarily the possibility of immunizing persons against the bacteria, pneumonia, streptococci, influenza bacillus and staphylococci, which are conceded by all to be the common causes of death in this disease." [*JAMA*. Jan. 4, 1919, **72**, 31].

While some of these pandemic pneumonia-directed vaccine efforts included some of the so-called Influenza (or Pfeiffer's) Bacillus, this seemingly was in reality a requisite inclusion based on "prevailing wisdom", i.e., insurance of a sort. Rosenow as well as prominent British authorities

Table i. Data in Chien 2010 & Incidence Ratios

DATA AS PUBLISHED IN CHIEN TABLE 3, FIGURES 2 & 3								Incidence Ratios		
	VACCINATED				NON-VACCINATED				per Totals		
Source	Total	Influ	Pneu	Died	Total	Influ	Pneu	Died	Influ	Pneu	Died
Civilian - vaccines with pneumococci											
Watters	1638	89	13	8	1599	471	88	40	5.42	6.93	5.12
Rosenow	143760	13666	745	276	345133	97253	7534	2951	2.96	4.21	4.45
Cadham/Civilian	52999	5203	300	85	85941	21285	1869	563	2.52	3.84	4.08
McCoy	390	119	23	10	390	103	17	7	0.87	0.74	0.7
Military - vaccines with pneumococci											
Cadham /Military	4842	282	17	5	2758	238	41	17	1.48	4.23	5.97
Leishman	15624	221	26	2	43520	2059	583	98	3.34	8.05	17.6
TOTALS	219253	19580	1124	386	479341	121409	10132	3676	2.84	4.12	4.36

Table i provides raw data for "VACCINATED" and "NON-VACCINATED" persons, "Military" and "Civilian" categories, for the five studies listed in Chien 2010 that provided vaccine inoculation totals and incidence data. As shown in the last three columns, "Incidence Ratios", vaccinated persons exhibited generally-huge advantages (over un-inoculated persons) in terms of incidence of influenza, pneumonia and deaths.

Table i Key:
-- Incidence ratios (IR) are calculated as IR = ARU/ARV. where ARU = unvaccinated attack rate, and ARV = vaccinated attack rate.
-- Thus for Cadham /Military, the Incidence Ratio IR for "Died", "per Total" is: (17/2758) / (5/4842) = 5.97; i.e. the unvaccinated died at 5.97 times the rate of the vaccinated.

Chien YW, KP Klugman, DM Morens, *J.Infect.Dis.* 202, Oct. 28, 2010, p. 1639-1648
Cadham FT, *The Lancet,* May 29 1919, 885-6 (¾ of 52999 civilian came from Rosenow)
Leishman WB, *The Lancet,* Feb. 14 1920, p. 366-8
Watters WH, *Bost.Med. & Surg. J,* Dec. 25 1919, p. 727-731
Rosenow EC, BF Sturdivant, *JAMA,* Aug. 9 1919, p. 396-401
McCoy GW, VB Murray, AL Teeter, *JAMA,* **71** No 24, Dec. 14, 1918, p. 1997

under Leishmann, who were doubtful about the relevance of Pfeiffer's bacillus, were compelled to include it in their initial mix of vaccine microbes. Some, such as Rosenow, subsequently dropped the Pfeiffer's bacillus out of the mix in the course of improving the vaccine being used. At the same time, it would appear that possible co-existence of the "Pfeiffer's bacillus" aka *Hemophilus influenzae*, in the presence of the generally-presumed causative influenza virus, might easily cause continued confusion.

Leaving aside such potential residual confusion, one might hope that Rosenow's pneumonia vaccine methodology would in any case be given consideration as an alternate to pneumonia vaccines being proffered by contemporary pharmaceutical companies.

In summary, its attributes:

-- one vaccine for both influenza and pneumonia;
-- huge quantities produced within 48 hours after isolation, pandemic or not;
-- consequential huge cost savings in research and production;
-- avoiding the complication of allergies to chicken-egg vaccines;
-- availability of an already-developed oral vaccine method;
-- implications for understanding epidemics and seasonality of infections;
-- viability of epidemic vaccine for years, implication for universal vaccine;
-- independence of Rosenow's pandemic work from that on "focal infection";
-- Price's 1923 Emendation – Pandemic Severity Mystery Solved?

One vaccine for both influenza and pneumonia

- *Rosenow's vaccine was effective against both the influenza and pneumonia of the pandemic.* Rosenow's results are supportive of and in concert with the idea, widely considered at the time, that both pandemic influenza and the associated distinctly-characteristic type of pneumonia may be caused by different phases of the same "pleomorphic" organism.

- *But isn't influenza caused by a virus, and pneumonia by bacteria?* Yes, but the virus associated with pandemic influenza and bacteria associated with pandemic influenzal-pneumonia are apparently intimately related -- different and reversible phases of the same microbe, depending on environment.

The term "virus" fundamentally denotes a small, filtrable size. The ability of some, if not all, microbes to change size and shape under varying environmental influences, or "pleomorphism", has been studied for well over a century (e.g., for early history, see Philip Hadley, *Jour. Infect. Dis.*1927, 1-312; and subsequent related articles, now available through Amazon.com as *Microbic Dissociation I-III,*). Specifically in the case of pandemic influenza, Olitsky [better known for work on polio with Sabin] and Gates (J Exp Med. 10/31/22) were among the first to show how the filtrable (viral) agent can be made to grow larger, to bacterial size, and revert to original smaller form, on appropriate culture media.

Rosenow: Over the years Rosenow conducted extensive tests demonstrating the intimate relation between implicated pneumonia (bacterial/streptococcal) and influenza (viral) microbes (from *A.M.A. Arch. Otolaryng.* 58: 609 622, Nov. 1953 – Appendix B of this compilation): *"The Streptococcus appears to be the toxicogenic, antigenic phase, and the virus the relatively non-toxicogenic, non-antigenic, but highly invasive phase."*

Large quantities of vaccine can be produced within 48 hours

- *Large quantities of vaccine can be produced quickly*, i.e., within 48 hours of isolation of the causative strain. The U.S. Department of Health and

Human Services has already committed more than a billion dollars to efforts to speed up the process of producing influenza vaccine, which currently takes months. Rosenow's vaccine involves the bacterial phase of the implicated organism, rather the smaller viral phase, works against influenza and pneumonia, and takes a mere couple of days to produce huge batches. Rosenow's methodology (*Am. Practitioner and Digest of Treatment*, 9(5), 1958, 755-761) is posted at http://instituteofscience.com/Ro-recdi.html .

Consequential huge cost savings in research and production

- *HUGE cost savings, annually -- BILLIONS.*

Avoiding the complication of allergies to chicken-egg vaccines

- *The Rosenow vaccine methodology does not involve chicken eggs*, thus avoiding the problem of egg allergies that afflicts many persons, as well as the time-consuming process of shipping hundreds of thousands of eggs to vaccine manufacturing plants, growing the virus in the eggs, extracting and killing the virus and distributing the vaccines.

Availability of an already-developed oral vaccine method

- *An oral version of Rosenow's vaccine yielded "striking results"* in preliminary tests in laboratory animals. "With its high concentration of hygroscopic sugars, bacteria are dehydrated, contaminants cannot grow, it does not require refrigeration, and dosage can be adjusted." (*Am. J. Clin. Path.* 8: 17-27, Jan. 1938, with FR Heilman)

Implications for understanding epidemics and seasonality of infections

- *Rosenow addressed the cause of epidemics and seasonality of respiratory infections* including influenza, as well as encephalitis and polio; he demonstrated how variations in the implicated causative organisms, directly attributable to variations in radiant energy, may cause seasonality. (*Postgrad. Med.* 7: 117-123, Feb. 1950; 8: 290-292, Oct. 1950.)

Viability of epidemic vaccine for years, implication for universal vaccine

- *Rosenow's pandemic vaccine was successfully used against influenza for several years afterwards*, having been preserved in glycerine-salt solution.

The late C.F. Williamson, Bacteriologist and Dean of the College of Arts and Sciences, U. of Miami, Oxford Ohio, had worked directly with Rosenow and was the last to have produced Rosenow's vaccines. According to Dean

Williamson, "for many years I supplied those to physicians who would give those prior to the season arriving, and with very good results." (Quote at 7:00 in a 1999 telephone interview with this writer; audio is posted at: https://www.youtube.com/watch?v=zqesi_Q88ok)

"The holy grail for flu, researchers say, is to find a universal vaccine that would render remaking the vaccine every year unnecessary. ... NIH's Dr. Anthony Fauci said he's optimistic a universal vaccine is five to 10 years away." [cnbc.com/2015/10/19/the-16-billion-business-of-flu.html]

Perhaps Rosenow's methodology might help accelerate this schedule.

Independence from Rosenow's work linking oral and systemic infections.

Further impetus for putting together this book was the apparent independence of Rosenow's Pandemic work vis-à-vis his early, seemingly-separate, legendary work with Frank Billings and Charles Mayo et al. that had already thoroughly documented the relationship between oral infections and systemic disease – the so-called doctrine of "focal infection". Frank Billings, former AMA President and generally-acknowledged father of American medical education, had considered his focal infection work to be the landmark achievement of his incredible career. Billings' 1916 book *Focal Infection* had featured Rosenow's 1915 *JAMA* article on the subject. But notwithstanding Rosenow's unimpeachable 3-decade-long career at the Mayo Foundation (1915-1944) and beyond, opposition by some dental and as well as some medical interests have continued to push back on the arguably-physiologically-sound science behind the focal infection concept. [For further discussion of historical opposition to Rosenow's focal infection legacy, see *Medicine's Grandest PhD*, available through Amazon.com.]

In any case, Rosenow's work on the 1918-9 pandemic seemingly opened a new vista for exposure – a chance to show his genius through a prism un-fettered by the continuing controversy over the role of oral foci in causing or contributing to systemic diseases. That said, a hospital study conducted by Weston Price DDS during the Pandemic but published later provides evidence that pre-existing oral infections may indeed have contributed to the severity of pandemic pneumonia and associated deaths.

Price's 1923 Emendation – Pandemic Severity Mystery Solved?

- So why did some suffer severe consequences in the 1918-9 pandemic, and others did not? This was the big take-away surprise of this research effort.

As indicated above, Rosenow's foundational work on pneumonia and pneumonia vaccines preceded, and was seemingly independent of, his well-known body of works implicating oral foci in a range of disease conditions. Thus it was hoped that the success of his pneumonia-related works, and his Pandemic contributions, could help shed fresh light on his monumental works overall.

Nonetheless, it was of great interest that, as this research progressed, "circumstantial" evidence seemed to be pointed to a virulent phase of a streptococcus (streptococcus viridans) commonly found in the mouth, albeit usually in a relatively non-virulent form, as the underlying organism responsible. The role of this organism in pandemic influenza-pneumonia seems to have been implicated first by Mathers (*JAMA* March 3, 1917, **68** (9):678-680, who was also an early victim) and confirmed in depth by Rosenow and others. The distinctive age of victims, i.e., adults in their prime, versus the age of victims of common forms of influenza (generally the very young or very old) is further suggestive that pre-existing oral infections may have contributed to the severity of the pandemic in some persons.

- *Weston Price's documentation of the correlation between oral infections and severity of pandemic complications:* Adding evidence to the hypothesis of an oral infection/ pandemic correlation is a study published by Weston Price in his 1923 book, "Oral Infections and Systemic Disease" (Volume I, Chapter xxi, p. 266-7), which reported:

" ... I made a careful study of influenza patients in five hospitals, three in the city [Cleveland] and two in Columbus, in the epidemic of 1918. This was a exceedingly difficult study to make for several reasons: First, the patients involved were frequently too ill to be questioned with sufficient care to bring out all the data; and second, it was not possible to make roentgenographic studies, and many cases of dental infections were undoubtedly overlooked, since only those were included which were sufficiently gross to be determined definitely by oral examination, palpation, etc. A study of **two hundred sixty influenza patients in five different hospitals, Figure 137**, disclosed that that when the patients were divided into two groups – those with, and those without clearly demonstrable dental infections – the **percentage of individuals developing serious complications** (in which we included pneumonia, empyema, carditis, severe neuritis and severe rheumatism) was found to be **in the group without dental infections 32 per cent, and in the group with serious dental infections 72 per cent.** Several factors should be carefully noted: In the pneumonias, the tendency to strangulation following coughing spasms, as a result of the bronchial exudates, produced violent inspirations which draw into the lung, fluids and infections from the mouth. This makes gingival infections a very marked contributing factor to the development of pneumonia. In general, however, the so-called locked infections (by which we mean those at root apices without opportunity for drainage in to the oral cavity, which therefore must

drain into the system, into the lymphatic and hematogenous circulations) are more to be feared since the system much of necessity become invaded from this source, with a breaking down of the local defense which has tended to wall off and defend the patients in times of their normal defense."
[Weston Price, *Dental Infections, Oral and Systemic*, 1923, Vol. I, 265-6]

Not proof positive, but certainly suggestive! This study by Weston Price, Rosenow's close associate for decades, was not available until 1923, thus not incorporated nor cited within Rosenow's 1919-1920 Pandemic series.

Table ii – from Weston Price, Oral Infections and Systemic Disease I, p. 267

ORAL INFECTIONS AND INFLUENZA COMPLICATIONS

Hospital	Date	No. of Flu Cases Studied	Flu Only	Flu with Various Complications	Flu with Pneumonia	With Oral Infection			Without Oral Infection		
						Total	Flu Only	Flu with Complications	Total	Flu Only	Flu with Complications
1 Lakeside, Cleveland Men's Ward	Nov. 30	20	13–65%	7–35%	7–35%	8–40%	2–25%	6–75%	12–60%	10–83%	2–17%
2 Lakeside, Cleveland Women's Ward	Dec. 1	6	1–17%	5–83%	5–83%	5–83%	1–20%	4–80%	1–17%	0	1–17%
3 St. Francis Columbus	Dec. 4-5	23	5–21%	18–78%	9–48%	18–22%	3–17%	15–83%	5–78%	2–40%	3–60%
4 Grant, Columbus Nurses	Dec. 5	50	41–82%	9–18%	2–4%	0	Held certificates from dentists		50–100%	41–82%	9–18%
5 Grant, Columbus Private Patients	Dec. 5	51	38–74%	13–26%	8–16%	0	None known		51–100%	38–74%	13–26%
6 City Hospital Cleveland	Dec. 7	26	·8–31%	18–69%	15–51%	23–88%	7–30%	16–70%	3–12%	1–33%	2–67%
7 Mt. Sinai Cleveland	Dec. 19	31	14–45%	17–54%	10–32%	21–68%	8–38%	13–62%	10–32%	6–60%	4–40%
8 Mt. Sinai Cleveland Nurses	Dec. 16	53	38–72%	15–28%	13–24%	0	Clean mouths		53–100%	38–72%	15–28%
Eight Sources		260	158–61%	102–39%	69–26%	75–29%	21–28%	54–72%	185–71%	136–68%	49–32%
Private Practice Patients		37	14–38%	23–62%	14–23%	37–100%	14–38%	23–62%	0		

But even without the Price emendation, the success of Rosenow's and the other Pandemic vaccines argues forcibly for renewed consideration in modern times. Swartz's 2004 endorsement of Rosenow's earlier pneumonia work, as well as Chien 2010's support for further investigation and reconsideration, are certainly welcome steps in this direction.

E.C. Rosenow's multi-faceted perspective on the pandemic was published as an eleven-part series, parts 1-4 in 1919 in the *Journal of the American Medical Association*, and parts 5-11 in 1920 in the *Journal of Infectious Diseases*. This series comprises the essential body of this present publication, as augmented by:
– Appendix A: Rosenow's summary 1929 article (*Minnesota Med.* **12**, 1929);
– Appendix B: His last dedicated influenza/pneumonia article, 1953, which discussed his substantial associated body of work on this subject over five decades (*A.M.A. Arch. Otolaryng.* **58,** Nov. 1953); and

– Afterword: A supplemental overview of the intimate relation of Rosenow's Pandemic work to the subsequent Post-Influenzal (Von Economo's) Encephalitis Lethargica ("sleepy sickness") epidemic, and this to the issue of the infectious etiology of various neurological conditions.

S. H. Shakman
Institute Of Science
InstituteOfScience.com / I-o-S.org
2014; Edited/revised February 16, 2018

---

*An Essential Clarifying Data Postscript:

As noted above and correctly listed by Chien 2010, half-million Rosenow-via-Mayo survey responses attest to substantial reductions in pneumonia (4.21:1), death (4.45:1) and influenza (2.96:1) incidence ratios resp. (see Table i). Ironically, Chien 2010 rejected this as "not consistent with our understanding of influenza etiology", and sought to characterize relative pneumonia and death rates more conservatively as (in essence) quotients of division by influenza rates (1.4-1.5:1).

Accordingly, given the continuing importance of Chien et al. 2010, as reflected in the authoritative position(s) of co-authors Klugman (B&M Gates Foundation) and Morens (Fauci/NIH), data therein and herein are further necessarily qualified as noted below. It is further suggested that this article be withdrawn as fundamentally misleading, due primarily to its having erroneously discounted the facts of favorable effects of vaccination against influenza. The authors and the J.Infect.Dis. are being informed of this suggestion; further details are being separately published in book form as **Public Health Dis-Service**, *available through Amazon.com. At the same time, the unadulterated data from Chien (Table i) have been thoroughly validated and provide unimpeachable testimony to the continuing and essential value of reference to E.C. Rosenow's Pandemic series as presented herein..*

Chien 2010 states: "We identified and retrieved full texts of 485 publications for assessment. ... 13 studies were included in the final analysis". However, Chien specifically excluded five of these from their assessment results – four (Hinton-Kane, Wadsworth, Duval-Harris, Barnes) which involved "influenza bacillis" only, and one (Ely) involving only streptococci.

Of the remaining eight studies, one (Minaker) did not provide pneumonia data and two (Cherry, and Eyre) did not provide total inoculation data, therefore precluding determination of incidence of pneumonia and death as called for in the title/scope.

For the remaining five studies (including Cadham which included both civilian and military components), incidence data provided by Chien 2010 have been duly verified by the original texts – in terms of numbers of subjects and incidence of influenza, pneumonia and deaths.

These five studies involve a total of **219,253** inoculations, including 143,760 in Rosenow's Mayo reports; plus 39,749 (¾ of Cadham's civilian total 52,999) prepared from bacteria from Rosenow; plus 390 McCoy (Rosenow vaccines from Chicago, inappropriately used in California). Thus, **183,899 of the total (84 %)** were in fact Rosenow vaccines.

Further, all of the Cadham 52999 civilian and 4842 military vaccines adhered to protocols observed by Rosenow. Adding these and McCoy's 390 to Rosenow's 143,760 vaccines, some **201,991 of the total 219,253 inoculations, i.e., 92% of the total assessed by Chien, were Rosenow vaccines or otherwise in accord with Rosenow protocols** – a decidedly positive endorsement.

###

STUDIES IN INFLUENZA AND PNEUMONIA

E. C. Rosenow
Mayo Foundation

An 11-part series

As originally published in the

Journal of the American Medical Association, 1919
Volumes 72 (31-4, 1604-9) and 73 (396-401)
and the
Journal of Infectious Diseases, 1920
Volume 26 (469-622)

PROPHYLACTIC INOCULATION AGAINST RESPIRATORY INFECTIONS DURING THE PRESENT PANDEMIC OF INFLUENZA
PRELIMINARY REPORT *

E. C. ROSENOW, M.D., ROCHESTER, MINN.

*From the Mayo Foundation.
*Read before the American Public Health Association, Chicago, Dec. 10, 1918.

In attempting to lessen the incidence and to reduce the severity of infections of the respiratory tract by vaccination, it is essential to consider the wide range of bacterial flora, the relative prevalence of each species, as well as the fluctuations in incidence and severity of these infections with changes in season. The well-defined tendency of bacteria of the same species to localize differently in different epidemics indicates peculiar infecting and antigenic powers. The short duration of immunity to infections following attacks adds greatly to the difficulty. However, owing to the high incidence and high mortality rate from infections of the respiratory tract during the present epidemic, a painstaking effort to raise the resistance of individuals by inoculation with appropriate vaccines appeared to be strongly indicated.

In considering prophylactic inoculations in this epidemic of influenza, we put aside the debated question as to the cause of the initial symptoms and considered primarily the possibility of immunizing persons against the bacteria, pneumonia, streptococci, influenza bacillus and staphylococci, which are conceded by all to be the common causes of death in this-disease. It was thought that it might be possible to raise to some degree, by artificial means, the immunity of persons to these micro-organisms to which they appear so susceptible, and thus to lower the incidence of the more serious respiratory infections, particularly pneumonia.

The bacteria found as the cause of the complications in this epidemic appear to have exalted and peculiar infecting powers. The mode of death and the findings in the lungs, for example, in the so-called acute bronchopneumonia following influenza, are quite unique and are strikingly similar, irrespective of the species of micro-organism present. Infection of the lung by hemolytic streptococci without empyema and without tonsillitis indicates peculiar localizing power of this micro-organism. The influenza bacillus appears to have acquired peculiar virulence. The frequency of staphylococci in the sputum and lung associated with pneumococci and streptococci far exceeds that which occurs in lobar pneumonia. A study of the various strains isolated has revealed commonly marked variations in cultural and other properties. Owing to these findings, it was the plan to prepare the vaccine not from saprophytized laboratory strains, as is too often the rule in vaccine therapy, but from strains freshly isolated from the sputum and lungs, and to incorporate the bacteria in the vaccine in about the proportion in which they are found, and before the more or less peculiar properties disappear. A bacteriologic study, made during the progress of the epidemic, showed a decided change in the bacterial flora, and hence new strains were added from time to time in order that the vaccine might represent as nearly as possible the bacterial flora of the disease at various stages of the epidemic.

Heretofore lobar pneumonia has been unusually prevalent for some months following epidemics of influenza. It was felt that this would be particularly apt to be the case following the present epidemic, since it began early in the season. It was decided, therefore, to include a series of the fixed types of pneumococci in the vaccine, although they were infrequently isolated, especially during the early part of the epidemic.

A study of the secretions from the nose and throat, of the sputum and lung exudate from the very beginning of the epidemic as it occurred in and about Rochester, revealed commonly, among other bacteria, a streptococcus having some distinctive features. Smears from the nose and throat and sputum at the onset of the attack show quite constantly large numbers of this organism in the form of gram-positive lanceolate diplococci occurring singly, but more often in rather long chains. The epithelial cells are frequently found packed with this micro-organism. On artificial cultivation of these exudates it presents morphologic and cultural features both of the pneumococcus and of Streptococcus viridans. It produces on isolation a rather moist, spreading, nonadherent, greenish colony on blood agar plates, and a diffuse cloud in glucose broth. On solid mediums it grows as a lanceolate diplococcus of quite uniform size, and usually is surrounded by a distinct capsule. In glucose broth it produces lancet-shaped diplococci in rather long chains. Smears from the older cultures often show extreme variations in size and shape. Injection of sputum into guinea-pigs is usually followed by death from peritonitis, the peritoneal exudate and blood showing this organism in pure or almost pure form. It is more virulent than the green-producing streptococci from the throats of normal persons, but is less virulent than pneumococci from lobar pneumonia. The strains do not usually ferment inulin. It does not autolyze readily and is not soluble in bile. Owing to these findings the vaccine was made to contain a heavy mixture of these strains.

The organism is undoubtedly the one found by the English investigators and designated by them as diplostreptococcus, and the one found by Mathers and for which Tunnicliff finds an increased opsonic content in the serum of convalescent patients. Immunologic and other studies to determine further the relations of this organism to influenza are under way and will be reported later.

Hemolytic streptococci were found next most frequently, particularly in fatal cases during the first half of the epidemic. Staphylococcus aureus and influenza bacilli appear to play a minor but definite role in the production of the complicating pneumonia in some cases. Hence, examples of strains of hemolytic streptococci, staphylococci and influenza bacilli were included in the vaccine.

PREPARATION OF THE VACCINE

The formula of the vaccine used during the earlier part of the epidemic, and exclusively in the cases in this report, is given in Table 1.

TABLE 1.—FORMULA OF VACCINE

Pneumococci, Types I (10 per cent.), II (14 per cent.) and III (6 per cent.)	30 per cent.
Pneumococci (Group IV and the allied green-producing diplostreptococci described	30 per cent.
Hemolytic streptococci	20 per cent.
Staphylococcus aureus	10 per cent.
Influenza bacillus	10 per cent.

The bacteria were grown for from eighteen to thirty-six hours at from 33 to 35 C., in 0.2 per cent, glucose broth. The broth was autoclaved at 20 pounds pressure for from one to two hours to insure freedom from living spores. The glucose was added in a sterile manner from a concentrated sterilized solution in water. It was found that the cultures of pneumococci and streptococci yielded approximately 1,000 million bacteria, and Staphylococcus aureus 2,000 million bacteria per cubic centimeter. Luxuriant growth (about 1,000 million per cubic centimeter) of the influenza bacillus was obtained by adding approximately 1 c.c. of laked human blood per liter of glucose broth. The strains were grown separately in the flasks. Smears were made before centrifugation of each flask to eliminate possible contaminations. The pneumococci and allied green-producing streptococci, the staphylococci and influenza bacilli were separated from the broth culture by centrifugation,[1] and then suspended in sodium chloride solution. At first 50 per cent, of the hemolytic streptococci were added in the form of the killed broth culture, and the other 50 per cent, in sodium chloride solution suspension after centrifugation. But owing to rather severe reactions, only 25 per cent, of the hemolytic streptococci are added in the form of the broth culture. The streptococci in the broth culture are killed by the addition of 0.5 per cent, cresol. The centrifugated bacteria are suspended in sodium chloride solution so that 1 c.c. represents approximately the growth from 50 c.c. of the broth culture, and are killed by the addition of from 1 to 1.5 per cent, purified cresol. The dense suspensions are diluted with an equal volume of sodium chloride solution after the cultures, made twenty-four hours after the cresol is added, have remained sterile for 48 hours. In some instances the suspensions became slightly contaminated with Bacillus subtilis, when heating to 60 C. for one hour was necessary to render them completely sterile. If this was not sufficient, the suspensions were discarded. At first, owing to the urgent demand for the vaccine, the use of extreme heat in the sterilization of the broth, negative aerobic and anaerobic cultures at the end of from forty-eight to seventy-two hours were considered sufficient as sterility tests. It is now the rule to hold the vaccine until all cultures and animal tests have proved negative for one week. Blood agar and glucose broth and glucose brain broth and litmus milk in tall columns are the mediums used for the sterility tests. The vaccine is finally made up by diluting the dense suspensions in the proper proportions with sodium chloride solution so that 1 c.c. contains approximately 5 billion bacteria. Purified cresol (0.3 per cent.) is used as a preservative. The initial dose for adults is 0.5 c.c. subcutaneously. This is followed in one week by 1 c.c. The third dose is given fourteen days after the first dose, and consists of 1.5 c.c. The doses in children are 0.1, 0.2 and 0.3 c.c. or more according to age. Owing to the relatively large doses, intervals shorter than one week between injections are considered inadvisable.

RESULTS

In most instances there is a moderate local reaction. Constitutional symptoms are usually mild or absent. Both local and general reactions are decidedly less than those following typhoid vaccines. Exceptionally severe reactions occur showing unusual individual susceptibility. The severer reactions are prone to occur in persons who give a history of recent exposure to the disease, or who already have beginning symptoms of it. In these persons, attacks may appear to be precipitated by the vaccination; but the course is usually short and relatively mild. Persons appear to be more sensitive to the vaccine during the incubation period than before or after the attack is established, or following recovery.

Physicians, nurses and employees of the several hospitals in Rochester were first inoculated. After it was determined that injections of the vaccine were followed by an increase in antibodies in the serum, that the inoculations appeared to be quite harmless, that there was no increased incidence of respiratory infection following the inoculations but an apparent decrease instead, it was decided to study its effects on a larger scale as the epidemic became acute. The vaccine was sent gratis for study by the Mayo Foundation to hospitals and physicians on request, on condition that reports of results be furnished.

The reports included in this paper are from physicians, hospitals and other institutions, chiefly from cities and towns within a radius of 200 miles from Rochester. In Table 2 is given a summary of the results obtained in a considerable number of inoculated and uninoculated control persons. The reports containing results in the vaccinated after the epidemic was on the decline are not included. The uninoculated represent such persons in institutions, colleges, factories, corporations and communities where the vaccine was used. Only those reports are included that contain accurate data as to the incidence and mortality among the uninoculated.

The age in both the inoculated and the uninoculated falls mainly between twenty and forty years. The observations were made from Oct. 15 to Dec. 8, 1918. It will be seen that there was no apparent negative phase following the first inoculation and that there was a progressive diminution of incidence and death from influenza and pneumonia following the successive inoculations. The total incidence of recognizable influenza, pneumonia and encephalitis in the inoculated is approximately one- third as great as in the control uninoculated. The total death rate from influenza or pneumonia is only one- fourth as great in the inoculated as in the uninoculated. No cases of meningitis occurred in the former, whereas in the latter there were 0.4 per thousand. These results were obtained by including all persons who developed influenza or pneumonia and all who died from the day of the first inoculation, and 7,667 persons, or about one fourth of the total number who received only one inoculation.

TABLE 2.—INCIDENCE OF ILLNESS AND MORTALITY FOR ONE THOUSAND PERSONS

	Inoculated					Uninocu- lated
	After First Inocu- lation	After Second Inocu- lation	Within 7 Days after Third Inocu- lation	Within 6 Weeks after Third Inocu- lation	Total	
Influenza............	23	10	9	14.6	56.6	229
Pneumonia..........	1.8	1	1	1.8	5.6	15.7
Meningitis..........	0	0	0	0	0	0.4
Encephalitis........	0.04	0	0.05	0	0.09	0.2
Deaths from influ- enza or pneu- monia............	0.03	0.08	0	0.19	0.9	3.4
Total number of inoculated and uninoculated persons..........	28,459	26,150	20,792	20,792	....	61,753

The total incidence and death rate in the uninoculated controls are well within the average, as they occur during the present epidemic and hence serve as a fair basis for comparison. Experiments in which alternate control persons were inoculated were not done because of difficulty to obtain consent, and because, after all, the results from prophylactic inoculation must be sufficiently favorable to be apparent under the conditions included in this report.

All but two of over seventy physicians who have used the vaccine report that the attacks of influenza, if contracted by the inoculated, are milder and of shorter duration, and that convalescence is more rapid than in the uninoculated. This agrees with our observations, and is in keeping with the lower death rate among the inoculated. This difference has been noted in communities in which the incidence and mortality rate were exceptionally high as well as where they were comparatively low. In view of this observation, granting that the initial symptoms in influenza may be due to an unknown virus, the lowered incidence of influenza among the inoculated may be only apparent. The attacks may have been so mild as to escape detection.

Among the nurses at St. Mary's Hospital, Rochester, where fourteen developed influenza within two days prior to the first inoculation, only one case developed subsequently during a period of six weeks. Similar apparent protection was afforded to the personnel of other hospitals following vaccination. At the State Hospital for the Insane at Rochester, with a total population of about 1,500, where one case of influenza had occurred before the inoculations were given, only three cases occurred following the date of the first inoculation for a period of six weeks. With the occurrence of the second wave of the epidemic, however, there occurred a mild outbreak of the disease. This would indicate that the immunity is of short duration.

Nearly all of the patients with influenza and pneumonia admitted for treatment in the hospitals in Rochester, where approximately one half of the population has been vaccinated, have been from the uninoculated group, excluding those patients who contracted the disease elsewhere.

In one hospital in which the nurses had been inoculated, no cases developed after the inoculations, although the nurses continued to care for patients with influenza. Owing to the scarcity of vaccine, some of the nurses, living under identical conditions, were not inoculated, and a high percentage of these contracted severe attacks.

Numerous instances have been observed in which protection appeared to be afforded to inoculated members of families of which all the uninoculated became ill. Similar results were obtained when conditions among the inoculated and uninoculated were comparable, such as in offices, factories and schools, where nearly all were inoculated, or where only a small percentage were inoculated. Illustrating results are as follows:

Of 1,000 persons employed by one company, 481, about one half, received one inoculation; 224 received two inoculations, and ninety-five received three inoculations. From October 28, the date of the first inoculation, to December 8, 138 cases of influenza occurred, only twenty of which were among persons who had had one or more inoculations. Of these, fourteen had had only one inoculation, and the remaining six had but two inoculations. There were thirteen deaths, only two of which followed influenza among the inoculated, and in these two cases only one inoculation had been given.

The mortality from bronchopneumonia in pregnant women has been especially high during the present epidemic. The vaccinations in a fairly large number of such persons appear to have afforded some protection against this complication. The bacteria included in the vaccine belong to the general group of microorganisms associated commonly with chronic infections, such as arthritis, sinusitis and bronchitis; hence some effect should follow its injection. Striking instances of improvement in these conditions have been noted but whether due to specific or nonspecific effects or whether the vaccine acts as an "exfoliative stimulus" according to Larson, liberating preformed specific antibodies, remains to be determined.

From the results obtained thus far, it appears possible to afford a definite degree of protection by prophylactic inoculation to persons against the more serious respiratory infections during the present epidemic of influenza. The duration of immunity is not known, but indications are that it is relatively short.

The vaccine should contain freshly isolated strains of the more important bacteria in approximately the proportions as found in the sputum and lungs in the disease, and since the relative proportions of the bacteria at hand differ so markedly in widely separated communities, judging by the reports, the formula of the vaccine should be made to conform as nearly as practicable to the respective flora of the disease in the communities in which the vaccine is to be used.

A saline vaccine was used as an emergency measure. Owing to the large number of different bacteria that need to be included and the large doses necessary, a lipovaccine, judging by the recent work of Whitmore, ought to possess definite advantages, since reactions should be less severe, the formation of antibodies more marked, and the resulting immunity more enduring.

I am constantly being asked with regard to the use of the vaccine in treatment. Since the severer complications in influenza, such as pneumonia, do not usually begin until the fourth day or later, the vaccine, if given at the onset of the disease might reasonably be expected to afford some protection. The initial prophylactic dose daily for one, two or three days, provided no unfavorable symptoms occur, is recommended. The results obtained are considered preliminary, and final conclusions cannot be drawn at this time. It is indicated that the vaccine used was at least harmless, that a certain degree of protection was afforded, and that prophylactic inoculation against the respiratory infections, so fatal during this epidemic, be studied on a large scale by many according to the principles herein laid down.

> 1. In connection with some work on poliomyelitis in which it became necessary to procure large quantities of the streptococcus, the ordinary large cup centrifuge proved inadequate. A number of centrifugal machines were tested to see if they might not facilitate greatly the clarification of broth in its preparation and to separate efficiently the bacteria from large quantities of liquid cultures. A number were found useful; but owing to the simplicity of construction and the ease with which bacteria may be obtained from the revolving bowl without contamination, the one manufactured by the Sharpies Separator Company, West Chester, Pa., was selected and has proved satisfactory for the purpose. By the use of the small laboratory size, it is possible, for example, to separate the bacteria from 50 liters of broth an hour. The revolving bowl and other utensils with which the broth comes in contact are autoclaved. A galvanized iron hood built over the machine makes it possible to sterilize the air in the hood with steam; and by siphoning the broth cultures from the bottles, large quantities of bacteria may be collected without contamination.

STUDIES IN INFLUENZA AND PNEUMONIA

II. THE EXPERIMENTAL PRODUCTION OF SYMPTOMS AND LESIONS SIMULATING THOSE OF INFLUENZA WITH STREPTOCOCCI ISOLATED DURING THE PRESENT PANDEMIC *

E. C. ROSENOW, M.D.
ROCHESTER, MINN.

* Presented before the Federation of American Societies for Experimental Biology, Baltimore. April 26. 1919.

During a study made some years ago[1] on the influence of environment on the pneumococcus-streptococcus group of micro-organisms, I noted marked changes in morphology, growth characteristics, infecting powers and immunologic reactions. Many of these changes appeared to be true mutations. Observations I have made since then, particularly during this epidemic, corroborate those findings and suggest the possibility that the present pandemic may be the result of infection by mutation forms of this group of micro-organisms. In studying the infecting power and other properties of streptococci when they are first isolated from tissues and foci of infection in various diseases including poliomyelitis, certain strains of streptococci which produce green discoloration on blood agar and which have peculiar infecting powers, specific immunologic properties and etiologic relationship have been found. In view of these facts, which are regarded as fundamental, it was thought possible that the peculiar clinical and pathologic picture of influenza, its accompanying pneumonia, and other lesions might be due to bacteria having peculiar infecting powers and other specific properties. The presence of a pandemic strain among the varieties of pneumococci and streptococci isolated by many observers was considered possible.

The somewhat peculiar green-producing streptococcus described in a previous paper,[2] has now been isolated quite constantly from a large series of cases of influenza. In making cultures from the blood, from the lung exudate, and from peribronchial lymph glands in patients who died from acute pulmonary edema and pneumonia, we were struck by the fact that the former was often sterile or contained few colonies and that the number of bacteria, particularly green- producing streptococci, were few in number in the latter as compared, for example, with that found in lobar pneumonia. Following intraperitoneal injections in guinea-pigs of

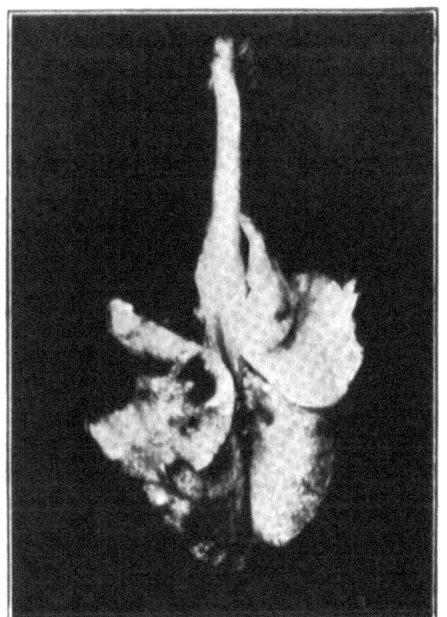
Fig. 1.—Lung of guinea-pig 761, injected intraperitoneally, showing hemorrhage, bronchopneumonia and emphysema. Total volume 12 c.c

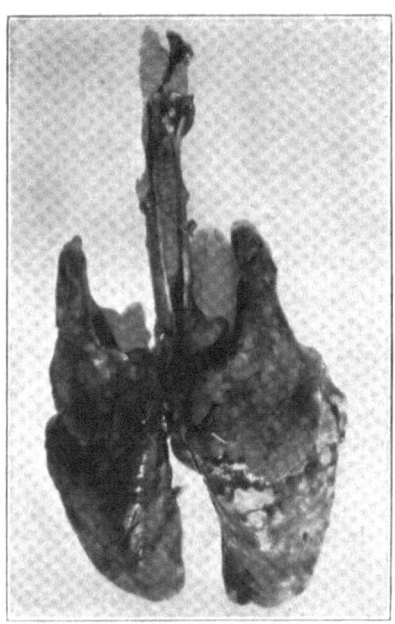
Fig. 2.—Lung of guinea-pig 851, injected intratracheally showing Coalescing bronchopneumonia of enlarged right. lower lobe Total volume 18 c.c.

the sputum and cultures, invasion by this organism was found in most instances, but, as in persons with influenza, the number of organisms in the blood was strikingly small and far less than that found in animals dead from intraperitoneal injections of type pneumococci. A special mechanism for the cause of death was thus indicated. In the animals it was found that the organism, when injected intraperitoneally or intravenously, tended to localize in the lung and to produce hemorrhages and bronchopneumonia, associated with a varying degree of emphysema (Fig. 1). This was not noted in animals dead from intraperitoneal injections of type pneumococci. The average volume of the lungs, the total displacement of water of guinea-pigs weighing about 350 gm., was found to be as follows: normal guinea-pigs killed with chloroform, 5.2 c.c.; guinea-pigs dead of intraperitoneal injections of type pneumococci, 6.7 c.c.; and guinea-pigs dead from intraperitoneal injection of sputum and green-producing streptococci from influenza, 12 c.c. Since localization tended

To be in the lung it was thought that direct application of the organism to the respiratory tract might afford better opportunity to study the peculiar infecting power of the bacteria found during this pandemic.

A simple method for intrabronchial injections of guinea-pigs was devised similar to that used in dogs by Lamar and Aleltzer and in rabbits by Winternitz and Hirschfelder. Discarded ureteral catheters cut at an angle of 45 degrees with the margins rounded are used to make the injections. The guinea-pig is wrapped in a towel, the head held in place by the handles of an inverted artery forceps. The mouth is held open by spring wire retractors and the tongue is depressed by a suitable small instrument. Under a strong reflected light, properly shaded, the catheter is inserted into the larynx with a quick stroke before the contraction of the muscles of the epiglottis can divert the tube into the esophagus. The animal's sharp, quick cough and total inability to use its voice, and the sensation of the catheters passing the tracheal rings, indicate that it has entered the trachea. The injections, varying from 0.1 c.c. to 2 c.c. in amount, are made slowly through the catheter with a syringe and needle.

By this method numerous experiments have been done with various strains of bacteria, including pneumococci, green-producing streptococci, hemolytic streptococci, staphylococci and influenza bacilli from persons with influenza as well as those from normal persons and other sources. The details of these experiments are reserved for subsequent reports; the purpose of this paper is to record a brief summary of the principal results obtained with strains of the green-producing streptococci and pneumococci belonging to Group IV from cases of influenza. By intrabronchial injection of these organisms a picture simulating influenza and pneumonia has been produced. Numerous animals have succumbed to acute pulmonary edema, to bronchopneumonia, to pneumonia involving whole lobes, and to acute hemorrhagic exudation in the pleura and pericardium together with marked or slight lung involvement.

The lungs of these animals, as in persons with influenza, were often voluminous. Many showed acute symptoms resembling anaphylactic shock and typical bronchial spasm a few minutes after intratracheal injection. The type of respiration in the animals that lived twenty-four hours or longer was often very different from that in the animals having respiratory embarrassment from extensive consolidation of the lung following injection of pneumococci from lobar pneumonia, or of mass cultures from throats of normal persons. In the former, the chest was often in almost complete expansion, the animals were irritable and restless, expiration was prolonged and difficult, and breathing was accomplished chiefly with the diaphragm. Injections of epinephrin and atropin in large doses often relieved the respiratory embarrassment. In the latter group of animals the respiration was normal in character, excursions of the chest were free and easy, and the animals were quiet, but the rate was often much increased, depending on the amount of consolidation. Injections of epinephrin and atropin were without effect. The lungs in the first group were often extremely emphysematous and contained much hemorrhagic edematous fluid (Fig. 2).

The massive bronchopneumonia was the rule in the animals that died late (Fig. 3). The rupture of alveoli, manifested as subpleural blebs, has been noted in animals showing extreme emphysema and hemorrhage. In a number, air was found in the mediastinal tissues, and several showed subcutaneous emphysema about the thorax. Sections of the lungs showed extremely narrow lumens of bronchi often filled with exudate. The mucous membrane appeared in great folds and the cartilages in the wall of the larger bronchi were often distorted as a result of the extreme spasm of the bronchial muscles (Fig. 4). The marked constriction of bronchi must have occurred before death and was not due to the fixation in 10 per cent, formaldehyd solution, since the total volume of lungs after fixation in formaldehyd solution (Kaiserling's solution) was found to be only about one-sixth less than that of the fresh lung.

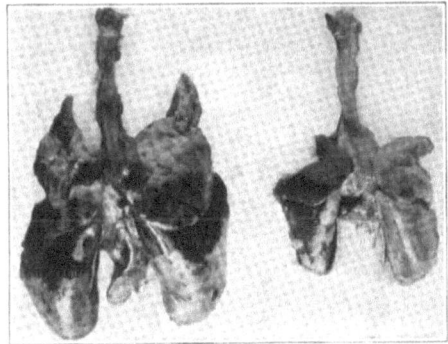
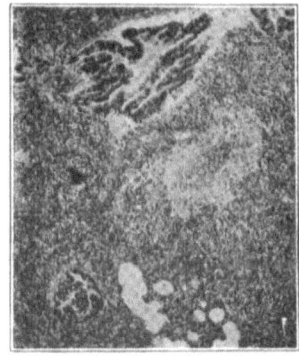

Fig. 3.—a, lung of guinea-pig 968, injected intratracheally, showing marked hemorrhagic edema and emphysema. Total volume, 22 c.c. --b, lung of guinea-pig of same weight dead from spontaneous pneumonia. Total volume 6.5 c.c.

Fig. 4.—Section of lung shown in Figure 3 a, showing marked dilation of alveoli, extreme contraction of bronchi, interstitial and alveola hemorrhage, and infiltration. Hematoxylin and eosin. X 70.

This picture is identical to that of the anaphylactic lung obtained by the usual methods, except that marked edema and hemorrhage occurred in the mucous membrane of the trachea and bronchi and in the interstitial tissue and the alveoli. The lungs of animals injected with type pneumococci, or with mass cultures from influenza and from normal persons, were not much larger than normal. The mucous membrane of the trachea and bronchi appeared normal. There was little hemorrhagic edema, but a variable amount of consolidation occurred, usually of the lobar type. The bronchi were not constricted and the dilatation of alveoli was absent. In addition to the picture in the lung, many of the animals aborted and many showed localization in the uterus. The picture of influenza was simulated in still other ways. There was delayed coagulation of the blood obtained from the heart and lung exudate in the animals, as in persons dead from influenza. Leukopenia usually occurred following injection of the strains. Leukocyte counts were made in 195 animals, following injections of numerous strains and their filtrates. Eighty-eight of these showed marked leukopenia, forty-one moderate leukopenia, thirty no change, thirty marked increase, and thirteen slight increase in leukocytes. The strains from patients showing marked leukopenia produced, usually, leukopenia in animals, while those from patients with leukocytosis usually produced leukocytosis in animals. Many animals (Table 1) showed leukopenia for a day or two; they appeared sick or prostrated; and, as recovery ensued, the leukocyte count increased. A persistent leukopenia was the rule in the animals that died.

In Table 1 are given the leukocyte counts in a series of animals following the injection of a number of strains, together with controls injected with type pneumococci. All but one of nine animals injected with Strain 2800 showed a marked or moderate leukopenia,while one showed slight leukocytosis. This difference in the behavior of an occasional animal was noted with other strains. The results as shown in Table 1 represent in a general way those obtained throughout these experiments. In some instances the cultures and their filtrates became so toxic that very small doses sufficed to cause hemorrhagic edematous frothy fluid to exude from the nose and mouth before death, and marked emphysema and hemorrhagic edema of the lung were found after death. One filtrate was so toxic that the instillation of 0.3 c.c. into the nostrils of a guinea-pig caused death in forty minutes from hemorrhagic edema and emphysema of the lung.

The freshly isolated strains from influenza and its accompanying lesions have been found to produce relatively large amounts of "anaphylatoxin" both in vitro and in vivo. The idea that the "virulence" of these bacteria may depend in part on their ability to produce "anaphylatoxin" is in accord with my[3] previous findings that virulent pneumococci and their filtrates produce a larger amount of this toxic substance than avirulent pneumococci. The picture in animals is clearly that of an anaphylactic intoxication, and suggests that the symptoms and lesions in man as recorded by numerous observers may likewise be due to this cause in which sensitization of the host to the bacterial proteins may or may not play a part. Findings as follows indicate . this mechanism : (1) the delay in the coagulation time of the blood, leukopenia and cyanosis; (2) the marked tendency to develop acute pulmonary edema with a distended lung and relatively immobile expanded chest, and extreme respiratory effort; (3) the voluminous king as found at necropsy; (4) the occurrence of the rupture of alveoli and consequent subcutaneous emphysema (bronchial spasm) ; (5) the frequency of abortion (contraction of unstriped muscle) and other uterine disturbances.

TABLE 1.—THE LEUKOCYTE COUNT FOLLOWING INJECTION OF GREEN-PRODUCING STREPTOCOCCI FROM INFLUENZA

No.	Dose in c.c. of Dextrose Broth Culture	Strain and Place of Isolation	Place of Injection	Before Injection	Leukocyte Count — Hours after Injection 24	48	72	After Death	Duration of Experiment in Days	Results
P. 959	0.1	2,800 sputum	Trachea	16,400	6,200	19,000	14,400	......	..	Recovery
P. 961	1.5	2,800 throat	Subcut. tissue	10,400	1,600	......	1,400	12,600	4	Death; subcutaneous cellulitis
P. 955	1.5	2,800 throat	Trachea	16,000	21,000	17,000	19,400	......	..	Recovery
P. 964	1.5	2,800* throat	Trachea	15,000	3,100	......	......	8,100	1	Death; hemorrhagic edema and emphysema of lung
P. 969	2	2,800* throat	Vein	12,000	4,200	......	......	4,400	2	Death; hemorrhagic edema and emphysema of lung
P. 981	1.5	2,800.2 blood	Trachea	8,000	2,000	6,200	12,000	......	..	Recovery
P. 995	1.5	2,800.2 blood	Trachea	9,600	6,200	14,000	......	......	..	Recovery
P. 1043	2	2,800.2² blood	Trachea	16,800	2,000	......	......	4,400	1.5	Death; hemorrhagic edema and emphysema of lung
P. 1056	2	2,800.4 blood	Trachea	12,000	6,800	5,000	8,000	8,000	3	Death; bronchopneumonia
P. 990	1	2,769² sputum	Trachea	7,400	2,200	2,500	......	......	4	Death; bronchopneumonia
P. 962	1.5	2,795.3 sputum	Trachea	16,200	......	28,000	17,000	6,500	4	Death; bronchopneumonia and hemorrhagic edema
P. 1004	1.5	2,839 throat	Trachea	18,000	......	2,600	......	2,600	2	Death; hemorrhagic edema and emphysema
P. 1019	1.5	2,839 throat	Trachea	22,400	5,400	......	......	5,400	1	Death; hemorrhagic edema and emphysema
P. 1174	1.5	2,981.2 stool	Trachea	18,000	6,800	9,400	......	9,400	2	Chloroformed; lobar pneumonia
P. 1023	1.5	Pneumococcus III	Trachea	6,600	4,400	7,800	......	......	..	Recovery
P. 1025	1.5	Pneumococcus III	Trachea	6,800	6,800	6,800	......	......	..	Recovery
P. 1026	1.5	Pneumococcus II	Trachea	5,400	5,400	9,000	......	......	..	Recovery
P. 1027	1.5	Pneumococcus II	Trachea	16,800	16,000	15,400	......	......	..	Recovery
P. 1031	1.5	Pneumococcus IV	Trachea	13,200	18,600	17,500	......	17,500	2	Death; lobar pneumonia

* The figure to the right and above the figures indicating the strain designates the animal passage; the one following the period, the subculture.

From this study it is clear that among the green- producing streptococci isolated by many observers in influenza and the accompanying pneumonia, a strain strains occur which possess marked and peculiar violence. By intratracheal injection of these strains the picture of influenza has been closely simulated.

PROTOCOLS ILLUSTRATIVE OF SOME OF THE RESULTS OBTAINED
PROTOCOL 1.—Guinea-pig 761, weighing 350 gm., was injected jntraperitoneally, Nov. 26, 1918, with 3 c.c. of the dextrose-brain-broth culture from a single colony of

the green- producing streptococcus isolated on blood agar plates from the sputum of a typical case (Strain 2611) of influenza November 27 the animal appeared quite well; November 28 it appeared sick, respirations had increased. November 29 it was found dead. Serofibrinous peritonitis and moderate emphysema of the lungs, a total volume of the lungs of 12 c.c., localized hemorrhagic edema and bronchopneumonia of the right apical, cardiac and diaphragmatic lobes were found. The lung was edematous on the cut surface, and the edematous areas were surrounded by marked emphysema (Fig. 1). The pleura was normal. November 30, blood agar cultures of the blood revealed a moderate number of green-producing streptococci and a few staphylococci; those of the lungs showed a large number of green-producing streptococci and a few staphylococci, while blood agar cultures of the peritoneal exudate revealed countless numbers of green-producing streptococci and many staphylococci.

PROTOCOL 2.—Guinea-pig 851, weighing 500 gm., was injected intratracheally, Dec. 28, 1918, with 0.5 c.c. of the dextrose- brain-broth culture of a green-producing streptococcus from the sputum of a case of typical influenza (Strain 2749) after one animal passage. Jan. 3, 1919, the animal died. Marked cloudy swelling of the myocardium, distention of the right ventricle, hemorrhages in the adventitia of the pulmonary artery, voluminous lungs weighing 20 gm., with, a total volume of 18 c.c., and marked hyperemia of the mucous membrane of the trachea and bronchi were found. The right diaphragmatic lobe was almost completely consolidated. The consolidation was clearly lobular in character, but numerous similar areas were completely coalesced. The left pleura was normal and the right was covered with a thick layer of adherent fibrin, particularly opposite the gray areas of consolidation (Fig. 2). There were no areas of softening; but a number of circumscribed areas of hemorrhage and edema in the emphysematous lobes were noted. Jan. 4, 1919, blood agar plate cultures of the blood showed a few colonies of the green-producing streptococcus; the pleural exudate, the pneumonic lung, the kidneys, and the mucous membrane of the nose showed countless numbers, while the edema fluid from the circumscribed areas in the emphysematous lung and the adrenals showed a few.

PROTOCOL 3.—Guinea-pig 968, weighing 380 gm., was injected intratracheally Jan. 14, 1919, at 3:30 p. m., with 2 c.c. of the dextrose broth culture of the hemorrhagic vaginal discharge from a fatal case (Strain 2800) of influenza. Blood agar plates of the culture injected showed countless numbers of green-producing streptococci and a moderate number of colon bacilli. At 7:30 p. m., the respiration was difficult and greatly increased.The animal was restless and irritable and coughed at intervals. At 7:40 p.m., the condition was worse; respirations were extremely rapid and labored, and a bloody fluid was noted about the nostrils. At 7:42 p.m., the animal had a violent attack of bronchial spasm, in which it threw itself about in the effort to breathe. It bled profusely from the nose and mouth, and died three minutes later. The lungs were heavy and enormously distended; their total volume was 22 c.c. (Fig. 3 a). Numerous large and small hemorrhages were found throughout all the lobes. The alveoli, in places, appeared at the rupturing point. There was a small amount of bloody fluid in the pleural cavities. A large amount of bloody frothy fluid escaped from the larynx, and the nostrils were filled with similar material. The cut surface of the lung was extremely moist, dark red, and a large amount of hemorrhagic frothy fluid escaped. There were two small hemorrhagic fetal masses, one in the vagina and the other at the bifurcation of the uterus. The uterine horns were hyperemia The placental mass surrounding the fetuses was hemorrhagic. A number of small hemorrhages were found in the mucous membrane surrounding the point of placental attachment. The amniotic fluid was clear and smears showed no bacteria.

January 16, the blood and mucus from both horns of the uterus were sterile. The lungs and kidneys showed a large number of green-producing streptococci and colon bacilli; the pleura showed colon bacilli, and the adrenal, spleen and liver .showed a few colonies of colon bacilli.

Sections of the lungs showed a striking picture of marked contraction of the bronchi, extreme dilatation of the smaller vessels, interstitial hemorrhage and cellular infiltration alternated with areas showing marked dilatation of alveoli. The dilated alveoli were often distended with edema fluid, blood corpuscles and leukocytes, or they were empty (Fig. 4). In the denser areas of hemorrhage and infiltration, the outline of the walls of the alveoli were wholly lost from edema and infiltration of interstitial tissue. The •denser areas of infiltration were situated around the bronchi. A large number of gram-staining diplococci and a few bacilli were found in the infiltrated areas both within the alveoli and the interstitial tissues.[4]

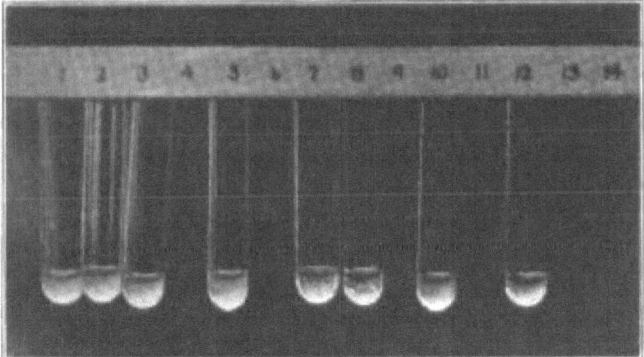

Fig. 5.—Photograph of experiment showing specific agglutination of streptococcus (Strain 3276) from influenza. Dilutions of serums 1-20. Tubes 1, 2, and 3 contain pneumococcus Types I, II and III serums; Tube 5 contains hemolytic streptococcus serum, Horse 9; Tubes 7 and 8 contain the monovalent serum following the injection of one strain of green-producing streptococcus from influenza, the former from a bleeding made March 3, the latter from a bleeding made May 4. Note the greater agglutination in the latter serum, Tube 8; Tube 10 contains normal horse serum; Tube 12, salt solution.

III. THE OCCURRENCE OF A PANDEMIC STRAIN OF STREPTOCOCCUS DURING THE PANDEMIC OF INFLUENZA *

* Presented before the Federation of American Societies for Experimental Biology, Baltimore. April 26. 1919.

The uniformity of symptoms in typical influenza suggests that the cause is a single bacterium having pandemic characteristics. The uniformity of the isolation of the somewhat peculiar green-producing streptococcus, previously described,[5] early in influenza and in the accompanying pneumonia, and the regularity of the invasion by this organism following the injection in guinea-pigs and mice, indicated early in the work that a pandemic strain might be found among this group of streptococci. The experiments following intratracheal injection, in which the picture of this disease is closely simulated, further indicate this possibility, and immunologic experiments were therefore instituted. I wish briefly to record here the main results obtained. The serum of convalescent patients has been found to agglutinate specifically some of the more sensitive strains. The increase in agglutinins has been noted as early as the third day of typical influenzal attacks The serum of cases that occurred early in the epidemic is found to agglutinate strains isolated then and kept in 50 per cent, glycerol as well as those isolated now and vice versa. The results given in Table 2 suffice to illustrate those obtained in a large series of cases. The amount of agglutination with the different strains varies greatly and some strains are not agglutinated at all.

A monovalent immune serum has been prepared in a horse with one of these strains isolated from the blood in a typical fatal case. The horse has been injected with increasing amounts, first with the dead bacteria and later with the living. The serum has developed marked agglutinating power (Fig. 5) over these strains, agglutination occurring in dilutions un to 1: 1,000 and 1: 10,000. The agglutinating power of various immune horse serums, as indicated in the tables, has been tested against numerous strains isolated from the sputum, throat, blood, and lung exudate. The well known methods for determining types of pneumococci, with minor modifications, were used. These included the animal inoculation method as worked out by Cole and the dextrose-blood-broth method as worked out by Avery. The various serums indicated in Table 3, were diluted 1: 10 and equal amounts of this and the broth culture or suspension (0.2 c.c.) were placed in each tube and mixed, incubated one hour, placed in the ice chest over night, and then readings were taken. This dilution was found, after a series of titrations, to be best suited for routine purposes. Specific agglutinations with the monovalent serum as indicated in Table 3 have thus far been obtained in sixty-five of a total of ninety-eight cases studied. Some of these strains, just as has been found to be the case with the streptococcus from poliomyelitis, lose their specific character promptly on cultivation, while others remain susceptible to specific agglutination months after isolation. This was anticipated in the beginning of the work, and dense suspensions of the freshly isolated strains were placed in 50 per cent, glycerol. This method was proved efficacious in studying the specific properties of the poliomyelitis strains, and has been found equally useful in this study. Many strains isolated in the beginning of the epidemic are agglutinated specifically by this serum prepared with a single strain isolated early this year (January, 1919), just as are the strains from typical influenza isolated since then. The cases studied came from widely separated communities- Most of the negative agglutinations occurred when the cultures were made during convalescence. The results in some typical cases, however, suggest the possibility of subgroups. The specific strain, according to this test, has been isolated from the sputum as early as the first day of influenza, from the sputum in the accompanying pneumonia, and from the blood and lung •exudate after death. It tends to disappear promptly during convalescence and is rarely found in normal throats. Strains of green-producing streptococci from a wide range of sources are rarely agglutinated by this serum. In studying the agglutinating power of various immune serums over strains from the sputum daily or on alternate days throughout the disease, it has been found that the strains are agglutinated specifically by this serum throughout the course in typical cases in which the patients recover without developing pneumonia or in which the pneumonia is of short duration. This is not usually true, however, of patients with protracted or recurring pneumonia, especially those who die (Strain 3276, Table 3). In these there may he a shifting of agglutination to pneumococcus serums, Types II or III, to hemolytic streptococcus serum, or, more often, they may not be agglutinated by any of the serums. Most of the specific strains, according to this test, do not ferment inulin and are not bile-soluble.

TABLE 2. – AGGLUTINATION EXPERIMENTS WITH HUMAN SERUMS

Serums from Influenza (Dilutions 1-10)	Day of Disease	Strains from Influenza						Control Strain 3323.3
		3271².3 Sputum	3296².2 Sputum	3331 Sputum	3333.2 Sputum	3333.2 Throat	3334.2 Sputum	
3074 (normal)	..	0	++	+	++	+	0	0
3075 (normal)	..	0	++	0	0	+	+	0
3076 (normal)	..	0	++	0	0	0	0	0
3282	..	++	++++	++	++	+++	++	0
3283	13	++	+++	++	+	+++	+	0
3331	6	++	+++	+	+++	+++	++	0
3332	5	++	+	+++	+	+++	++	+
3334	5	+++	++	++	++	++	++	0
3338	7	++	++++	++	+	++	0	0
3339	2	++	++++	++	++	++	++	0
3348	4	+++	+++	++	+++	++	+	0
3348	10	++	++++	+++	+++	++	++	0
3349	3	++	+++	+	+++	++	++	0
3349	9	++	+++	+++	+++	+++	0	0
NaCl	..	0	0	0	0	0	0	0

The results obtained in this series of experiments are illustrated, in the main, in Table 3. It will be noted that the primary cultures (Strains 3208, 3297, 3301, 3302, 3276) and the peritoneal washings from mice (Strains 3225,² 3226,² 3227,² 3231²) were agglutinated specifically by this serum (Horse 15) in every instance as were the cultures from single colonies after animal passage (Strains 320S².2, 3276².2). The

TABLE 3. AGGLUTINATION OP STREPTOCOCCI FROM INFLUENZA BY IMMUNE HORSE SERUMS

* The figures to the right and above the figures indicating the strain indicate the animal passage, those to the right of the period indicate the culture generation.

result in the third column (Strain 3208.2) shows that it is not always possible to fish the specific strain when the sputum or other material is plated directly. Many strains of the green-producing streptococcus from influenza have acquired hemolytic power in my hands and resemble closely the hemolytic streptococci isolated from some of the cases, especially after death. The close relationship of the green-producing strains to hemolytic streptococcus is indicated, moreover, by the fact that the hemolytic streptococcus serum commonly manifests decided agglutinating power over them (Table 3). The agglutination experiments show that the green-producing strains of streptococci from influenza are immunologically identical or closely related. If this is true, single highly agglutinable strains should absorb the specific agglutinins from the serum for all the rest. This has been found to be the case in a large number of tests. Strains isolated in the beginning of the epidemic absorb the agglutinins so that a large number of strains isolated recently are no longer agglutinated. The results with a number of these strains are given in Table 4. It will be noted that while the specific strain absorbed the agglutinins, Type II pneumococci, which were not agglutinated, removed few or no antibodies.

The symptoms and lesions of influenza have been closely simulated in guinea-pigs by the intratracheal application of green-producing streptococci from influenza. The existence of a pandemic strain among the green-producing streptococci or diplostreptococci in influenza is shown by the immunologic studies summarized in this paper.

TABLE 4. SPECIFIC AGGLUTININ-ABSORPTION BY THE STREPTOCOCCUS FROM INFLUEZA

Mixtures (Dilution of Serum 1-40)	Strains											
	3208*.2	2900*.2	2874.13	3238*	3203.4	3382.3	337.0.4	3389	3407.2	3404	3412	3415.2
Serum Horse 15	4+	3+	3+	2+	2+	3+	2+	2+	4+	2+	2+	3+
Serum Horse 15 after treatment with pneumococcus II	3+	2+	3+	2+	2+	2+	2+	2+	3+	2+	2+	3+
Serum Horse 15 after treatment with streptococcus from Influenza	0	0	0	+	+	0	0	0	+	0	0	+
Normal horse serum	0	0	0	0	0	0	0	0	0	0	0	0
NaCl solution	0	0	0	0	0	0	0	0	0	0	0	0

1. Rosenow, E. C.: Transmutations Within the Streptococcus-Pneumococcus Group, J. Infect. Dis. 4:1-32, 1914
2. Rosenow, E. C.: Prophylactic Inoculation Against Respiratory Infection During the Present Pandemic of Influenza, Preliminary Report, J. A. M. A. 72: 31, 1919.
3. Rosenow, E.C.: On the Toxicity of Broth, of Pneumococcus Broth Culture Filtrates, and on the Nature of the Proteolytic Enzyme Obtainable from Pneumococci, J. Infect. Dis. 11 : 286 292, 1912.
4. In addition to the references already given, the following will be found of interest:
Lamar, R. V., and Meltzer, S. J.: Experimental Pneumonia by Intra- bronchial Insufflation, J. Exper. Med. 15: 133, 1912.
Winternitz, M. C., and Hirschfelder, A. D.: Studies upon Experimental Pneumonia in Rabbits, Parts I and II, J. Exper. Med. 17: 657, 1913.
5. Rosenow, E. C.: Prophylactic Inoculation Against Respiratory Infection During the Present Pandemic of Influenza.—Preliminary Report, J. A. M. A. 78:31-34 (Jan. 4) 1919.

STUDIES IN INFLUENZA AND PNEUMONIA

IV. FURTHER RESULTS OF PROPHYLACTIC INOCULATIONS *

E. C. ROSENOW, M.D.
AND
B. F. STURDIVANT, M.D.
ROCHESTER, MINN.

*From the Division of Experimental Bacteriology, Mayo Foundation.
*This paper and that of Dr. G. W. McCoy which follows are part of a symposium on "Influenza." The remaining papers and the discussion will appear next week.
*Read before the joint meeting of the Section on Pharmacology Therapeutics, the Section on Pathology and Physiology and the Section on Preventive Medicine and Public Health at the Seventieth Annual Session of the American Medical Association, Atlantic City, N.J., June, 1919.

To determine the value of vaccination against disease, it is essential that the disease shall be one which a relatively large number of persons will develop unless protected, and that it be accompanied by serious consequences. These conditions were amply fulfilled during the pandemic of influenza. Moreover, the vaccine should contain the killed bacteria that produce symptoms and which are at least contributory to the cause of death. We have attempted, so far as possible, to fulfill this requirement by making a careful bacteriologic study of the disease, and by incorporating into the vaccine the important bacteria isolated. The epidemic was severe, and the need and the demand for vaccination were great; a large number of cases were available for bacteriologic study and to supply the proper strains for the vaccine. Vaccinations in large numbers during the past ten years with bacteria belonging to the group found in influenza have at least proved harmless, and in the case of pneumonia, prophylactic vaccinations have been successfully carried out by Wright,[1] Lister,[2] and Cecil and Austin.[3] A splendid opportunity to study the effect of prophylactic inoculation was at hand. Owing to the foresight of the founders of the Mayo Foundation, necessary funds to meet the emergency were available. A large amount of the vaccine has been prepared and sent gratis on request to numerous physicians on condition that reports of the results be returned.

In a previous report,[4] the reasons for the use of a mixed vaccine containing, as far as possible, freshly isolated strains were discussed. It was pointed out that the streptococci, especially green-producing streptococci from influenza, have certain peculiar properties. The preliminary results, as reported from the use of this vaccine, indicate that considerable protection is afforded against influenza and especially against the accompanying pneumonia. Vaccinations were begun soon after the onset of the epidemic. The period of observation was six weeks. It is our purpose in this paper to emphasize essential points in the preparation of the vaccine, to present further results from its use, and to record certain immunologic experiments.

COMPOSITION AND PREPARATION OF THE VACCINE

Influenza bacilli were isolated in large numbers at the outset of the epidemic, but they were rarely found later in the epidemic. The small fraction of influenza bacilli included in the first few batches of vaccine were therefore omitted, and the vaccine was made to contain a proportionately higher percentage of the green- producing streptococci. In other respects, the original formula has been adhered to. The formula as used in almost all cases covered by the present report is given in Table 1.

TABLE 1.—FORMULA OF VACCINE

Pneumococci, Types I (10 per cent.), II (14 per cent.), and III (6 per cent.)	30 per cent.
Pneumococci Group IV and the allied green-producing diplostreptococci described	40 per cent.
Hemolytic streptococci	20 per cent.
Staphylococcus aureus	10 per cent.

The preparation of the medium, the method of cultivating and collecting the bacteria, and the procedure of standardizing the dose and killing the bacteria are described in the preliminary report.[4] The vaccine, it will be remembered, was made to contain approximately 5 billion bacteria for 1 c.c. Later, the concentration was made twice as great, and the quantity of liquid was reduced to one-half. The injections were given subcutaneously one week apart. The first dose of the concentrated vaccine (0.25 c.c.) contained 2.5 billion, the second (0.5 c.c.) 5 billion, and the third (0.75 c.c.) 7.5 billion bacteria. Considering the large size of these doses and the reactions obtained, the injections should not be given oftener than once a week in order not to overstimulate the mechanism of immunity.

The tendency of streptococci to undergo changes and to lose specific properties has been repeatedly emphasized by one of us. It was thought important that freshly isolated strains should be included in the vaccine. In Table 2 are given the culture generations of all the strains that have been used throughout the epidemic. The fermentation power was tested of fifty-seven strains of the green-producing streptococci included in the vaccine; only twenty-seven fermented inulin, and only eight were bile soluble.

TABLE 2.—CULTURE GENERATION OF BACTERIA FROM INFLUENZA AS USED IN THE VACCINE

Cultures	Green-Producing Streptococcus	Hemolytic Streptococcus	Staphylococcus
Third generation or below	58	18	18
Fourth to tenth generation	95	20	8
Eleventh to twentieth generation	21	0	0
Total	174	38	26

The advantages which should come from the use of a lipovaccine, particularly when a series of strains needs to be included, have already been pointed out, and a simple method for the preparation in oil of a vaccine of the formula given in Table 1 has been developed and submitted for publication. A further study of the sputum and other material shows that of all the bacteria isolated, the somewhat peculiar green-producing streptococcus or diplostreptococcus is the most important. This organism is present in large numbers at the very outset of symptoms of influenza and of the accompanying pneumonia; it is commonly present after death. If the sputum or mass cultures are injected intraperitoneally into animals, they die, usually from invasion of the green-producing streptococci or pneumococci. If injected intratracheally in guinea-pigs the picture of influenzal pneumonia is closely simulated. Immunologic experiments with the serum from a horse injected with one strain indicate that most of the strains are immunologically alike. The serum of cases of influenza develops agglutinating power over these strains.

AGGLUTINATING POWER

In Table 3 it is shown that the vaccine used possessed well marked antigenic powers. The strains S 1, S 3, $2598^2.2$, 2604.2, 3048.3, and $2874^2.3$ were green-producing streptococci or pneumococci; 2575.2, a hemolytic streptococcus, and $2608^3.2$, a staphylococcus from cases of influenza. It will be noted that agglutinins appear in the serum on the tenth day and persist for six weeks. Table 3 shows, moreover, that the bacteria in the vaccine (492) used as the antigen in the first column were susceptible to agglutination. This vaccine was prepared three months previously and was kept in the ice chest. Most of the strains used as antigen in the experiment recorded in this table were not included in the vaccine used to immunize the persons whose serums were tested. All the green- producing streptococci were agglutinated, however, by the monovalent horse serum.

TABLE 3.—AGGLUTINATING POWER OF SERUM OF PERSONS INOCULATED WITH SALINE VACCINE

In Table 4 are given the results following the injection of a single dose of the lipovaccine (from 25 to 75 billions) in three persons. It may be noted that the amount of agglutination is greater than that following the injection of the saline vaccine, but here, as in the case following the injection of the saline vaccine, not all strains are equally susceptible to agglutination, and some are not agglutinated at all.

TABLE 4 AGGLUTINATING POWER OF SERUM, PERSONS INOCULATED WITH LIPOVACCINE

Serums (Dilutions 1:20)	3,271a.8	3,296a.2	3,331	8,332.2	3,334.2	3,334.2	3,342
3,074 normal	0	++	+	+	0	++	0
8,074 4 days after lipo-vaccine	+	+++	++	++	+	++	0
8,074 10 days after lipo-vaccine	+++	++++	+++	++	++	+++	0
8,074 6 weeks after lipo-vaccine	++	+++	++	+	+	++	0
3,075 normal	0	++	0	0	+	0	0
3,075 4 days after lipo-vaccine	++	+	0	0	+	++	0
3,075 10 days after lipo-vaccine	+	++++	+	+	++	++	0
8,076 normal	0	++	+	0	0	0	0
3,076 4 days after lipo-vaccine	+	+++	+	0	+	0	0
3,076 10 days after lipo-vaccine	++	+++	++	0	+	0	0
3,076 6 weeks after lipo-vaccine	+++	++++	+	0	++	0	0
NaCl	0	0	0	0	0	0	0

Table 5 shows the agglutinating power of various immune horse serums over strains of green-producing streptococci from influenza, strains included in the vaccine. The serum from Horse 15, immunized with one strain from the blood of a patient who died, has marked agglutinating power over most of the strains. Of the thirty-three strains tested in this manner, twenty-five were agglutinated specifically by this serum. The results indicate clearly that among the green-producing streptococci, including Group IV pneumococci in influenza, there are strains which have a specific relationship, and that we were fortunate in successfully separating them from the ordinary Streptococcus viridans and including them in the vaccine long before the results of immunologic experiments were available.

The apparent protection against attacks of influenza noted in the preliminary report, difficult to understand at that time, now becomes rational.

METHOD OF SECURING DATA

In most instances the reactions were mild, about one person in each 100 reacted more severely. Some reacted severely to all three inoculations, others only to one or two. Persons coming down with a cold or with symptoms of influenza are often hypersensitive. Marked diffuse redness resembling erysipelas about the site of inoculation, with swelling and, later, marked induration, has occurred occasionally. In no instance were the symptoms alarming. The number of severe reactions is sufficiently large, however, to prevent general vaccination except at the time of an acute emergency.

This is in accord with the experience of Cecil and Austin,[3] noted during prophylactic inoculations with pneumococci. An outline for records of persons vaccinated was sent with each batch of vaccine and later a questionnaire. The questionnaire asked for the date of the onset of the epidemic, the date when the vaccine was first used, the week of the height of the epidemic, the week in which the greatest number of vaccinations were given, and the duration of the epidemic. The number of cases of influenza from the time the vaccinations were begun until the end of the epidemic, or up to May 1, and the number of deaths which occurred among the vaccinated and unvaccinated in the same period, in the practices of the physicians supplied with the vaccine, were asked. The reports of the use of the vaccine after the epidemic had disappeared were excluded. The period of observation in most instances was from four to five months.

In determining a safe criterion as to the value of the vaccine, we have purposely been unfair to the vaccinated group. The protection afforded among the vaccinated patients was measured from the day of the first vaccination, whereas, judging by the agglutination experiments, it should be calculated from about one week after the third injection.

There is another reason why we have arbitrarily decided to make our calculations from the day of the first vaccination. A procedure, calculated to protect against an epidemic disease, such as influenza, should have sufficient protective value when given after the onset of the epidemic to be measurable, for it is practically impossible to anticipate these epidemics and, moreover, persons will not present themselves for vaccination until the epidemic is at hand.

TABLE 5. – AGGLUTINATING POWER OF VARIOUS IMMUNE HORSE SERUMS OVER STREPTOCOCCI INCLUDED IN THE VACCINE

Serums (Dilutions 1:20)	2,347.19	2,349.18	2,350.16	2,531.14	2,532.4	2,534.11	2,557.2	2,604.2	2,618².2	2,684.16	2,696³.3	2,719²	2,769	2,800².2	2,825
Pneumococcus Type I	0	0	0	+	0	0	0	0	0	0	0	0	0	0	0
Pneumococcus Type II	++	0	0	+	0	+	0	0	0	++	0	0	0	0	0
Pneumococcus Type III	0	0	0	+	0	+	0	0	0	0	0	+++	0	0	0
Horse 9	++	++	0	+	0	++	0	0	0	0	0	+++	0	0	++
Horse 15	++++	++	++++	++++	+++	++++	0	+++	++++	++	++++	++	0	++	+++
Normal horse	0	0	0	+	0	+	0	0	0	0	0	0	0	0	0
NaCl	0	●	0	0	0	0	0	0	0	0	0	0	0	0	0

TABLE 6. – AS REPORTED IN QUESTIONNAIRES FROM ALL SOURCES

Groups	Total Number	Incidence for 1,000 Persons									
		Disease				Deaths					
		Influenza	Acute Edema of Lungs	Pneumonia	Empyema	Acute Edema of Lungs	Pneumonia	Empyema	Meningitis	Encephalitis	Total Deaths
Vaccinated once	20,936	118.2	3.1	8.7	0.29	0.14	2.6	0.07	0.18	....	3.0
Vaccinated twice	23,348	97.0	0.77	3.04	0.17	0.47	1.9	0.04	0.21	....	2.62
Vaccinated 3 times	93,478	87.9	0.8	4.4	0.18	0.18	1.2	0	0.05	....	1.43
Not vaccinated	345,133	281.8	4.4	21.0	0.83	1.7	2.37	0.07	0.15	0.03	8.55

The questionnaire was arranged so as to yield information regarding the incidence of influenza, acute edema of the lungs, pneumonia and empyema, and the deaths from acute edema of the lungs, pneumonia, empyema, meningitis, and encephalitis among the vaccinated and the unvaccinated. Separate reports including the foregoing points were asked for from institutions and in the cases of pregnant women. The impressions gained from the use of the vaccine regarding the severity of the disease if contracted following vaccination, and the effect, if any, which the vaccine had on certain chronic infections, such as bronchitis, sinusitis, myositis, and arthritis were asked for.

Many physicians were so overwhelmed during the height of the epidemic that accurate records could not be kept, and accordingly the reports containing accurate data are proportionately few. The reports of 530 physicians were fairly complete, however, and these are summarized in Table 6. It is realized that there must necessarily be errors in the morbidity figures as reported to us, ji.it as in the case of reports to boards of health. It is generally agreed that as influenza became more prevalent and less severe, a proportionately smaller number of cases were reported, and that all morbidity figures reported are well below the actual figures. The error, however, among the vaccinated and unvaccinated groups in the reports to us, should be approximately the same, and hence the figures should be comparable. Mortality figures, on the other hand, may be considered as fairly accurate.

RESULTS OF INOCULATION

The total number of unvaccinated persons recorded in Table 6 represents the sum of the estimated clienteles of the various physicians reporting the cases, and averages about 1,200 for each. It will be noted that the incidence of influenza, of acute edema of the lungs, of pneumonia following influenza, and the number of deaths from all causes among the vaccinated are consistently lower than that among the unvaccinated. Moreover, the incidence of disease and deaths is lowest in the group of 93,476 persons who were vaccinated three times. The reports included in this table were from many states, but the largest number came from Iowa, Minnesota, and Wisconsin. Thirteen thousand, six hundred and fifty persons inoculated and 2,083 who died were grouped according to age by decades. The curves indicating the percentage in each run roughly parallel.

The largest number of inoculations were given and the largest number of deaths occurred between the ages of 11 and 40 years. The percentages of the former in these three decades were 23, 19, and 21, of the latter 13, 29, and 23, respectively. Through the cooperation of the Board of Health of Minnesota we were able to check the results as reported to us with the morbidity and mortality figures as reported to them. Reports on a considerable number of vaccinations were received from Brown, Chippewa, Clay, Dodge, Fillmore, Goodhue, Houston, Itasca, Lesueur, Lyon, Mower, Olmsted, Rice, Stearne, Steele, Wabasha, Waseca, Watonwan, and Winona counties. The total estimated population of these counties is 472,584. The total number of cases of influenza in these counties reported to the board of health from the beginning of the epidemic until May 1 is 30,763, or sixty-five for each thousand. This is admittedly a low figure. The total mortality rate as reported to the board of health during this time is 4.2. The mortality rate, excluding the deaths which occurred in the respective counties prior to the date of the first vaccinations, is 3.2 (Table 7). The figures in the table indicating the cases and the

TABLE 7.—RESULTS AS REPORTED IN QUESTIONNAIRES FROM NINETEEN COUNTIES IN MINNESOTA EXCLUSIVE OF THE MAYO CLINIC

Groups	Total Number	Disease				Incidence for 1,000 Persons		Deaths			Total Deaths
		Influenza	Acute Edema of Lungs	Pneumonia	Empyema	Acute Edema of Lungs	Pneumonia	Empyema	Meningitis	Encephalitis	
Vaccinated once...	4,828	115.1	0.4	8.28	0	0	0.2	0	0	0	0.2
Vaccinated twice..	4,029	88.3	0.74	3.7	0.47	0.47	1.9	0	0.47	....	3.2
Vaccinated 3 times	17,532	102.8	0.17	4.3	0.22	...	0.62	....	....	....	0.8
Not vaccinated....	36,100	373.5	1.35	20.4	0.6	1.4	4.0	0.13	0.16	0.02	6.35
As reported to State Board of Health............ (Estimated population)	472,584	65.3	....	....	....	....	....	....	....	....	3.2*

* Exclusive of deaths which occurred prior to the use of the vaccine and exclusive of Mayo Clinic cases.

deaths as reported to us are believed to be more accurate. The mortality rate, exclusive of that of the Mayo Clinic, in the 17,532 persons vaccinated three times is only one fourth of that reported to the board of health. Moreover, the total number of deaths among the vaccinated, including the persons inoculated only once and twice, is 1.6 for 1,000, or half the mortality rate as reported to the board of health during the same period of time. When we consider the fact that the deaths in each group were counted from the time the first vaccinations were given, which is really unfair to the vaccine, and the fact that our figures include all pneumonias, while those of the board of health include only the influenzal pneumonias, there seems little doubt that the difference must be due to the protection afforded by the vaccine. The figures given in Table 8 for Olmsted County, where about one third of the population was vaccinated, exclusive of the Mayo Clinic and the state hospital, are similar to those obtained elsewhere. The incidence of disease and the death rate among those vaccinated three times are well below that of those not vaccinated.

TABLE 8.—RESULTS IN OLMSTED COUNTY EXCLUSIVE OF MAYO CLINIC & STATE HOSPITAL FOR INSANE

Groups	Total Number	Disease				Incidence for 1,000 Persons		Deaths			Total Deaths
		Influenza	Acute Edema of Lungs	Pneumonia	Empyema	Acute Edema of Lungs	Pneumonia	Empyema	Meningitis	Encephalitis	
Vaccinated once...	2,424	100.2	0	6.1	0	0.41	2.8	0	0	0	3.2
Vaccinated twice..	1,021	291.8	2.9	0	1.9	0	4.8	0	1.9	....	6.7
Vaccinated 3 times	9,300	41.0	0.18	3.9	0.43	....	0.43	0.21	....	....	0.64
Not vaccinated....	8,700	248.0	3.2	13.1	0.45	0.9	2.6	0.45	0.12	....	4.0

The results obtained in institutions in which the conditions among the vaccinated and the unvaccinated were comparable are summarized and given in Table 9 in order still further to check the figures. The number of persons in most of the institutions included (fifty- three in all) was small. The opportunity for accurate observation was, therefore, favorable. The institutions included factories, personnel of hospitals, schools, and offices. The proportion of the vaccinated and unvaccinated varied between wide limits. The period of observation in the two groups was the same. The incidence of disease and the number of deaths in almost all instances were lower in the vaccinated than in the unvaccinated group. The total average, as given in Table 9, compares favorably with that of the others. The death rate among the vaccinated is decidedly lower than among the unvaccinated.

The results given in the tables are in agreement with the numerous reports received by which it appeared that the vaccine had afforded striking instances of protection. In a few cases no protection seemed to be afforded, but in most of these the vaccinated persons contracted the disease a long time after the inoculations. It is fully realized how difficult-it is to judge just how much protection was conferred in many of these, instances, and how much of the apparent protection was merely coincidental. But a careful study of the reports from 303 physicians, some of which were the result of careful observation, forces the conviction that real protection, especially against pneumonia, was afforded. In some of these instances most of the observations were made within six weeks to two months after the vaccine was given.

TABLE 9.—RESULTS OF PROPHYLACTIC INOCULATION IN INSTITUTIONS WHERE THE CONDITIONS AMONG THE VACCINATED AND UNVACCINATED WERE COMPARABLE

Groups	Total Number	Incidence for 1,000 Persons — Disease			Deaths		
		Influenza	Acute Edema of Lungs	Pneumonia	Empyema	Acute Edema of Lungs	Pneumonia
Vaccinated 3 times	8,806	31	0.1	1.0	0.2	0	0.5
Not vaccinated	9,388	200	0.5	12.0	0.6	0.4	5.5

It was thought that the injection of large doses of a mixed vaccine might have some effect on certain chronic infections, especially of the respiratory tract. A summary of the reports shows that 961 persons with chronic bronchitis were benefited and that thirty-eight were made worse. The reports show that 127 persons with chronic sinusitis were benefited and four made worse. Improvement was noted in 121 persons having myositis and in 129 with arthritis, while in one of the former and in twenty-two of the latter the symptoms were aggravated. These figures are not considered to be especially significant but worthy of record. They are in accord with our own observations.

RESULTS OF PROPHYLACTIC INOCULATION IN PREGNANCY

The results of vaccinations in pregnant women as reported in the questionnaires are summarized in Table 10. The incidence of disease and that of miscarriages and the mortality rate are consistently lower among those vaccinated than among those not vaccinated. The mortality (20 per cent.) of the unvaccinated pregnant women who developed influenza is somewhat lower than that reported from similar statistical studies by Bland[5] and by Harris.[6] They report a mortality of 37.7 per cent, and 27 per cent., respectively. The mortality of 12 per cent, in the 997 pregnant women inoculated in our series is in sharp contrast and calls for a further trial of this measure.

Almost from the beginning of the epidemic of influenza, patients who registered at the Mayo Clinic were advised to be vaccinated. From October 1 to May 1, 55,189 patients registered. Of these, 2,542 were vaccinated once, 1,030 twice, and 1,850 three times, a total of 5,422.

TABLE 10.—RESULTS OF PROPHYLACTIC INOCULATIONS IN PREGNANCY

		Disease — Incidence for 1,000 Persons — Deaths										
		Acute				Acute						Mortality of Those
Groups	Total Number	Influenza	Edema of Lungs	Pneumonia	Empyema	Miscarriage	Edema of Lungs	Pneumonia	Empyema	Meningitis	Total Deaths	Who Developed Influenza
Vaccinated 3 times	997	109.3	17.0	27.0	....	14.0	2.0	12.0	....	....	14.0	12 per cent.
Not vaccinated....	3,556	294.6	17.7	80.4	0.22	46.2	12.3	46.2	0.54	0.82	59.9	20 per cent.

A reliable morbidity and mortality rate for each thousand of the vaccinated and unvaccinated could not be determined because such a large percentage of patients remained in Rochester for too short a time.

TABLE 11.—RESULTS IN CASES OF INFLUENZA ADMITTED TO HOSPITALS IN ROCHESTER

Groups	Cases of Influenza	Incidence of Pneumonia	Deaths from Pneumonia, per Cent.
Vaccinated once.................	59	39	10
Vaccinated twice................	24	95	12
Vaccinated three times..........	57	21	5
Not vaccinated..................	609	57	22

It was thought that a study of the cases of influenza admitted to the hospitals might, however, be worthwhile. Of these, 749 were undoubted cases of influenza, and were analyzed from various standpoints. Fifty-nine of the patients were vaccinated once; twenty-four, twice, and fifty-seven, three times, while 609 were not vaccinated. The incidence of pneumonia and the deaths from pneumonia in these groups are recorded in Table 11. The average interval between the vaccinations and the onset of influenza was nine days in those vaccinated only once, twenty-six days in those vaccinated twice, and forty-five days in those vaccinated three times. The average temperature was more than one degree higher in the unvaccinated than in the vaccinated, and the average duration of fever nearly two days longer. The percentage incidence of pneumonia in those vaccinated three times was 21; in those not vaccinated, 57, while the percentage of deaths from pneumonia was 5 in the former group and 22 in the latter. The mortality from pneumonia of those vaccinated only once and those vaccinated twice is also well below that of the unvaccinated. The mortality figure in the unvaccinated is abnormally high because only the patients with relatively severe attacks were admitted to the hospitals.

The greater tendency to the development of pneumonia in influenza among the unvaccinated group as observed in this series is in keeping with the lower incidence of this complication (4.7 per cent.) in 11,325 cases of influenza in which the vaccine was given after the onset of the symptoms, as compared with the incidence (8.7 per cent.) in 41,788 cases in which the vaccine was not used. The average mortality in the cases in which the vaccine was used in treatment was 1.4 per cent.; in those not treated it was 2.1 per cent.

From these results considerable weight may be attached to the opinion of nearly all the 430 physicians who have used the vaccine and who have reported on this point, an opinion in agreement with our own observations, that is, that the attacks of influenza if contracted following vaccination are milder and of shorter duration.

SUMMARY

The immunologic and animal experiments reported[7] elsewhere indicate that the mixed vaccine used by us contained the important bacteria as they occur in influenza and the accompanying pneumonia, and that a relatively large number of strains of the green-producing streptococci which appear to have a specific relationship to the initial attack were included. The reports included results obtained under the most varied conditions, from many communities covering a wide range of territory. In some communities the mortality rate was excessively high, in others comparatively low. The number of persons inoculated is sufficiently large to make the statistical figures fairly accurate. The period of observation was from three to seven months. The incidence of influenza and pneumonia as reported to us is probably far from exact, but the percentage of error should be about the same in the vaccinated and unvaccinated groups. Indeed, if a difference exists, the number of cases reported among the vaccinated might be expected to be proportionately higher because, even though no protection was promised, the fact that influenza occurred after the vaccinations were taken would naturally lead to a higher percentage of reports to the physician who gave the inoculations. The average incidence of influenza and pneumonia in the group inoculated three times is about one-third that of the uninoculated group.

The average mortality rate in the uninoculated, as reported to us, approximates the mortality rate (5.4 per cent.) of sixteen large cities of the United States as given in Public Health Reports for February 7. The average mortality rate in the group inoculated three times is about one-fifth that of the uninoculated. A definite, although a smaller degree, of protection appeared to be afforded to those who took only one or two inoculations. From a study of a series of hospital cases of influenza it is found that the tendency to the development of pneumonia in the vaccinated is about one third as great as among the unvaccinated, and that the mortality in the former is about one fifth as great as in the latter. The number of completed vaccinations in pregnant women is not large enough to give exact figures, but the results indicate clearly that a definite degree of protection was afforded in this group of individuals.

It appears from all the facts at hand that by the use of a properly prepared vaccine it is possible to rob influenza of some of its terrors.

The preliminary results from the use of more than 500 doses of this vaccine suspended in oil, the immunologic studies and the results from the use of pneumococcus lipovaccine reported by Fennel[8] and by Cecil and Vaughan[0] suggest strongly that both the degree of protection and the duration of the immunity may be materially increased by the use of lipovaccine over that reported in this paper from the use of the saline vaccine.

1. Wright, A. E.; Morgan, W. P., et al.: Observations on Prophylactic Inoculation Against Pneumococcus Infections and on the Results Which Have Been Achieved by It, Lancet X: 1-10 (Jan. 3) 1914..

2. Lister, F. S.: Prophylactic Inoculation of Man Against Pneumococcal Infections and More Particularly Against Lobar Pneumonia; Including a Report on the Results of the Experimental Inoculation with a Specific Group Vaccine, of the Native Mine Laborers Employed on the Premier (Diamond) Mine and the Crown (Gold) Mines in the Transvaal and the de Beers (Diamond) Mines at Kimberley — Covering the Period from Nov. 1, 1916, to Oct. 31, 1917, Publications ot » South African Institute for Medical Research, Johannesburg, So Africa, W. E. Horton and Company, Ltd., 1917, pp. 1-30.

3. Cecil, R. L., and Austin, J. H.: Prophylactic Inoculation Against Pneumococcus, J. Exper. M. 28:19-41 (July 18) 1918.

4. Rosenow, E. C.: Prophylactic Inoculation Against Respiratory Infections: Preliminary Report, J. A. M. A. 72: 31-34 (Jan. 4) 1919.

5. Bland, P. B.: Influenza in Its Relation to Pregnancy and Labor, Am. J. Obst. 79:184-197 (Feb. 19) 1919.

6. Harris, J. W.: Influenza Occurring in Pregnant Women, J, A. M. A. 72:978-980 (April S) 1919.

7. Rosenow, E. C.: The Experimental Production of Symptoms and Lesions Simulating Those of Influenza with Streptococci Isolated During the Present Epidemic, Study II, J. A. M. A. 73:1604-1608 (May 31) 1919. The Occurrence of a Pandemic Strain of Streptococcus During the Pandemic of Influenza, Study III, ibid. pp. 1608-1609.

8. Fennel, E. A.: Prophylactic Inoculation Against Pneumonia, J. A. M. A. 71:2115-2120 (Dec. 28) 1918.

9. Cecil, R. L., and Vaughan, H.: Results of Prophylactic Vaccination Against Pneumonia at "Camp Wheeler, J. Exper. M. 29:457-4S3 (June) 1919.

STUDIES IN INFLUENZA AND PNEUMONIA

STUDY V. OBSERVATIONS ON THE BACTERIOLOGY AND CERTAIN CLINICAL FEATURES OF INFLUENZA AND INFLUENZAL PNEUMONIA

E. C. ROSENOW

Division of Experimental Bacteriology, The Mayo Foundation, Rochester, Minnesota.

The bacteriologic studies of the epidemic of influenza of 1889-1890,[13] of lesser outbreaks prior to the pandemic of 1918,[15] and the preliminary studies of the pandemic by others have shown that while influenza bacilli occur commonly the organisms of the pneumococcus-streptococcus group are constantly associated with this disease. In the course of my studies on this group of organisms and the diseases due to them I have been impressed repeatedly by the marked changes they undergo at times, particularly in infecting powers and immunologic reactions. In some instances these changes appeared to be true mutations.[25] It was thought possible that the peculiar picture presented in influenza, such as the marked prostration, cyanosis, leukopenia, and its almost simultaneous appearance over wide areas might be due to variants or mutation forms of organisms commonly present in the respiratory tract of man. Accordingly, as the epidemic reached Rochester a comprehensive plan of study, taking into consideration this possibility, was determined on. The results obtained form the basis of the series of experiments that I report. Preliminary statements, including a description of the somewhat peculiar green-producing streptococcus isolated quite constantly,[22] of immunologic studies,[24] and of the extraordinary invasive power of the streptococci from influenza on intratracheal application,[23] have been published.

In this paper are recorded the more important bacteriologic findings obtained throughout the four epidemic waves of influenza which occurred in Rochester during the autumn and winter of 1918-1919, and these findings correlated with certain clinical features of the disease.

The epidemic of 1918 began in Rochester during the latter part of September. An emergency hospital was opened and when this became inadequate certain parts of other hospitals were set aside for the care of influenza patients. The source of the material studied was, in the main, from patients admitted to these hospitals, most of whom had come to the Mayo Clinic for the treatment of some other condition or to accompany patients. A large number of cultures, however, were made from persons residing permanently in Rochester who had contracted influenza. A large proportion of the first group came long distances from widely separated communities, and many developed symptoms before or soon after their arrival. Some no doubt were infected en route or before leaving home; hence, the cases studied represent a heterogeneous group and the findings accordingly may be regarded as quite representative of the epidemic.

TECHNIC

Cultures were made from throat swabs prepared in the usual manner, from sputum, anterior nares, lung exudate, trachea and bronchi, peritracheal lymph gland, pleural fluid, the blood after death, and in some instances, from the blood during life. The sputum was collected in sterile, wide-mouthed glass vials and taken to the laboratory while fresh. Cultures were made on the surface of blood-agar plates directly or after washing in sodium chlorid solution, and into tall columns of dextrose broth, dextrose-brain broth or dextrose-blood broth. Owing to the mucoid and serous character of the sputum in influenza washing the sputum was quite unsatisfactory since it led to too great a dilution and hence the plates were made routinely by spreading a rather large amount of the unwashed sputum (about 0.1 cc) directly over the plates by means of triangular-shaped spreaders made from flat nicrome wire. The material was spread over the whole surface of the plate, part of the plate was heavily, and part lightly inoculated. The plates were incubated twenty-four hours at from 33 to 35 C. and then read. If influenza bacilli were not present the plates were incubated for an additional twenty-four or forty-eight hours. The air in the incubator was kept saturated with moisture by means of an open dish of water and by reducing the amount of ventilation to the minimum. The results of the cultures on the plates were recorded according to the numerical scale of 1 to 4; 1 indicating from 1 to 10 colonies; 2 from 11 to 100 colonies; 3 from 101 to 1,000 colonies and 4, 1,000 colonies and above, of the different bacteria. After death material was collected in sterile pipets by the pathologist in charge and brought directly to the laboratory for examination. The cultures of this material were made in the same manner as those from the sputum. Smears from throat and sputum during life, and of material after death were made, stained for bacteria and examined, in some cases in order to check the results of the cultures, and to study the proportion and character of the cells and their behavior toward the bacteria present. In order to check the results of cultures and direct examination of the exudate still further, and to determine which of the bacteria nearly always present had the greatest invasive powers in influenza, the sputum and exudates of some of the cases were injected intraperitoneally and intratracheally into guinea-pigs and intraperitoneally into white mice. Smears and cultures of the peritoneal or lung exudate and blood of these animals were made according to the method just described.

At first plain agar, made from beef extract and peptone, to which 5 per cent. of defibrinated human blood was added, was used, but since influenza bacilli were not detected on these plates, the so-called "hormone" or "vitamine" agar was substituted. The medium was carefully titrated to $+0.6$ per cent. to phenolphthalein, and cleared by the use of a centrifugal machine. Usually, however, it was slightly opalescent from fat which was not wholly removed from the meat. One and seven-tenths per cent. agar was added instead of from 2 to 2.5 per cent. as is usually done. To this medium, cooled to about 60 C. approximately 4 per cent. of defibrinated human blood was added before it was poured into the plate. The plates were not usually incubated previously so that the surface of the agar was not hard and dry, but soft and moist. The advantages of this medium over the plain agar medium for growing influenza bacilli were striking. Large numbers of typical influenza bacillus colonies developed from the sputum of patients when few or none had been detected previously on plain-blood agar. In order to make sure that the lack of growth of bacilli on the plain blood-agar used previously was not due to their absence, but to a difference in the medium, parallel cultures on the two mediums were made of the sputum of 8 cases of typical influenza occurring at the outset of the first wave. All hormone-blood-agar plates showed countless numbers of influenza bacilli which grew in symbiosis with the green-producing streptococcus or pneumococcus, hemolytic streptococcus, and staphylococcus colonies, whereas the plain blood-agar plates showed few or no colonies of influenza bacilli. The colonies were usually found in the heavily inoculated part of the plate and surrounding colonies of green-producing streptococci and staphylococci, but were found also in other parts of the plate. Cultures from throats of some of these patients yielded similar results although influenza bacilli were present in larger numbers. Because of these findings, this medium was adopted for routine platings throughout the study. During the latter part of the work the special mediums for the isolation of influenza bacilli such as Avery's oleate agar [1] and of "chocolate" blood-agar plates were also used.

RESULTS

Cultures were made of the sputum or from the exudate of the throat of 571 patients with influenza or influenzal pneumonia during life, of the lung exudate, peribronchial lymph glands, or the blood after death in 107 cases. In 309 of the group of 571 and in 65 of the 107, both the clinical history and pathologic findings left no doubt as to the diagnosis. In the remaining 262 cases complete histories were not available for final analysis, but the diagnosis of influenza or influenzal pneumonia was made by the physician in charge at the time of the attack. The findings after death in 42 of these were clearly those of influenza, and since the bacteriologic findings in all were similar to those in the undoubted cases the diagnosis of influenza may be considered quite accurate.

TABLE 1

RESULT OF CULTURES OF MATERIAL FROM INFLUENZA AND INFLUENZAL PNEUMONIA

Bacteria	Material Cultured, Blood-Agar Plates					
	Sputum During Life (571 Cases)			Lung Exudate after Death (107 Cases)		
	Predominating or in Pure Culture, Percentage	Not in Predominating Numbers, Percentage	Total Percentage	Predominating or in Pure Culture, Percentage	Not in Predominating Numbers, Percentage	Total Percentage
Green-producing streptococci or pneumococci	41	54	95	18	37	55
Hemolytic streptococci	1	29	38	23	54	77
Staphylococci	17	55	72	10	40	50
Bacillus influenzae	5	8	13	0	5	5
Micrococcus catarrhalis	0	6	6	0	3	3
Bacillus mucosus	0.8	1	1.8	4	7	11
Bacillus coli	0	0.8	0.8	3	15	18

The results obtained are summarized in Table 1. The figures giving the number of instances in which the various bacteria were found are omitted from the table and only those indicating the percentage are given, thus making direct comparisons readily possible. Fractions of a per cent. below 0.5 are dropped, to those 0.5 or above, one is added. The tabulations shown represent cases and not specimens. In many cases the sputum was cultured repeatedly during the course of the initial influenzal attack and during the influenzal pneumonia which followed. The figures in the first and fourth columns indicate the percentage incidence in which the different bacteria were present in predominating numbers or in pure culture; in the second and fifth columns the percentage incidence in which the bacteria were present, but not in predominating numbers; and in the third and sixth columns the total percentage incidence to the occurrence of the different bacteria in the sputum and lung exudate respectively.

Green-producing streptococci (some of which fermented inulin) were isolated from the sputum in predominating numbers or in pure culture in 41 per cent., and not in predominating numbers in 54 per cent., a total of 96 per cent. of the 571 cases studied; they were isolated from the lung exudate after death in predominating numbers or in pure culture in 18 per cent., and in smaller numbers in 37 per cent., a total of 55 per cent. of the 107 cases in which necropsies were made. Hemolytic streptococci occurred in the sputum in predominating numbers or in pure culture in 9 per cent., and not in predominating numbers in 29 per cent., a total of 38 per cent. of the cases studied during life; they occurred in the lung exudate in predominating numbers or in pure culture in 23 per cent., and not in predominating numbers in 54 per cent., a total of 77 per cent. of the cases after death. Staphylococci were isolated in varying numbers from the sputum in 72 per cent. and from the lung exudate in 50 per cent. of the cases. The influenza bacillus was isolated from the sputum in 13 per cent., and in predominating numbers in 5 per cent.; it was isolated from the lung exudate in 5 per cent. of the cases, never in predominating numbers. Micrococcus catarrhalis was found in the sputum in 6 per cent., and in the lung exudate in 3 per cent. of the cases, always in small numbers. The Bacillus mucosus was found in the sputum in 1.8 per cent., and in the lung exudate in 11 per cent. The colon bacillus occurred in the sputum in 0.8 per cent., and in the lung exudate in 18 per cent. of the cases.

The figures represent only in a general way the relative importance of a series of different types of bacteria isolated during life and after death. Thus the incidence of staphylococcus in predominating numbers in the sputum in 17 per cent. of the cases should not be taken to mean that this organism was the cause of the attack in this percentage of cases, because in many only one or two cultures were made, often late in the disease when staphylococci had become relatively numerous. The lowering in total incidence of green-producing streptococci of from 96 per cent. in the sputum to 55 per cent. in the lung exudate, and the increase in incidence of hemolytic streptococci of from 38 per cent. in the sputum to 77 per cent. in the lung exudate may be regarded as expressing roughly the importance of these two types of streptococci as causes of death in influenzal infection. Instances occurred in which the bloody fluid from the lungs of patients who died from acute hemorrhagic edema showed large numbers of green-producing streptococci or hemolytic streptococci in pure culture, as well as mixtures of these two types of streptococci. Cultures made from throats of patients who could not raise sputum at the onset of the attack and in some as controls of sputum cultures, showed similar results to those obtained from the sputum. Throat cultures at the beginning of influenza often showed large numbers of the green-producing colonies, in pure or almost pure form.

The number of colonies of the different bacteria which developed on the blood-agar plates was recorded according to the numerical scale of 1 to 4. It was thought worth while to determine the figure expressing the average incidence by days of the three main varieties of bacteria (green-producing streptococci, hemolytic streptococci, and staphylococci) which were isolated in influenza and in influenzal pneumonia throughout the four epidemic waves. This was done by adding the figures representing the number of colonies of each organism and dividing this sum by the total number of specimens of sputum cultivated on the different days. There was no noteworthy difference in the average incidence of the various bacteria for influenza and for the first five days of influenzal pneumonia; hence these cases are considered together. The number of green-producing streptococci averaged highest each day for the first five days, the average figures being 3.7, 3.4, 3.6, 3.6 and 3.4, respectively. The average figures for the first five days for staphylococci were 2.0, 2.4, 2.2, 3.0 and 2.4. The average figures for hemolytic streptococci were 1.2, 1.6, 1.8, 1.7, and 2. In numbers staphylococci occupied the middle position and hemolytic streptococci the lowest position, but there was a tendency to an average increase in staphylococci and hemolytic streptococci during the later stages of the disease. The figures representing the average incidence of the different bacteria after the fifth day varied between wide limits. Thus the figures expressing the average increase of green-producing streptococci occupied the middle position on the sixth, seventh, eighth, tenth, and eleventh days; hemolytic streptococci, the lowest position on the sixth, seventh, eighth, tenth and eleventh days, the highest position on the ninth and twelfth days; staphylococci, the highest position on the sixth, seventh, eighth, tenth, and eleventh days, and the middle position on the ninth day. It becomes apparent, therefore, that the time in the attack when the cultures are made must be considered in order properly to interpret their meaning.

Marked variations in the type of bacterial flora were often noted at different stages of the disease during life and after death, and at different periods in the epidemic waves. In almost all instances of undoubted cases of influenza green-producing streptococci, together with a variable number of staphylococci or Micrococcus catarrhalis were the predominating flora at the outset of the influenzal attack throughout the epidemic waves. In most of the patients who recovered without developing pneumonia and in many who developed nonfatal or fatal attacks of pneumonia during the earlier part of the waves, this flora persisted. Later in the epidemic waves, however, there was a tendency for the green-producing streptococci to be displaced by hemolytic streptococci. This tendency to an increase in hemolytic streptococci in the later stages of the disease was noted especially in the patients who succumbed to the infection. Thus, in 21 fatal cases in which repeated cultures were made of the sputum during life and in which the lung exudate was cultured after death, green-producing streptococci predominated in the sputum during life in 16, and hemolytic streptococci in 5, while in these same cases hemolytic streptococci predominated in 11, and green-producing streptococci in 10, in the lung exudate after death. There was a shifting, therefore, from a predominant green-producing streptococcal flora to a hemolytic streptococcal flora in 6 of these fatal cases. The sputum usually became bloody as this occurred; the blood count showed no noteworthy change. The interval from the time of the sputum cultures to the time of the lung culture in these 6 cases was 1, 2, 4, 12, 12, and 4 days, respectively, or an average of 5.8 days. In some of the patients who recovered, on the other hand, the green-producing streptococcal flora again became predominant as the symptoms disappeared. This shifting of bacterial flora occurred both in cases of influenza without demonstrable lesions in the lung, as well as in influenzal pneumonia, but it occurred more often in the latter condition. The lack of agreement in the flora was noted not infrequently in cultures from the blood, from the lung, and from the pleural and other exudates after death. At times this occurred simultaneously in groups of patients who contracted the disease at about the same time. The blood after death proved to be sterile in about one-third of the cases cultured, and in the others green-producing streptococci or hemolytic streptococci alone or with staphylococci were isolated in about an equal number of cases. Green-producing streptococci were, at times, found in pure culture in the blood when the lung and other exudates showed few or no green-producing streptococci, but hemolytic streptococci with or without staphylococci. The cases which showed empyema usually yielded a predominating number of hemolytic streptococci.

The lack of agreement in the type of streptococcus colonies isolated from material after death, as noted in some cases, is well illustrated in the cultures from a case of fulminating influenzal bronchopneumonia and ulcerative laryngitis. The necropsy was performed soon after death. Cultures from the larynx, bronchial tubes and lung exudate showed large numbers of moist, spreading, slightly hemolyzing streptococci, a few typical hemolytic streptococcus colonies, and a moderate number of staphylococci, while blood-agar-plate cultures from dextrose broth inoculated with the blood from the heart showed pure growth of moist, spreading, nonhemolyzing green-producing colonies of streptococci. The morphology and character of the colony of the slightly hemolyzing streptococci and the green-producing streptococci from the blood were identical. In another case of influenzal bronchopneumonia with huge right and slight left empyema and beginning pericarditis, the cultures showed large numbers of hemolyzing streptococci and staphylococci from the pneumonia, a few hemolyzing streptococci and staphylococci from the left pleura, staphylococci from the pericardium, and larger numbers of green-producing streptococci and a few staphylococci in the pus from the right pleural cavity.

Staphylococci were rarely found in large numbers in the sputum early in the disease, but there was in general a tendency to an increase in the numbers of these organisms during the later stages, especially of influenzal pneumonia. In many instances the green-producing streptococcal flora noted at the outset when the sputum was mucoid in character was later partially or wholly displaced by staphylococcal flora, as the sputum became more purulent in character. This occurred especially during the later stages of the epidemic waves and in groups of patients who became ill at about the same time. Usually no particular change was noted in the patient's condition as staphylococci became more numerous in the sputum. Staphylococci were often found in predominating numbers or in pure culture in the pus from abscesses in bronchopneumonic areas in cases in which hemolytic or green-producing streptococci were the predominating organism in the pneumonic exudate remote from these abscesses. In such instances it was impossible to evaluate the exact rôle played by these organisms. In some cases, however, there could be little doubt that they were the cause of death just as was the case in the series of staphylococcal pneumonia that developed during the influenza epidemic at Camp Jackson, as reported by Chickering and Park.[6] In these there was a rapid change for the worse in the patient's condition as the staphylococci appeared in large numbers in the sputum and as the sputum became bloody, although purulent in character. The leukocyte count remained at about the same level or became lower as death occurred from acute hemorrhagic edema, or acute bronchopneumonia in from one to three days. The lung exudate after death showed enormous numbers of micrococci in groups in smears and staphylococci in enormous number usually in pure or in almost pure form in cultures. The freshly isolated organisms from some of these cases were found to be extremely virulent for animals. Intratracheal injection into guinea-pigs produced violent symptoms associated with leukopenia, and frequently death occurred from acute hemorrhagic bronchopneumonia, hemorrhagic edema, and voluminous lungs. The picture in these animals was quite different from that following injection of freshly isolated strains of staphylococcus from furunculosis, and from the abscesses in the lungs of some patients who died later. In the latter, symptoms were slight or absent, leukocytosis developed, recovery was the rule, and while areas of bronchopneumonia were found acute hemorrhagic edema never developed.

Influenza bacilli were isolated from the sputum in large numbers only during the early part of the first wave and almost not at all after that. These organisms were present in only a small number of cases after death, and when found were always in small numbers. That the absence of this organism in the cultures was due to their absence in the material cultured and not to their inability to grow on the medium used is certain. The medium which we used throughout the different waves was found quite efficient for cultivating this organism from swabs of the nasopharynx of influenza patients and from normal persons by Dr. Williams and Dr. Hatfield, working in our laboratory during the fourth wave. It is true, however, that cultures made at the same time on the special mediums which they used for isolating influenza bacilli showed this organism in a somewhat higher percentage of cases. We were especially interested in whether or not influenza bacilli were present in the exudate of the lower respiratory tract, the point of chief

attack, but cultures of sputum at this time again showed influenza bacilli in only a few cases, and in these in small numbers. Smears of the sputum, lung exudate, and tracheal mucus failed to show influenza bacilli when they were absent in cultures.

The results of the injection into animals (mice and guinea-pigs) of the sputum and lung exudate directly or of the primary mass culture in dextrose-blood broth served as an additional check on the cultures, for it was thought that growth of influenza bacilli, if of great significance in the production of symptoms in the disease in our cases, might occur in animals known to be susceptible to these organisms. Moreover, it was thought that a fairly accurate knowledge of the degree of invasive power of the different bacteria might be obtained in this way. A study was, therefore, made of the relative numbers of the different bacteria in the sputum and primary cultures in dextrose broth of sputum which was injected into animals and their relative numbers from the peritoneal and lung exudates of the animals that died. Sixty-eight animals succumbed to the intraperitoneal or intratracheal injection of sputum or of primary cultures from sputum and from lung exudate. Green-producing streptococci were the predominant organisms in the material injected in 68 per cent. of the animals, while after death this organism predominated in the blood, peritoneal or lung exudate in 78 per cent. of the animals. In most of the others hemolytic streptococci, and in a few, staphylococci, were the predominating organisms. Influenza bacilli were not isolated in a single instance, notwithstanding the fact that some of the specimens of sputum injected contained this organism in large numbers. The blood-agar plates made from the peritoneal exudate usually showed a mixture of streptococci and staphylococci in about the same proportions as in the material injected, while the blood nearly always contained pure cultures of streptococci, usually of the green-producing variety. In some animals, however, striking deviations from this rule occurred. Staphylococcus colonies in varying numbers often developed from the peritoneal exudate when the blood-agar plate from the material injected showed only streptococcus colonies. In some instances green-producing streptococci were isolated from the blood of these animals in pure culture, or together with hemolyzing streptococci when pure cultures of hemolyzing streptococci were injected, and vice versa. These findings were noted also when the cultures injected were derived from single widely separated colonies and at the same time in series of animals including several species.

The respiratory infections were of quite different types during several weeks prior to the occurrence of the first epidemic wave, at the height of the waves, as the waves subsided, and for several weeks following. Prior to the first severe outbreak mild attacks of pharyngitis and bronchitis with little fever and with slight or no constitutional symptoms occurred. Cultures from these cases showed a green-producing streptococcal flora in the sputum and throat. At the height of the epidemics, especially the first wave, marked prostration, cyanosis and leukopenia, high fever, and marked tendency to lung involvement with slight injection of pharynx and tonsils dominated the picture. Deaths from acute hemorrhagic edema were relatively common. As the waves subsided the symptoms became less marked, leukopenia was less persistent, deaths from respiratory involvement occurred later, and the lung showed relatively more true consolidation, but symptoms referable to infection of the nose and throat were more pronounced. In such cases it was often difficult to make the diagnosis, and cultures in some showed hemolyzing streptococci from the beginning of the attack. Still later well marked pharyngitis, often associated with follicular tonsillitis, absence of leukopenia or even leukocytosis, became prevalent. Involvement of the lung was now rare and deaths from pneumonia no longer occurred. Cultures from the throat and tonsils of patients in the latter condition showed hemolytic streptococci to be the chief organism.

The technic of making the cultures was uniform throughout the four waves, and the results were recorded according to the scale of 1 to 4, thus affording opportunity to study the changes in the character of the colonies of the different species and changes in their relative numbers as the epidemic waves appeared and disappeared. Each of the four epidemic waves studied ran its course in about six weeks, and the crest was reached in about two weeks; accordingly the results of sputum cultures from cases of influenza and influenzal pneumonia, and the fatal cases, were arranged into three groups of two weeks each, and the average of the three main types of bacteria (green-producing streptococci, hemolyzing streptococci, and staphylococci) determined. The first period comprised the first two weeks, the second the third and fourth weeks, and the third the fifth and sixth weeks of the four waves. The figures representing the average incidence of green-producing streptococci for the three periods of the four waves were 2.6, 2.3 and 2.7; for hemolyzing streptococcus 1.1, 1.4, and 1.4; and for staphylococci 1.8, 2.1, and 2.4, respectively. According to these figures it is evident that the green-producing streptococcus in the sputum averaged the highest throughout the epidemic waves, and that the hemolyzing streptococcus and staphylococcus while comparatively few early in the epidemic became relatively more numerous as the waves subsided. In the case of cultures after death the figures representing the average for green-producing streptococci for the three periods were 1.5, 2.6 and 1.0, for hemolyzing streptococcus 1.1, 1.7 and 2.5, and for staphylococcus 1.1, 1.1 and 2.1, respectively. According to these figures, the green-producing streptococcus was the chief cause of death during the first four weeks of the waves, and the hemolyzing streptococcus and staphylococcus during the fifth and sixth weeks, or as the waves were subsiding.

MORPHOLOGY, CULTURAL CHARACTERISTICS AND FERMENTATIVE POWERS OF THE STREPTOCOCCI FROM INFLUENZA

Green-Producing Streptococci. — The somewhat peculiar green-producing streptococcus isolated during the first wave has been described (Study 1). The further results, throughout the subsequent waves, have in the main corroborated the earlier findings, although greater differences in cultural characteristics have been noted than were at first apparent. From a study of a large number of cases we have found green-producing streptococci, including pneumococci, to be the most common organism present in influenzal infection. The strains when first isolated usually produced rather moist, spreading, non-adherent greenish colonies on blood-agar plates and a diffuse cloud in glucose broth. Smears of young cultures from these mediums showed gram-positive oval shaped diplococci of quite uniform size, singly, in pairs, and usually in fairly long chains. These were of about the size of pneumococci and were often indistinguishable from them, although chain formation was usually more marked and the capsule less distinct. Smears from older cultures, especially in the deeper layers of tall columns of glucose-brain broth, often showed diplococci of extreme variations in size and shape. During the first wave the colonies were quite moist, usually resembling type III pneumococci, although less mucoid in character; in the subsequent outbreaks, especially during the later stages, they were usually not so moist and were often indistinguishable from pneumococcus colonies. The more moist spreading type of colonies, some resembling Pneumococcus mucosus, were isolated, however, during these waves in some instances. This was true particularly early

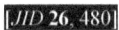

in each wave, in severe cases occurring in groups of persons who contracted influenza soon after arriving in Rochester, and who came from the same locality, as well as in individual families residing in Rochester and in the surrounding country. The chief distinguishing characteristics of these strains as of those in the first wave, however, were their marked and peculiar invasive power on intratracheal injection. As the

TABLE 2

The Variability in Fermentative Power of Green-Producing Streptococci from Influenza

Date of Test	Strain	Dextrose	Lactose	Maltose	Saccharose	Raffinose	Mannite	Salicin	Inulin	Control
9/25/18	2539.6	+4	+4	+4	+4	+4	0	+4	0	0
3/ 6/19	2539.8	+3	+2	+2	+4	+4	+	+2	0	0
3/ 4/19	2341.17	+3	+3	+3	+4	+4	0	+3	+	0
12/30/19	2341.20	+2	0	+	+	0	0	0	0	0
3/ 3/19	2347.12	+3	+3	+2	+4	+4	+	+	+	0
11/14/19	2347.23	+3	+3	+4	+4	+3	0	0	0	0
3/ 3/19	2349.12	+3	+3	+3	+4	+4	0	+2	+2	0
11/14/19	2349.18	+4	+3	+4	+4	+3	0	0	0	0
3/ 6/19	2531.8	+3	+2½	+3	+4	+	0	0	+2	0
11/ 4/19	2531.12	+3	+3	+3	0	0	0	0	0	0
3/ 6/19	2532.0	+3	+3	+3	+4	+4	0	+3	+2	0
11/ 4/19	2532.8	+3	0	+2	+2	+	+3	+3	0	0
3/15/19	2620.3	+3	0	+3	+4	0	0	+4	0	0
3/15/19	2620.3	+2	+	+2	+4	0	0	+3	0	0
3/10/19	2724.8	+3	+2	+2	+4	+4	0	0	0	0
11/18/19	2724.11	+	+3	+3	+3	+3	0	0	0	0
3/12/19	2789.4	+3	+3	+2	+4	0	0	0	0	0
12/17/19	2789.8	+3	+	+2	+2	0	0	0	0	0
3/12/19	2748.8	+3	+3	+3	+3	+4	0	+3	0	0
5/ 8/19	2748.10	0	+	+2	+3	+4	0	+	+3	0
11/22/19	2748.11	+3	+	+2	+	0	0	0	0	0
3/12/19	2762.6	+3	+3	+	+4	+4	0	+4	+3	0
11/22/19	2762.8	+	+3	+2	+	+2	+2	0	0	0
3/12/19	2763.6	+3	+3	+3	+3	+4	+2	+4	0	0
10/22/19	2763.14	+4	+	+3	+	0	0	0	0	0
11/22/19	2763.9	+3	+3	+2	+	+3	0	+	0	0
3/12/19	2770².7	+3	+4	+3	+3	+4	0	+3	0	0
3/12/19	2770².7	+3	+3	+3	+3	+4	0	+2	0	0
5/ 8/19	2770².9	+2	+2	+2	+4	+4	+	+4	+2	0
3/19/19	2818.6	+3	+3	+3	+4	+4	+4	+3	+3	0
10/22/19	2818.9	+3	+2	+3	+3	+1	+2	+3	0	0
3/26/19	2824.6	+3	+2	+2	+3	+4	0	0	0	0
11/ 6/19	2824.14	+3	+2	+2	+4	0	0	+3	0	0
3/26/19	2825.6	+3	+3	+3	+4	0	0	0	0	0
4/18/19	2825.11	+3	0	0	+2	0	0	+4	+	0
11/10/19	2825.3	+4	+	+3	+4	0	0	0	0	0
4/16/19	3365.2	+3	+3	+3	+4	+4	0	+3	0	0
4/16/19	3365.2	+4	+3	+3	+4	+4	0	+3	+3	0
11/14/19	3365.7	+3	+3	+3	+3	+	0	+	0	0

epidemics subsided and the infections became milder the colonies of green-producing streptococci from sputum became smaller, and less moist, capsule formation was slight or absent, the chains were longer, and growth in glucose broth was more granular or occurred only at the bottom of the tubes. The virulency of these, determined by intraperitoneal injections into mice and intratracheal injections into guinea-pigs was of a lower order. This difference in character of growth was

TABLE 3
THE VARIABILITY IN FERMENTATIVE POWER OF HEMOLYTIC STREPTOCOCCI FROM INFLUENZA

Date of Test	Strain	Dextrose	Lactose	Maltose	Saccharose	Raffinose	Mannite	Salicin	Inulin	Control
3/15/19	2541.3	+3	0	+2	+4	0	0	+3	0	0
12/12/19	2541.6	+3	+2	+3	+3	0	0	+3	0	0
3/15/19	2559.5	+3	0	+	+4	0	0	+4	0	0
12/12/19	2559.8	+4	+2	+3	+3	0	0	+3	0	0
3/6/19	2557.14	+3	+3	+2	+4	0	0	+3	0	0
3/6/19	2557.14	+3	+3	+3	+4	0	0	+3	0	0
12/16/19	2557.16	+3	+3	+3	+4	0	0	0	0	0
5/8/19	2774.10	+2	0	0	+3	0	0	+2	+3	0
12/19/19	2774.13	+3	+2	+3	+4	0	0	0	0	0
3/19/19	2821.6	+4	+2	+3	+4	0	0	+4	0	0
10/23/19	2821.12	+4	+	+3	+	0	0	+2	0	0
3/21/19	2815.6	+3	0	+2	+4	0	0	+	0	0
12/17/19	2815.28	+3	+2	+2	+3	0	0	0	0	0
3/26/19	2826.6	+2	0	+3	+4	0	+4	0	0	0
10/26/19	2826.5	+4	+3	+	+3	+2	+2	0	0	0
3/26/19	2851.3	+3	+2	+4	+3	0	0	+3	0	0
3/26/19	2851.4	+3	+3	+3	+3	0	+4	0	0	0
12/19/19	2851.6	+3	0	+3	+3	0	0	+2	0	0
4/8/19	2902.3	+3	+3	+2	+4	0	0	0	0	0
11/24/19	2902.4	+3	+3	+3	+2	0	0	+4	0	0
4/16/19	3358.2	+3	+3	+3	+3	0	+4	+4	0	0
12/22/19	3358.6	+4	+	+2	+	0	+2	+3	0	0
4/29/19	3387ª.3	+2	+4	+2	+3	+3	0	+3	0	+
11/14/19	3387ª.5	+4	+3	+4	+3	0	0	+4	0	0
4/29/19	3395.5	+2	+4	+3	+3	+4	0	+3	0	0
12/19/19	3395.9	+2	+	+	+	0	0	0	0	0
4/29/19	3398.4	+3	+3	+2	+3	0	+2	+3	0	0
5/24/19	3398ª.5	+4	+2	+2	+4	+4	0	+3	0	0
1/3/20	3398.7	+2	0	0	+	0	+2	0	0	0

noted in strains isolated directly from the sputum as well as from the animals that succumbed to injections of sputum. Distinct as these differences were in cultural features, immunologic studies (Study III) showed most of them to be identical, especially those isolated early in the attack. In making cultures from the sputum and lung exudate on blood-agar plates small indifferent colonies of streptococci resembling influenza bacilli were frequently noted. This resemblance was often so marked that examination of smears stained with a Gram stain were necessary to differentiate them. These often acquired the power to produce green on blood agar after one or more cultivations in tall tubes of glucose broth. Moreover, colonies which appeared to be transition forms between green-producing and hemolytic streptococci were frequently noted, especially in the sputum of patients as the epidemics were subsiding. After cultivation on artificial mediums the strains often showed marked changes. The colonies became dry, and smaller; and often diffuse growth in glucose broth no longer occurred, but instead a growth with granular sediment resembling Streptococcus viridans. In some instances indifferent colonies developed and in many instances they acquired hemolytic power. This was of all grades from a narrow zone peripheral to an inner green zone to well marked hemolytic zones beginning immediately around the colony.

Hemolytic Streptococci.—The infections of the lung by hemolytic streptococci, as they occurred during the pandemic of influenza usually without empyema, without tonsillitis and without leukocytosis, but with leukopenia, indicated peculiar infecting powers not possessed by hemolytic streptococci found so commonly in normal throats and tonsils in acute follicular tonsillitis, and in the pneumonia empyema epidemic of 1917-1918. This has been found actually to be the case. Strains from the sputum and lung in cases of acute hemorrhagic edema reproduced this condition associated with leukopenia in guinea-pigs on intratracheal injections; whereas strains of hemolytic streptococci from simple pharyngitis caused leukocytosis (reported elsewhere), but never acute hemorrhagic edema of the lung. Culturally, there was often a distinct difference between these strains and those isolated from cases of empyema and the throats of persons suffering from pharyngitis and tonsillitis. The colonies were more moist, less opaque, often spreading in character, quite as the colonies of green-producing streptococci, and the hemolytic zone was not so wide, not so clear, and the margin less sharply defined. Freshly isolated strains from acute cases produced diffuse growth in glucose broth, while hemolytic streptococci from the pus in cases of longer duration like those from other sources, usually grew granular with flocculent sediment. Morphologically, these strains were at times indistinguishable from the green-producing streptococcus, the smears showing elongated diplococci singly and in chains of various lengths. After cultivation on artificial mediums for a time these peculiar properties tended to disappear, in some instances abruptly, and were no longer distinguishable from the hemolytic streptococcus obtained from other sources. In some instances the hemolytic streptococci acquired the power to produce green colonies.

The tendency of the green-producing streptococci to acquire hemolytic powers, and to a lesser degree the tendency of the hemolytic streptococci to acquire the power to produce green colonies was so marked that it was found necessary in agglutination experiments to plate the cultures actually agglutinated in order properly to interpret the results obtained. The tendency of hemolytic streptococci to lose their hemolyzing powers was especially marked in freshly isolated cultures when grown in tall tubes of glucose-brain broth. This frequently occurred in cultures derived from single colonies from plates showing large numbers of the organism in question in pure form. The cultures which were put aside for study were made on blood-agar slants from single colonies, or from a group of colonies well separated from other bacteria. The tendency to mutations in these cultures may best be illustrated by giving the results of subcultures when this point was especially noted. Thus of a total of 623 cultures, green-producing streptococci bred true to type in 348 instances, and hemolytic streptococci in 168, a total of 516. In the remaining 115 cultures, green-producing streptococci yielded hemolytic streptococci in 45 instances, indifferent streptococci in 27, and staphylococcus colonies in 22, while hemolytic streptococci yielded green-producing streptococci in 9 instances, indifferent streptococci in 7, and staphylococci in 5. In most instances the changes in type occurred abruptly, under various conditions, but especially when old cultures on blood-agar and dextrose-brain broth were transferred. The instability of the streptococcus strains from influenza often made it difficult to obtain the proper proportions of the different strains in the vaccine which was used for prophylactic inoculations. The routine procedure consisted of transferring single colonies or a group of colonies of the different bacteria to bottles containing 150 c c of 0.2 per cent. glucose broth, incubating these over night, making smears, plating a loop full, and inoculating about 30 c c with a bulbed pipet into large bottles containing about 3,500 c c of glucose broth. Smears and blood-agar plates were again made of the latter. It frequently happened that while the plating from the small bottles of broth showed pure growths of the type inoculated, the plating from the large bottle often showed a partial or totally changed streptococcus flora, and not infrequently showed staphylococcus colonies as well, in spite of great precautions taken to avoid accidental contamination. Owing to these findings, further studies were made on this point. The findings in Case 3101 and the behavior of the strain isolated will suffice to illustrate results obtained along this line:

Case 3101, a man, aged 32, became sick Feb. 28, 1919, with severe headache, aching all over the body, marked prostration and chilly sensations, but no distinct chill. The next day he was admitted to the hospital with a temperature of 104, pulse 90, and respiration 20. The throat was slightly infected, and moderate dullness and decreased breath sounds over the base of both lungs were found. The temperature ranged between 100 and 104 until March 5. March 6 the temperature was higher and scattered areas of dullness with râles were elicited. March 7 the patient became cyanotic, extremely short of breath, and expectorated large amounts of bloody, frothy material. He grew rapidly worse in spite of venesection (400 cc) and transfusion of 250 cc of convalescent human blood, and died March 8. The leukocyte count on March 3 was 10,600; March 4, 9,000; March 5, 9,500; March 7, 9,100. March 2 and 6 the sputum was mucopurulent and showed large numbers of green-producing streptococci, slightly hemolyzing streptococci, and staphylococci. March 7, the day the patient became worse, the sputum showed no change in flora, but a blood culture yielded a pure growth of hemolytic streptococci. March 8 the sputum contained enormous numbers of hemolytic streptococci and staphylococci, but no longer green-producing streptococci nor slightly hemolyzing streptococci. One guinea-pig was injected with the twenty-four hour primary culture from the blood in glucose-brain broth. The animal was ill for a time and lost 30 gm. in weight, and then recovered. A second guinea-pig was injected March 9 with 2 cc of the glucose-brain broth culture made from a single colony of hemolytic streptococcus on a blood-agar plate inoculated with the culture injected into the first guinea-pig. The plate showed a pure culture of hemolytic streptococcus. The guinea-pig lost in weight, and respirations were increased. It was chloroformed two days after injection and two large areas of consolidation in the right diaphragmatic lobe were found. From these areas pure cultures of green-producing streptococci, but no hemolytic streptococci were obtained. The tube of glucose-brain broth inoculated with the blood, which showed on plating a hemolytic streptococcus in pure form, was placed in the ice chest until September 8, when a glucose-brain-broth culture and a plating on blood-agar were made. The blood-agar plate yielded one colony of hemolytic streptococcus. From this colony a blood-agar plate and a tall tube of glucose-brain broth were inoculated (September 13). The former showed pure cultures of hemolyzing streptococci. The latter developed abundant growth, but the tube was not opened until November 28, at which time two blood-agar plates were made; both showed many colonies of hemolyzing streptococci as well as green-producing streptococci. From this plate single hemolyzing and green colonies well separated from other colonies were inoculated December 1 into one tube of glucose-brain broth each. Both tubes developed abundant diffuse growth, and platings on blood-agar December 2 showed pure cultures of green-producing streptococci. In both instances intra-tracheal injection into 3 guinea-pigs of the growth in the tube inoculated with hemolytic streptococcus colonies resulted in the production of acute bronchopneumonia with death of two on the third day while the third animal recovered after three days of illness. Green-producing streptococci were isolated in large numbers from the two that died. Hemolytic streptococci in the tube of glucose-brain broth when fresh were injected intratracheally into one guinea-pig. It developed bronchopneumonia and from the lung lesions pure cultures of green-producing streptococci were isolated. The tube of glucose-brain broth inoculated (September 9) showed diffuse growth, and a blood-agar plate September 10 contained pure culture of typical hemolytic streptococci. A single colony was used to inoculate a blood-agar plate and a tube of glucose-brain broth. The former yielded a pure culture of hemolytic streptococci; a plating of the latter September 13 also showed a pure culture of the hemolytic streptococcus, but a plating made November 28, after incubation at 35 C. since September 9 showed countless numbers of indifferent colonies of streptococci and moderate numbers of slightly hemolytic streptococci. The tube of glucose-brain broth inoculated with a single colony September 10 developed diffuse turbidity and September 12 yielded countless hemolytic streptococcus colonies on blood-agar plates. A blood-agar plate made of this same tube November 28 showed countless staphylococcus colonies with no hemolytic or green-producing streptococcus colonies. December 2 intratracheal injection into two guinea-pigs of this culture containing staphylococci caused leukopenia, increased respiration for a time, and death on the eleventh day. There was no lung involvement and the organism was lost. The culture in glucose-brain broth made from a single colony of hemolytic streptococci September 13 was injected intratracheally into one guinea-pig and intraperitoneally into a mouse. The guinea-pig had marked increased respiration for a number of days, and died nineteen days after the injection from interstitial bronchopneumonia. The mouse lived thirteen days, and then died. Cultures of the blood of both yielded hemolytic streptococci.

The infecting power and immunologic conditions of the organisms as changes occurred have been studied extensively. The details of these experiments will be reported elsewhere, but it may be stated that high and peculiar invasive powers of the changed forms have been noted repeatedly, and that as cultural properties changed immunologic reactions usually became different also.

FERMENTATIVE POWERS OF THE STREPTOCOCCI

The fermentative powers of the streptococci over the usual test sugars have been determined in a large number of strains. The method which we have found most efficient and convenient for this study is a modification of the Hiss serum water medium. This modification consists of the Hiss serum water medium with the addition of 0.5 per cent. agar, just sufficient to jell, 1 per cent. of the different test sugars, and Adraid's indicator instead of litmus. The medium is placed in small tubes, 3 inches by 3/8 of an inch, about 2 c c into each tube, and steamed in the usual manner on three successive days. Inoculations are made by stabbing the medium with a loop containing organisms from fresh cultures on blood-agar. The tubes are incubated for seventy-two hours, and then read. Negative reactions can be determined easily since if growth has taken place a streak along the line of inoculation can readily be made out. A negative result is not recorded unless a distinct growth has taken place. The degree of acidity is indicated with one or more + signs according to the depth of red color produced.

Altogether, we have tested the fermentative power of 254 strains of the green-producing streptococci soon after isolation. Of these, 94 per cent. fermented dextrose; 90 per cent. lactose; 93 per cent. maltose; 78 per cent. saccharose; 49 per cent. raffinose; 35 per cent. mannite, 67 per cent. salicin, and 38 per cent. inulin. After cultivation for from six to nine months on blood-agar, 139 strains were again tested. The results in dextrose, lactose, maltose and saccharose were practically the same as with the freshly isolated strains, but the number fermenting raffinose, mannite, salicin and inulin was decidedly less in each, the percentage being 22, 16, 45 and 17, respectively. Tests of the fermentative power of 119 strains of hemolyzing streptococci soon after isolation resulted as follows: 91 per cent. fermented dextrose, 71 per cent. lactose, 87 per cent. maltose, 82 per cent. saccharose, 19 per cent. raffinose, 16 per cent. mannite, 79 per cent. salicin, and 8 per cent. inulin. After prolonged cultivation a general lowering of fermentative powers was noted in 70 strains tested. This was especially marked in the case of lactose and salicin. The instability of these strains as noted on blood-agar and other mediums was noted also with respect to their fermentative powers. The results obtained from a study of a large series of strains by testing each strain on different dates are well illustrated by the summaries in tables 2 and 3. It becomes apparent at once from a study of these tables that a classification of the streptococci, especially the green-producing streptococci, on the basis of their fermentative reactions would have little real meaning, since they frequently acquire or lose, quite without regard to rule, the power to ferment important carbohydrates.

GENERAL DISCUSSION AND SUMMARY

From a bacteriologic study of a large series of cases of influenza and influenzal pneumonia throughout four epidemic waves, green-producing streptococci (including pneumococci) were found to occur more constantly and in larger numbers than any other organisms commonly associated with this disease. This flora predominated alike in the cases of influenza without lung involvement, in those of lung involvement in the initial febrile attack as well as in those in which influenzal pneumonia developed after a quiescent interval following influenza. This was especially true early in the attacks throughout the epidemic waves, and the flora usually persisted and was the chief cause of death during the early part and during the height of the epidemic waves. Moreover, the agglutination experiments with a monovalent immune horse serum have shown that most of the strains isolated early in the disease are immunologically alike, whereas later they become more heterogeneous, just as do the specific strains after cultivation on artificial mediums.

During the latter part of the outbreaks hemolytic streptococci became relatively more numerous, especially late in the disease, and death was often the result of invasion by these organisms. A similar increase in the number of staphylococci occurred, and in some instances these appeared to be the immediate cause of death. The change in the type of the disease and the character of the lesion in the lung, which were noted during each of the epidemic waves, appeared to be due more to a change in the virulence of the organisms than to a change in the type of flora. Thus well marked instances of acute hemorrhagic edema occurred, but almost wholly at the height of the epidemic waves in which each of these organisms was found in pure culture or in mixture in various proportions.

The influenza bacillus was found in the sputum in the early part of the first wave only in a few cases and always in association with streptococci, while throughout the remaining three waves it was isolated only occasionally. The criticism which has been raised by those who believe the influenza bacillus to be the cause of influenza, that the methods used by those who fail to isolate this organism are inadequate, does not apply to this study, because the medium used throughout this study was proved effective for the growth of the influenza bacillus. Special mediums were employed during the latter part of the study, smears failed to show the organism, and influenza bacilli were not found in the animals injected directly with sputum and lung exudate. Hence it is certain that in the majority of cases studied this organism played little or no rôle in the production of symptoms. Its presence in large numbers in some cases in the early part of the first wave and its almost complete absence in sputum and lung exudates subsequently indicate that the difference in the frequency of isolation of this organism by various workers is in general, as emphasized by

MacCallum and others, a measure of its prevalence in the particular epidemics studied, and that many epidemics of typical influenza occur that are not due to this organism. Moreover, when found it is usually associated with organisms of the pneumococcus-streptococcus group (Park, Williams, Dick and Murray).

The finding of a preponderance of the pneumococcus-streptococcus group of organisms reported herewith is in accord with the results obtained by the pneumonia unit at Camp Lewis, by Blanton and Irons, Friedlander, McCord, Sladen and Wheeler, Stone and Swift, Jordan, Hirsch and McKinney, Dunn, and many others.

It has been demonstrated repeatedly in this study that the peculiar infecting power of streptococci from influenza does not depend on their power to ferment certain carbohydrates, and that the fermentation reactions are variable. Hence the difference in the relative number of instances in which green-producing streptococci, hemolytic streptococci, or Group 4, or even type pneumococci were isolated by the different workers during the pandemic does not necessarily mean that the different strains did not have the infecting power peculiar to influenza, just as has been found to be the case in our hands. A striking example in support of this idea occurred at Camp Grant in which type II pneumococci of extreme virulency were found to be the cause not of lobar pneumonia, but of acute bronchopneumonia typical of influenza during an extremely fatal epidemic as described by Hirsch and McKinney.

The changes observed in morphology, cultural characteristics, fermentative and immunologic reactions in the green-producing streptococci indicate that the organism described by the English observers and designated by them as diplostreptococcus, the green-producing streptococcus found by Mathers as described by Tunnicliff, the diplococcus epidemicus described by Bernhardt and by Segale, the diplococcus mucosus described by Stephan, and the pleomorphic streptococcus described by Wiesner in influenza, are identical with the green-producing streptococcus isolated in this study, or modifications thereof. Moreover, the marked changes or true mutations that have occurred in the culture tube under controlled conditions indicate that the change in the bacterial flora at different stages of the disease in the individual and in the epidemic waves may not always be the result of superimposed infections from the upper respiratory tract as is now generally believed.

BIBLIOGRAPHY

[1] Avery, O. T.: A Selective Medium for B. Influenzae Oleate-Hemoglobin-Agar, Jour. Am. Med. Assn., 1918, lxxi, 2050-2051.

[2] Bernhardt, G.: Zur Aetiologie der Grippe von 1918, Med. Klin., 1918, xiv, 683-685.

[3] Blanton, W. B. and Irons, E. E.: A Recent Epidemic of Acute Respiratory Infection at Camp Custer, Mich., Jour. Am. Med. Assn., 1918, lxxi, 1988-1991.

[4] Brem, W. V., Bolling, G. E. and Casper, E. J.: Pandemic "Influenza" and Secondary Pneumonia at Camp Fremont, California, Jour. Am. Med. Assn., 1918, lxxi, 2138-2144.

[5] Camp Lewis Pneumonia Unit: The Relation of Bronchopneumonia to Influenza, Jour. Am. Med. Assn., 1919, lxxii, 268-269.

[6] Chickering, H. T. and Park, J. H.: Staphylococcus aureus Pneumonia, Jour. Am. Med. Assn., 1919, lxxii, 617-626.

[7] Dunn, A. D.: Observations on an Epidemic of Bronchopneumonia in Omaha, Jour. Am. Med. Assn., 1918, lxxi, 2128-2130.

[8] Friedlander, A., McCord, C. P., Sladen, F. J., and Wheeler, G. W.: The Epidemic of Influenza at Camp Sherman, Ohio, Jour. Am. Med. Assn., 1918, lxxi, 1652-1656.

[9] Goodpasture, E. W.: The Significance of Certain Pulmonary Lesions in Relation to the Etiology of Influenza, Am. Jour. Med. Sc., 1919, clviii, 863-870.

[10] Hirsch, E. F. and McKinney, M.: An Epidemic of Pneumococcus Bronchopneumonia, Jour. Infect. Dis., 1919, xxiv, 594-617.

[11] Influenza Committee of the Advisory Board to the D. G. M. S., France: A Report on the Influenza Epidemic in the British Armies in France, 1918, Brit. Med. Jour., 1918, ii, 505-509.

[12] Jordan, E. O.: Observations on the Bacteriology of Influenza, Jour. Infect. Dis., 1919, xxv, 28-40.

[13] Kinsella, R. A.: The Bacteriology of Epidemic Influenza and Pneumonia, Jour. Am. Med. Assn., 1919, lxxii, 717-720.

[14] MacCallum, W. G.: Pathology of the Pneumonia Following Influenza, Jour. Am. Med. Assn., 1919, lxxii, 720-723.

[15] Mathers, G.: The Bacteriology of Acute Epidemic Respiratory Infections Commonly Called Influenza, Jour. Infect. Dis., 1917, xxi, 1-8.

[16] Medalia, L. S.: Influenza Epidemic at Camp MacArthur: Etiology, Bacteriology, Pathology, and Specific Therapy, Boston Med. and Surg. Jour., 1919, clxxx, 323-330.

[17] Neufeld, F., and Papamarku, P.: 'Zur Bakteriologie der diesjährigen Influenzaepidemic, Deutsch. med. Wchnschr., 1918, ii, 1181.

[18] Nuzum, J. W., Pilot, I., Stangl, F. H., and Bonar, B. E.: Pandemic Influenza and Pneumonia in a Large Civil Hospital, Jour. Am. Med. Assn., 1918, lxxi, 1562-1565.

[19] Park, W. H.: Bacteriology of Recent Pandemic of Influenza and Complicating Infections, Jour. Am. Med. Assn., 1919, lxxiii, 318-321.

[20] Park, W. H.: The Bacteriology of Influenza and Its Complications, Med. Rec., 1919, xcvi, 215.

[21] Potter, A. C.: Bacteriology of the Present Epidemic of Influenza, Journal-Lancet, 1918, xxxviii, 708-709.

[22] Rosenow, E. C.: Prophylactic Inoculation Against Respiratory Infections, Jour. Am. Med. Assn., 1919, lxxii, 31-34.

[23] Rosenow, E. C.: Studies in Influenza and Pneumonia. II. The Experimental Production of Symptoms and Lesions Simulating Those of Influenza with Streptococci Isolated During the Present Pandemic, Jour. Am. Med. Assn., 1919, lxxii, 1604-1608.

[24] Rosenow, E. C.: Studies in Influenza and Pneumonia. III. The Occurrence of a Pandemic Strain of Streptococcus During the Pandemic of Influenza, Jour. Am. Med. Assn., 1919, lxxii, 1608-1609.

[25] Rosenow, E. C.: Transmutations Within the Streptococcus-Pneumococcus Group, Jour. Inf. Dis., 1914, xiv, 1-32.

[26] Segale, M.: Azione dei filtrati di "Str. pandemicus" in rapporto alla dottrina della filtrabilita del virus grippale, Policlinico, 1919, xxvi, 289-290.

[27] Stephan, R.: Ueber einen neuen Infektionserreger bei epidemischer Influenza, München. med. Wchnschr., 1917, lxiv, 257-260.

[28] Stone, W. J., and Swift, G. W.: Influenza and Influenzal Pneumonia at Ft. Riley, Kansas, from Sept. 15 to Nov. 1, 1918, Jour. Am. Med. Assn., 1919, lxxii, 487-493.

29. Tunnicliff, Ruth: Phagocytic Experiments in Influenza, Jour. Am. Med. Assn., 1918, lxxi, 1733-1734.

[30] Wiesner, R. R.: Streptococcus pleomorphus und die sogenannte Spanische Grippe, Wien. klin. Wchnschr., 1918, xxxi, 1101-1104.

[31] Williams, Anna W.: The Etiology of "Influenza," Proc. New York Path. Soc., 1918, xviii, 83-90.

STUDIES IN INFLUENZA AND PNEUMONIA

VI. THE LEUKOCYTIC REACTION IN INFLUENZA AND INFLUENZAL PNEUMONIA

E. C. ROSENOW

Division of Experimental Bacteriology, The Mayo Foundation, Rochester, Minnesota.

Leukopenia, or absence of leukocytosis, has come to be regarded as an important aid in the diagnosis of influenza, and a persistent leukopenia as of bad prognostic import. The cause of the leukopenia has been the subject of much speculation. It is thought by many observers that an unknown virus produces the initial leukopenia, and that this virus interferes with the leukocytic response when secondary infection by streptococci or pneumococci is believed to occur as pneumonia develops.

No matter what the cause of influenza may be, the absence of leukocytosis is a striking phenomenon. The exact leukocytic reaction, however, throughout the initial influenzal attack and in influenzal pneumonia in fatal and nonfatal infections has not been determined, nor has a systematic study of the leukocytic reaction in animals been made following injections of the different species of bacteria that are so commonly isolated in influenza. It was therefore thought worth while to determine the leukocytic curves in the spontaneous disease and in experimental animals in which the dosage and type of organism introduced could be accurately controlled and might throw light on the question as to the cause of leukopenia in influenzal infection and determine more accurately the prognostic significance of the lack of leukocytic reaction in this disease.

In figure 1 the curves indicate the average leukocyte counts by days in influenza and influenzal pneumonia in man, and experimental influenzal pneumonia in guinea-pigs, according to fatal and nonfatal infection. There were no deaths from influenza without lung involvement among the cases included in part 1 of figure 1. The dotted line represents the count in the cases in which fatal attacks of influenzal pneumonia later developed. The average count for the first six days in influenza was about 6,500, and was approximately the same in the fatal

Received for publication Feb. 28, 1920.

and nonfatal cases. From the seventh to the tenth day the count rose somewhat in the patients who recovered, while it dropped in those who later developed influenzal pneumonia from which they succumbed. It will be noted that, contrary to the general belief, the average leukocyte count when influenzal pneumonia developed was no higher than during the initial influenzal attack. The count in the nonfatal infections then gradually rose, while in the fatal infections it rose for two days and then gradually declined. This finding is in accord with that of Haase

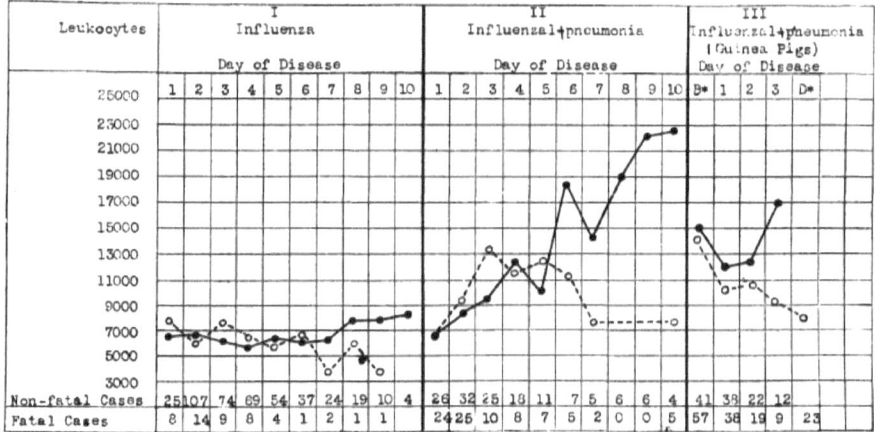

Fig. 1.—Average leukocyte count by days in influenza and influenzal pneumonia in guinea-pigs according to fatal and nonfatal infection. —denotes the average leukocyte count in nonfatal infection; — — average leukocyte count in fatal infection; * B, before injection; * D, after death.

and Wohlrabe [1] who also found that there is a tendency of the leukocyte count to rise in the later stages of influenza and influenzal pneumonia.

Marked individual differences were noted in the leukocytic response in guinea-pigs following injection of bacteria from patients with influenza. If a series of animals was injected with the same dose of a given strain, nearly all showed a drop in the number of leukocytes; the drop in some was slight, in others it was marked, and occasionally an animal showed leukocytosis. There was no definite relation between

---

[1] Haase, N., and Wohlrabe: Ueber das Blutbild bei Influenza, Deutsche. med. Wchnschr., 1918, 44, p. 1383.

the mortality rate and the initial leukopenia, but a persistently low count occurred more often in the fatal infections. In part III of figure 1 the average leukocyte count by days in nonfatal infections shows a decided drop for two days following injection and then a rise, while in the fatal infections there was a progressive diminution. These curves are believed to be accurately representative, since they include, as indicated, the average of a large series of animals and correspond roughly with the curves in the spontaneous disease. The leukocyte count in apparently normal guinea-pigs varies greatly, but counts made repeatedly show that it tends to remain at a given level

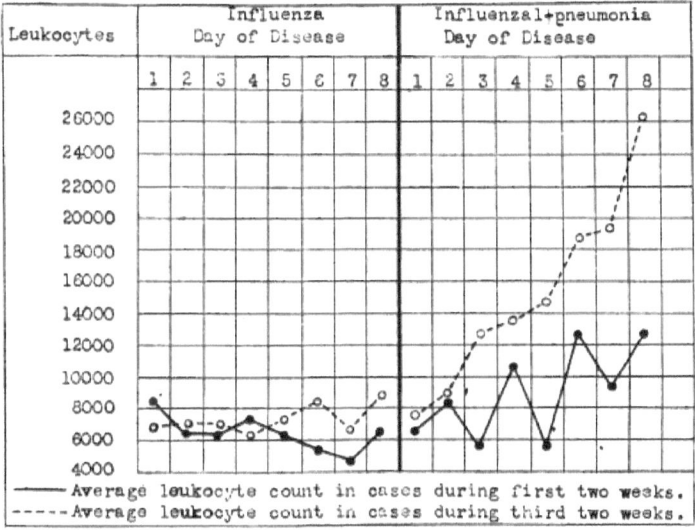

Fig. 2.—Average leukocyte count by days according to time in epidemic waves.

over a period of some days. The injections were made in various ways with sputum, primary cultures, exudates and pure cultures of green-producing streptococci from the sputum or lungs in undoubted cases of influenzal infection.

It has been our observation that the most typical cases of influenza and the highest mortality rate occurred at the height of epidemic waves. It was thought worth while, therefore, to group the cases with leukocyte counts according to the time in epidemic waves (figure 2), and to learn whether the average leukocyte count might not be lower in the cases at the height of epidemic waves as compared with that in the cases as the epidemic waves subsided. It was found that each of the four waves of influenza that occurred in Rochester during the fall of 1918 and winter and spring of 1919 ran its course in about six weeks, and that the crest of the wave was reached in about two weeks in each. Each wave was therefore arbitrarily divided into two-week periods for study. The average counts by days of patients developing influenza and influenzal pneumonia during the first two weeks and the third two weeks were determined and traced in figure 2. The average count for the first five days of the influenzal attack in the two groups was about the same; after that the count was decidedly lower in the group contracting the disease during the first two weeks of each wave than during the third two weeks. The average count during influenzal pneumonia was about the same during the first two days and no higher than at the outset of influenza, but after that the rise in leukocytes was decidedly less during the first two weeks than during the third two weeks of each wave. The mortality rate in the first two weeks was definitely higher than in the third two weeks.

In table 1 are given the leukocytic reaction and other findings in guinea-pigs injected with material, first, from patients showing marked leukopenia, and second, from patients showing no reduction or a moderate increase in the leukocyte count. It will be seen that the average leukocyte count in the five patients (table 1, part I) showing leukopenia was 4,340. Two of these died. Four had influenzal bronchopneumonia, and one (case 2,981) showed symptoms of intestinal influenza. All of the 19 animals injected with material from this group of patients showed reduction in the leukocyte count on the day after injection. In some instances this was very marked (P 961, P 981, P 1,069), while in others it was relatively slight. The average diminution in the leukocyte count was 58%. The average reduction 48 hours after injection was 36%. The reduction occurred over a wide range of dosage, 0.1 c c to 1.5 c c. It followed subcutaneous as well as intratracheal injections of green-producing streptococci isolated from the throat, sputum, lungs, blood, and stool. The cultures of streptococci injected were in the first to the fourth generation, and some were derived from single green colonies on blood-agar plates. Injection of a filtrate of a fresh culture of green-producing streptococci also showed reduction in leukocytes (P 996, P 997). This is in accord with the findings following injection of other filtrates (table 2). The mortality in this group of animals was 47%. The reduction in leukocytes twenty-

TABLE 1

LEUKOCYTIC REACTION IN GUINEA-PIGS FOLLOWING INJECTIONS OF MATERIAL FROM INFLUENZA AND INFLUENZAL PNEUMONIA

I. Cases Showing Marked Leukopenia

Number	Leukocyte Count	Result	Guinea-Pigs Injected					Leukocyte Count			Findings
			Number	Material Injected			Place	Before Injection	Twenty-Four Hours after Injection	Forty-Eight Hours after Injection	
				Dose in c c	Organisms in Glucose Broth Culture or Sputum	Culture Generation					
2,800	2,800	Death	P951	1.5	Hemolytic streptococcus, throat	3	Trachea	26,000	21,000	19,200	Marked increased respiration; subnormal temperature; death sixth day from bronchopneumonia; acute peritonitis apparently secondary to colitis; green streptococci from blood
			P955	1.5	Green streptococcus, throat	2	Trachea	16,000	11,000	17,000	Sick; marked increase in respiration for two days; weight from 450 gm. to 320 gm.; recovered
			P959	0.1	Sputum, green streptococcus	0	Trachea	16,400	6,200	19,000	Fever; increased respiration for three days; recovered
			P961	1.5	Green streptococcus, throat	2	Subcutaneous tissue	10,400	2,400	1,600	Fever; increased respiration for two days; weight from 420 gm. to 320 gm.; death fourth day of bronchopneumonia and hemorrhagic edema; green streptococci from blood, lung, and uterus
			P971	1.5	Green streptococcus, lung	1	Trachea	11,000	9,000	27,000	Fever for two days; recovered
			P973	1.5	Green streptococcus, blood	1	Trachea	17,600	10,600	25,000	Remained well
			P981	1.5	Green streptococcus, blood	2	Trachea	8,000	2,000	6,350	Respirations slightly increased for two days; recovered
			P983	1.5	Green streptococcus, blood	3	Trachea	8,500	4,600	5,400	Increased respiration for a time, then better; death on eighteenth day from marked lesions in stomach and throughout intestinal wall; green-producing streptococci and B. coli from blood, uterus, stomach, and intestinal contents
			P984	1.5	Green streptococcus, blood	2	Trachea	8,800	4,400	9,600	Respirations increased for several days
			P993	1.0	Green streptococcus, blood	3	Subcutaneous tissue	26,000	12,000	9,300	Subnormal temperature; death in 48 hours; emphysema (13 c c), edema and hemorrhage of lungs; subcutaneous cellulitis; countless green streptococci
			P994	1.5	Green streptococcus, blood	2	Trachea	6,800	4,500	15,200	Subnormal temperature; death on seventh day from bronchopneumonia
			P995	1.5	Green streptococcus, blood	2	Trachea	9,600	6,300	14,400	Increased respiration for a few days, then better; death from bronchopneumonia eighteenth day after injection; hemorrhagic pleuritis, myocardial degeneration; countless green streptococci
			P996	1.5	Green streptococcus, blood (filtered)	2	Trachea	11,000	5,000	5,400	Remained well

											Remained well
2,770	3,800		P997	1.5	Green streptococcus, blood (filtered)	2	Trachea	15,600	9,800	8,200	Remained well
		Death	P1056	1.5	Green streptococcus, blood	4	Trachea	12,000	6,600	5,000	Increase in temperature and respiration for three days; recovered
		Recovery	P870	0.1	Green streptococcus, sputum	1	Trachea	17,000	8,900	5,800	Diffuse coalescing bronchopneumonia; death on seventh day from hemorrhagic pleuritis; green streptococci from blood, lung and pleura
2,873	6,200	Recovery	P1069	1.5	Green streptococcus, sputum	2	Trachea	11,600	4,200	9,400	No noteworthy symptoms
2,951	5,400	Recovery	P1174	1.5	Green streptococcus, sputum	2	Trachea	18,000	6,800		Increased respiration for two days; recovered
3,598	3,500	Recovery	P1261	1.5	Green streptococcus, stool	1	Trachea	11,800	7,000	5,800	Death in 48 hours; diffuse coalescing bronchopneumonia and acute myocardial degeneration; large number of green streptococci from blood, lung, pleural and peritoneal fluid
Average	4,340							18,000	7,500	11,570	Total: 19 animals injected; 9 died

II. Cases Showing No Reduction or Moderate Increase in Leukocyte Count

2,616	3,300	Death	P755	3.0	Green streptococcus, lung	0	Peritoneal cavity	15,000	12,000	9,400	Recovered
2,619	7,700	Recovery	P749	0.3	Sputum, green streptococcus	0	Peritoneal cavity	5,600	10,850	6,600	Recovered
			P750	0.3	Sputum, green streptococcus	0	Peritoneal cavity	14,400	4,600		Increased respiration; expiratory difficulty; relieved with epinephrin; death 48 hours after injection; emphysema; hemorrhagic edema; bronchopneumonia; serofibrinous peritonitis; green streptococci from blood and peritoneal fluid
2,620	11,100	Recovery	P752	0.3	Sputum, green streptococcus	0	Peritoneal cavity	25,500	20,500	6,800	Recovered
2,621	14,500	Recovery	P751	0.3	Sputum, green streptococcus	0	Peritoneal cavity	6,600	12,750	15,300	Recovered
2,798	12,500	Recovery	P957	1.5	Hemolytic streptococcus	2	Trachea	16,000	19,000	16,500	Increased respiration; death sixth day from hemorrhagic pleuritis; countless numbers of green streptococci in pleural fluid and lung
2,887	11,000	Death	P1109	5.0	Hemolytic streptococcus	2	Stomach	12,000	7,400		Remained well
			P1110	2.0	Hemolytic streptococcus	2	Trachea	7,600	6,000	11,100	Increased temperature and respiration rate for two days; recovered
3,295	11,300	Recovery	P1258	1.5	Primary culture, sputum, green streptococcus	1	Trachea	11,000	12,000		Death in 24 hours from acute hemorrhagic edema and hemorrhagic pleuritis; pleural fluid, lung, and blood showed countless numbers of staphylococci
3,297	13,000	Recovery	P1260	1.5	Primary culture, sputum, green streptococcus	1	Trachea	11,200	10,800		Death fourteenth day from bronchopneumonia due to green streptococcus
Average	11,300							12,490	11,580	10,960	Total: 10 animals injected; 4 died

four hours after injection was practically the same in the fatal and non-fatal infections, whereas forty-eight hours after injection the leukocyte count was usually lower in the animals that died as a result of the injection than in those that recovered (P 961, P 983, P 870, P 1,261).

Injections were made of material from 8 patients with undoubted influenza but who showed no reduction, or even a slight increase, in leukocytes at the time the animal experiments were performed (table 1, part II). The symptoms of these patients were the same as of those in the former group, although not so severe. The average leukocyte count was 11,300; two of these patients died. Four of the patients had influenza without lung findings, and 4 influenzal pneumonia (1 complicated with empyema) at the time of the animal injections. The leukocyte counts in the 10 animals injected with material from these patients averaged 12,490 the day before injection. Six of the animals showed slight reduction in leukocytes and 4 showed a slight increase twenty-four hours after injection; the total reduction in leukocytes was only 9%. The total average reduction of leukocytes in forty-eight hours after injection was also slight (11%). It is thus evident that injections of material from the patients showing marked leukopenia caused a greater reduction in leukocytes (58%) twenty-four hours after injection than the material (9%) from patients showing little or no reduction.

In table 2 is summarized the incidence of the occurrence of leukopenia, leukocytosis, and no change in the leukocyte count of guinea-pigs following injections of material from patients with influenza (part I), and in a control series with material from sources other than patients with influenza (part II). Injections of sputum, primary cultures from sputum, pure cultures of green-producing streptococci and hemolytic streptococci from patients with influenza were followed by the occurrence of leukopenia in a high percentage of the animals injected and to a lesser degree (33%) following injection of influenza bacilli. Moreover, injection of filtrates from sputum, lung emulsions, and broth cultures likewise was followed by a reduction in leukocytes in 65% of 26 animals injected. The total average of 99 animals in which leukocyte counts were made following injection of material from influenza which showed leukopenia was 57%; leukocytosis, 12%, and no change in the leukocyte count, 29%.

Sharp reductions in leukocyte counts were noted also following injection of staphylococci from the lungs or sputum of patients with

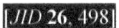

influenza. This in some instances was as marked as following the injection of the green-producing streptococcus from the same case. Thus, 2 guinea-pigs were injected intraperitoneally with these strains isolated from single colonies on a blood-agar plate inoculated with the peritoneal fluid of a guinea-pig that died from injection of sputum. The one injected with Staphylococcus aureus showed 9,200 leukocytes before injection; twenty-four hours after injection, 3,200; and forty-

TABLE 2

THE LEUKOCYTIC REACTION IN GUINEA-PIGS INOCULATED WITH MATERIAL FROM PATIENTS WITH INFLUENZA AND FROM OTHER SOURCES

I. Material from Patients with Influenza

Injection	Place of Injection	Animals	Percentage of Animals Showing		
			Leuko-penia	Leuko-cytosis	No Change
Sputum	Trachea	5	80	0	20
Sputum	Peritoneal cavity	5	40	20	40
Primary culture of sputum	Trachea	9	78	11	11
Green-producing streptococci	Trachea	41	46	17	34
Green-producing sterptococci	Peritoneal cavity	4	75	0	25
Hemolytic streptococci	Trachea	6	83	17	0
Influenza bacilli	Trachea	3	33	0	67
Filtrates from lung emulsions and broth cultures	Trachea	26	65	7	27
Total		99	57	12	29

II. Material from Sources Other Than Patients with Influenza

Hemolytic streptococci from a patient with simple nasopharyngitis and leukocytosis	Trachea	3	0	67	33
Sputum and cultures of green streptococci from a patient with simple tracheitis, nasopharyngitis and leukocytosis	Trachea	7	29	57	14
Type pneumococci from patients with lobar pneumonia	Trachea	9	11	22	67
Broth (controls)	Trachea	6	16	17	67
Total		25	16	36	48

eight hours after injection, 6,000. It died of peritonitis and pancreatitis with moderate emphysema of the lungs, and a few small, localized hemorrhages, with a leukocyte count of 3,240, and large numbers of hemolytic staphylococci in the blood and peritoneal fluid. The one injected with the green-producing streptococcus showed 6,000 leukocytes before injection; twenty-four hours after injection, 4,800, and forty-eight hours after injection, 3,600. This animal also died in three days with serofibrinous peritonitis, beginning pericarditis, acute pancreatitis, and moderate emphysema of the lungs, showing a few small circumscribed hemorrhages and large numbers of green-producing streptococci in pure culture in the blood, together with a moderate number of staphylococcus aureus in the pericardial and peritoneal fluid. The blood-agar plate of the material injected in each of these animals showed pure cultures of staphylococci and green-producing streptococci, respectively.

The percentages following injection of material from sources other than influenza patients are quite different. In this group the first case was that of a patient with a severe attack of nasopharyngitis and sinusitis, in which the throat was extremely red and the tonsils absent, and in which much mucopurulent material, at first tinged with blood, came from the nose and throat. The attack began with marked chilliness, but no distinct chill, and was followed by fever for a number of days and a leukocytosis of 14,000 on the first day. The patient recovered without developing symptoms of infection of the trachea or bronchi. The hemolytic streptococcus in the second culture generation isolated from the throat produced, on intratracheal injection, leukocytosis in 67% of the animals. The patient, it should be noted, developed no symptoms suggesting infection of the trachea or bronchi and the streptococcus caused no deaths on intratracheal application. This finding is in sharp contrast with the results of injection of the hemolytic streptococci from influenza in which leukopenia occurred in 83% and leukocytosis in only 17% of the animals injected, and in which death from hemorrhagic edema, hemorrhagic pleuritis, or bronchopneumonia occurred in a high percentage of animals injected (figure 1).

The results in the second case are also in sharp contrast to those obtained with material from patients with influenza. In this case the patient awoke in the morning with marked soreness in the upper part of the chest and a painful cough by which thick, mucopurulent material was raised. The day following, the cough and soreness in the chest continued and typical symptoms and signs of a nasopharyngitis had developed, with sneezing and abundant mucous discharge associated with redness of the mucous membranes of the nose and throat. There was little general aching, slight fever, and a leukocytosis of 13,500 on the second day. Recovery was practically complete on the fourth day. Intratracheal injections of the sputum and cultures of the green-producing streptococcus in the primary culture from the nasopharynx, and the same organism in the third culture generation isolated from the sputum on the second day was followed by leukocytosis in 57% of the animals. There was leukopenia in 29% and no change in leukocytes in 14%. None of the animals died of acute hemorrhagic pulmonary edema or hemorrhagic pleuritis. Three developed mucopurulent discharge from the nose in which the streptococcus injected was present in large numbers.

The intratracheal application of type pneumococci isolated originally from lobar pneumonia and proved virulent on intraperitoneal injection just prior to intratracheal injection was followed by leukocytosis in 22%, leukopenia in 11%, and no change in the leukocyte count in 67% of the animals injected. The relatively few instances of leukopenia following injection of the cultures from sources other than influenza usually occurred in animals that succumbed from overwhelming infection. Most of the intratracheal injections consisted of broth cultures of the different bacteria. Control injections of broth in the same dosage were followed by temporary leukopenia in 16%, leukocytosis in 17%, and no change in 67% of the animals injected. In the experiments in which filtrates of the cultures were injected the broth and culture filtrates were of the same batch. The occurrence of leukopenia in 65% of the animals injected with filtrates in contrast to 16% of those injected with broth represents roughly the "leukotoxin" formed by the growth of the streptococci in the broth. Filtrates of pneumonic lungs also possessed this power to a marked degree. In most instances 0.2% glucose-broth cultures and filtrates of cultures in this medium were injected. The broth cultures usually developed an acidity to phenolphthalein of from 1.5 to 2.5%. A series of experiments was made in which parallel intratracheal injections of 0.5 c c for each 100 gm. of body weight of cultures of acid reaction were given, and the same cultures injected after neutralization with sodium hydroxid. There was no noteworthy difference in the two sets of animals, in the leukocytic reaction, in the immediate respiratory symptoms, or in the late results from infection. Moreover, the "leukotoxin" or the property in broth culture filtrates which causes leukopenia and the symptoms of anaphylactic shock is not destroyed by heating to 60 C. for thirty minutes. (See experiments with filtrates.)

The degree of leukopenia following intratracheal injection of these cultures was found to be roughly proportional to the severity of respiratory embarrassment in the animals. In the case of extremely toxic cultures, a sharp reduction has been noted within a few hours after intratracheal application, and even after intranasal insufflation. In some instances the reduction in the leukocyte count did not occur for several days and then with the occurrence of death, with voluminous hemorrhagic and edematous lungs showing few leukocytes in the alveolar exudate, due to streptococci, a sharp drop in leukocytes was sometimes noted. On the other hand, in the animals that died late and that showed leukocytosis, the lungs were not so voluminous, the areas of consolidation were more firm, less moist on the cut surface, peribronchial in location, and the alveolar exudate was rich in leukocytes. These animals also often showed purulent bronchitis and tracheitis.

The leukopenia following direct inoculation of sputum was no greater and occurred no oftener than following injection of pure cultures of the streptococci. The latter were usually derived from single colonies and were in the first to the eleventh culture generation. The animals that succumbed following injection of sputum nearly always showed green-producing streptococci, and injection of pure cultures of these produced marked leukopenia often to a greater degree than those in the first animal passage.

This finding indicates that the reduction in leukocytes following injection of the material from patients with influenza may not be due to an unknown virus, but to peculiar properties of the streptococci or other bacteria at hand in this disease. These streptococci have the power by growth in vitro and in vivo to produce a soluble filterable substance. The filtrates from broth cultures and from influenzal lungs and sputum when applied intratracheally in guinea-pigs have the power, among other properties, to cause sharp reduction in leukocytes. The reduction in leukocytes has occurred with regularity only in the animals injected with influenza strains and not following injection of streptococci in like dosage from similar conditions showing leukocytosis, or type pneumococci. The average degree of leukopenia in the animals was roughly proportional to that found in the patients from whom the strains were isolated, and the leukocyte curves in fatal and nonfatal infections in the animals correspond roughly to those noted in the spontaneous disease in man. The conclusion seems warranted, therefore, that the leukopenia in influenzal infection in man may be due to peculiar properties of the bacteria which are now generally regarded as secondary invaders and not to an unknown virus. Moreover, according to our findings, a persistent, marked leukopenia, or an increasing leukopenia in influenza predisposes to influenzal pneumonia and in the latter indicates a bad prognosis.

STUDIES IN INFLUENZA AND PNEUMONIA

VII. A STUDY OF THE EFFECTS FOLLOWING THE INJECTION OF BACTERIA FOUND IN INFLUENZA IN NORMAL THROATS, IN SIMPLE NASOPHARYNGITIS, AND IN LOBAR PNEUMONIA

E. C. ROSENOW

Division of Experimental Bacteriology, The Mayo Foundation, Rochester, Minnesota.

CONTENTS

Introduction.
Technic of intratracheal injection.
Incidence of occurrence of voluminous lungs, hemorrhagic edema or bronchopneumonia, and pleuritis following intraperitoneal and intratracheal injection of sputum, lung and other exudates, and cultures from patients with influenza in relation to mortality.
Protocols of experiments following injection of material from influenza.
Control experiments with cultures from the throats of normal persons during and after the epidemic. The detection of the carrier state.
Control experiments with cultures from throat and sputum of patients with simple nasopharyngitis and tracheitis and with cultures from the nose of normal guinea-pigs.
Control experiments with type pneumococci from lobar pneumonia.
Protocols of cases of influenza and influenzal pneumonia and animal experiments. Similarity in localization of micro-organisms.
Experiments with filtrates of lung emulsions and cultures.
Experiments indicating the transmission of influenzal infection by contact.
Symptoms and gross lesions following intratracheal injection of influenzal material.
Microscopic anatomy of the lungs.
Lesions of the female generative organs and of tissues other than those of the lung.
Experiments on the mechanism of respiratory embarrassment in influenzal pneumonia.
Relation of mortality in guinea-pigs to virulency of the organisms isolated in fatal and nonfatal infection in patients.
General discussion and summary.

INTRODUCTION

It is my purpose to record in this paper the results obtained from the injection in various ways into animals of material obtained from patients with influenza and influenzal pneumonia and from sources other than influenza, to give the important facts in a series of cases of influenza in which the findings in the patients and the results from the injections of animals are correlated, to describe and illustrate the gross and microscopic changes that followed the injection of the bacteria

Received for publication Feb. 23, 1920.

from influenza, and to compare these changes with those noted in influenzal infection as it occurred during the epidemic of 1918 to 1919.

In a previous report [21, 22] it was pointed out that the streptococci from patients with influenza when injected intraperitoneally into mice and guinea-pigs possessed high virulency, that following these injections, lesions of the lungs and pleura occurred frequently, and that the animals often showed respiratory embarrassment during life and voluminous, emphysematous, and sometimes hemorrhagic lungs after death (case 2607, guinea-pig 737; table 2).

These findings in the experiments with streptococci suggested that the direct application of influenzal material to the normal, uninjured mucous membrane of the trachea and bronchi of animals might result in the production of lesions more marked than those following intraperitoneal injection, and should this be true, it might be possible to throw light on the mechanism of infection in this disease, and to compare the lesions obtained under controlled conditions of dosage and type of micro-organism in animals with those in man. The experiments on intraperitoneal injection and many clinical findings such as the relatively immobile, expanded thorax, the wheezing râles, the dyspnea, cyanosis, and leukopenia suggest strongly that influenza may be in part an anaphylactic reaction. The voluminous lung noted so commonly after death is another argument for this view. The guinea-pig, known to respond more like man than any other animal with respect to anaphylactic reactions, was selected as probably the most suitable in which to study the pulmonary and other lesions following the injection of influenzal material.

Technic of Intratracheal Injection

The technic of intratracheal injection should be such as to make it quite impossible to injure materially the lining of the trachea and bronchi. Discarded ureteral catheters cut at an angle of 45 degrees with margins rounded have been found to fulfill this requirement. The guinea-pig is wrapped in a towel; the head is held in place by the handles of an inverted artery forceps. The mouth is held open by spring wire retractors, and the tongue is depressed by a suitable small instrument. Under a strong reflected light, properly shaded, the catheter is inserted into the larynx with a quick stroke before the contraction of the muscles of the epiglottis can divert the tube into the esophagus. The animal's sharp, quick cough and total inability to use its voice, and the sensation of the catheter's passing the tracheal rings, indicate that it has entered the trachea. The catheters are sterilized by boiling and in order to avoid the possibility of transmitting accidental infection from one guinea-pig to another, a separate, freshly sterilized catheter was used for each animal in this series. Care was exercised to use only healthy, vigorous, and active animals from stock that was free from epidemic disease. At first the dose of culture given was very small, and the results in consequence were too irregular to permit accurate analysis. Later the dose was increased; 0.1 c c of the sputum or exudate and 0.5 c c of the glucose-blood or brain-broth culture for each 100 gm. of body weight were used in the experiments reported unless it is otherwise indicated. The cultures for injection were incubated at from 33-35 C. for from eighteen to twenty-four hours in tall columns of glucose-brain broth or glucose-blood broth. Control cultures of the material injected were always made on blood-agar plates. This was found necessary not only in order to prove the viability of the organisms injected, but also in order to determine the type that had grown in the particular culture. As has been pointed out heretofore,[20] the most important organism found in the sputum in influenza was a gram-positive, often lanceolate diplostreptococcus which produces greenish colonies on blood-agar plates. The colonies are larger, flatter, and more moist than those of Streptococcus viridans, often indistinguishable from pneumococcus colonies. In this report I shall designate this organism, including the strains that ferment inulin, as a "green-producing streptococcus" or "green streptococcus" to distinguish it from Streptococcus viridans.

Control experiments were first made to determine the harmlessness of intratracheal injection of varying amounts of salt solution and sterile broth. All guinea-pigs injected with salt solution (1 with 6 c c; 3 with 3 c c, and 1 with 2.5 c c) remained well. They showed a slight increase in respiration immediately after injection. All were free from symptoms the following day and remained so. Fifteen guinea-pigs were injected with glucose broth, glucose-blood broth, or glucose-brain broth (4 with 3 c c; 3 with 2.5 c c, 7 with 1.5 c c, and 1 with 1 c c). They showed relatively slight respiratory disturbance immediately after injection. Some, especially those injected with meat infusion-peptone-glucose-blood broth, showed mild symptoms of anaphylaxis. They coughed, scratched the nose with their paws; and were irritable for a short time after injection. All were well the day after injection, and all but two remained well subsequently. The one which had been injected with 1.5 c c died thirteen days later from an old bronchopneumonia that showed Bacillus bronchisepticus. The other, which had been injected intratracheally with 3 c c glucose broth, died ten days later with bronchopneumonia and a moderate amount of bloody fluid in the pleural cavities. Cultures from the blood showed a few colonies of green-producing streptococci, and from the pleural fluid, staphylococci and B. bronchisepticus. The culture in glucose-brain broth of the green-producing streptococci from the blood was injected intratracheally in 3 guinea-pigs. Two had slightly increased respirations for two days and then recovered. The other had no symptoms; it was chloroformed three days after injection and showed no lesions. None of the guinea-pigs showed leukopenia. The average leukocyte count before injection was 9,600, twenty-four hours after injection 9,100, and forty-eight hours after injection, 12,200.

INCIDENCE OF OCCURRENCE OF VOLUMINOUS LUNGS, HEMORRHAGIC EDEMA OF BRONCHOPNEUMONIA, AND PLEURITIS FOLLOWING INTRAPERITONEAL AND INTRATRACHEAL INJECTION OF SPUTUM, LUNG AND OTHER EXUDATES, AND CULTURES FROM PATIENTS WITH INFLUENZA IN RELATION TO MORTALITY

The more marked effects of intratracheal injection over intraperitoneal injection of material from patients with influenza became apparent at once. The symptoms of respiratory embarrassment were more pronounced and the lungs more voluminous. In table 1 the average volume and weight of the lung of a series of guinea-pigs injected intratracheally, and of normal guinea-pigs are given (fig. 1). The volume of the lungs in cubic centimeters, as measured by displacement of water for normal guinea-pigs weighing about 350 gm., and killed with chloroform, was 6.5 c c, or approximately one-fiftieth or 2% of the weight of the animals expressed in grams. The average volume of the lungs of guinea-pigs that had died from causes other than pneumonia was found to be about normal. The average weight of the lungs was found to be 3.3 gm., or about 1% of the body weight. It is evident from table 1 that the more toxic or virulent the culture, the more severe the reaction in the lung, and the earlier the death occurred following intratracheal injection, the greater was the volume and weight of the lung. Thus the volume and weight were approximately three and four times the normal in the guinea-pigs dying in two and one-half hours and two days after injection, respectively, and in those that died in three days the average volume of the lung was less than twice that and the weight about two and one-half times that of the average normal.

TABLE 1

RESULTS OF INTRATRACHEAL INSUFFLATION OF CULTURES FROM INFLUENZA AS SHOWN BY VOLUME AND WEIGHT OF LUNGS

	Average Weight of Animals, Gm.	Average Volume of Lungs, C C	Average Weight of Lungs, Gm.
Guinea-pigs living an average* of 2.5 hours	410	19	13
Guinea-pigs living an average of 2 days	390	17	14
Guinea-pigs living an average of 3 days	340	10	8
Normal guinea-pigs (controls)	350	6.5	3.3

* The averages of 6 guinea-pigs in each series are given.

The increase in lung volume was about the same following the injection of sputum, primary culture of sputum, pure cultures of freshly isolated strains of green-producing streptococci, hemolytic streptococci and staphylococci (usually in the second or third generation). The average volume of the lung of a large number of guinea-pigs after intratracheal injection of influenzal material was 15 c c, and after intraperitoneal injection 10 c c; after injection of type pneumococci it was 10 c c and 7 c c, respectively.

From table 2 may be obtained a general picture of the differences in the results obtained in the mortality and incidence of lesions of the lungs in guinea-pigs injected intratracheally and intraperitoneally with material from patients with influenza, with cultures from normal throats during the epidemic and after it had subsided, with type pneumococci, and with sputum and cultures from patients with simple nasopharyngitis and tracheitis. The total average mortality following injection of material from 111 cases of influenza in 192 animals was

TABLE 2

MORTALITY AND INCIDENCE OF LESIONS OF THE LUNGS IN GUINEA-PIGS INJECTED WITH MATERIAL FROM INFLUENZA; WITH CULTURES FROM NORMAL THROATS DURING AND AFTER THE EPIDEMIC; WITH TYPE PNEUMOCOCCI AND WITH SPUTUM AND CULTURES FROM PATIENTS WITH SIMPLE NASOPHARYNGITIS AND TRACHEITIS

Material Injected	Place of Injection	Number of Strains	Number of Animals			Percentage of Mortality	Percentage Showing		Pleuritis
			Injected	Recovered	Died		Voluminous Lungs	Hemorrhagic Edema or Pneumonia	
Sputum............	Trachea....	16	17	5	12	70	64	62	54
	Peritoneum	38	48	15	33	68	25	8	14
Primary culture.....	Trachea....	17	31	16	15	48	36	55	15
	Peritoneum	12	13	7	6	46	22	22	11
Green-producing streptococci.......	Trachea....	19	33	17	16	48	73	54	26
	Peritoneum	12	16	7	9	56	58	17	42
Hemolytic streptococci..............	Trachea....	9	17	7	10	59	53	71	44
	Peritoneum	4	6	2	4	67	67	0	0
Staphylococci.......	Trachea....	6	11	5	6	55	71	43	43
Total for influenza (111 cases)........	....	133	192	81	111	58	55	46	28
Primary culture of throats of normal persons during epidemic of influenza..............	Trachea....	4	12	7	5	42	17	17	0
Primary culture of throats of normal persons months after epidemic had disappeared..	Trachea....	15	15	12	3	20	0	20	0
Type I, II, III, and IV pneumococci from lobar pneumonia............	Trachea....	14	20	14	6	30	30	35*	35
	Peritoneum	14	18	0	18	100	6	0	28
Sputum and cultures from patients with simple nasopharyngitis and tracheitis.....	Trachea....	2	10	8	2	20	0	20	0

* Lobar pneumonia.

58%. The total average incidence of voluminous lungs was 55%; of hemorrhagic edema or bronchopneumonia, 46%, and of pleuritis, 28%. The killing power of the influenza strains was only slightly lower when they were applied to the normal mucous membrane of the trachea and bronchi than when they were injected intraperitoneally. The results of control experiments with type pneumococci were quite different in this respect; their killing power was 100% on intraperitoneal injection, whereas only 30% of the animals died following intratracheal injections of the same dose. The average incidence and the degree of lesions of the lung and pleura were higher, as would be expected, following intratracheal injection than following intraperitoneal injection.

The property in these strains which caused symptoms resembling anaphylaxis, voluminous lungs with acute hemorrhagic edema of lungs and leukopenia, and the general virulency, tended to disappear promptly on artificial cultivation, especially if the organisms were cultivated under aerobic conditions. To illustrate:

The volume of the lungs in 2 guinea-pigs was 20 and 12 c c, respectively (average 16 c c), following injection of the primary culture from the blood of a patient with influenza containing a pure culture of the green-producing streptococcus while that in 2 guinea-pigs injected with the same strain in glucose broth after one plating on blood agar was 12 and 10 c c (average 11 c c), and the hemorrhage and edema of the lung were much less marked. Different strains differed markedly in the loss of this power, depending to some extent on the method of cultivation. Aerobic cultivation on blood agar destroyed these peculiar properties rapidly, while by rapid transfers of glucose-brain broth from tube to tube they might be retained for many generations. The typical picture has followed injection of strains in the eleventh culture generation. The tendency of some of the strains to localize and produce a certain type of lesion was striking, often corresponding to the type of lesions found in the patient. Thus, in a case of death from hemorrhagic edema of the lung with pseudolobar pneumonia and hemorrhagic pleuritis (case 2800), the cultures from the throat in the first and second culture generation produced hemorrhagic edema of the lung and hemorrhagic pleuritis in two guinea-pigs injected into the trachea (g. pigs 947 and 956), and in one injected into the stomach (g. pig 948). The same strain injected about three months later when in the sixth subculture had lost much of its virulency, but it still localized in the same manner and produced bronchopneumonia with localized abscesses in the lung and adhesive pleuritis resulting in perforative peritonitis (g. pig 1311).

Experiments with Lung and Other Exudates.—During the course of the experiments the effects of injecting directly the lung exudates of patients and of lung emulsions, peritoneal, and pleural exudates from animals was also studied. Contrary to expectations, the symptoms and lesions following direct injection were less acute than those following injection of the cultures made from these exudates and following the injection of sputum and cultures of streptococci from the sputum and throat. The mortality following direct intratracheal injection of the exudates from 16 cases into 19 guinea-pigs was only 42% as compared, for example, with a mortality of 70% following injection of sputum. The mortality in the 19 guinea-pigs was almost wholly due to injection of peritoneal and lung exudates in guinea-pigs dead from injection of sputum or cultures. Most of the animals that died showed bronchopneumonia, and only a few acute hemorrhagic edema. This relatively low mortality was not due to a lesser number of viable organisms injected because plate cultures often showed a larger number of living bacteria than were present in the sputum or cultures. Under the conditions of a more forced experiment, intraperitoneal injection, the mortality in 11 guinea-pigs injected with 11 strains was higher (64%). Moreover, the theory that these bacteria when soaked in blood or lung exudate tend to lose their bite, as it were, when applied to the normal pulmonary epithelium is further borne out by the fact that the virulency and incidence of acute hemorrhagic edema were higher following injection of cultures from the sputum and throat than of cultures from the blood. Thus, in one case (case 2,800) the mortality following intratracheal injection of the throat and sputum strains was 64%, while following injection of the strain isolated from the blood it was 33%.

Intratracheal Injections of Influenza Bacilli. — Recently isolated strains from the throats of 5 undoubted cases of influenza — 4 in the second, and 1 in the sixth culture generation — were injected intratracheally into 5 guinea-pigs. The dose was 0.5 c c for each 100 gm. body weight of a dense salt suspension from rich growths on chocolate blood agar. The amount of culture injected ranged from the growth of from 1-5 slants. In 3, leukocyte counts were made; 1 of these showed a drop from 12,000 before injection to 6,800 twenty-four hours after injection and 8,000 seventy-two hours after injection. The others showed no change in the leukocyte count. All the animals recovered. Besides slightly increased respiration immediately after injection there was no noticeable effect, and all the animals seemed quite well without increased respiration or rise in temperature 24 hours after injection. The virulency of 2 of these strains was proved in a mouse. Injection of 0.4 c c of a mixture of 3 of the strains killed the mouse in 24 hours. The animal showed enormous subcutaneous hemorrhages in the right groin adjacent to the point of the intraperitoneal injection, and there were hyperemia of lungs and a number of subpleural hemorrhages, but no gross evidence of peritonitis. The cultures from blood and peritoneal fluid on chocolate and blood-agar plates yielded countless numbers of influenza bacilli. In connection with these experiments with pure cultures of influenza bacilli should be considered the fact that intraperitoneal injections of sputum into mice and intraperitoneal and intratracheal injections into guinea-pigs were never followed by invasion by influenza bacilli as determined by cultures, direct examination of smears, and microscopic examination of

TABLE 3

PREDOMINATING ORGANISM IN SPUTUM AND PRIMARY CULTURES FROM SPUTUM INJECTED IN ANIMALS AND FOUND IN THE ANIMALS THAT DIED

Material Injected	Place of Injection	Strains	Incidence of Predominating Organism in						
			Material Injected			Animals Cultured	Animals That Died		
			Green-producing Streptococci, per Cent.	Hemolytic Streptococci, per Cent.	Staphylococci, per Cent.		Green-producing Streptococci, per Cent.	Hemolytic Streptococci, per Cent.	Staphylococci, per Cent.
Sputum	Trachea or peritoneum of guinea-pigs	54	71	20	9	29	81	4	15
Primary culture from sputum	Trachea or peritoneum of guinea-pigs	29	59	24	17	22	73	14	13
Sputum	Peritoneum of mice	19	69	21	10	17	82	12	6
Total		102	68	20	12	68	78	9	13

sections stained for influenza bacilli as recommended by MacCallum.[17] In some of the sputums thus injected large numbers of influenza bacilli were demonstrated in smears and by cultures before injection. Thus in the lung of the guinea-pig shown in figures 5, 10 and 11 the sputum injected contained large numbers of influenza bacilli, but they were absent in the peritoneal exudate, blood and lung tissue. The invasive power of freshly isolated influenza bacilli (virulent to mice on intraperitoneal injection) and of those in the sputum itself when applied to the tracheal mucous membrane in guinea-pigs was found to be slight as compared with the invasive power of the streptococci. It is possible that tracheal injection of adapted strains or those whose virulency is enhanced by animal passage through intraperitoneal injection might acquire the power to invade the lung and produce bronchopneumonia and possibly hemorrhagic edema of the lungs.

The Comparative Invasive Power of the Bacteria from Patients with Influenza. — The high invasive power of the green-producing streptococcus became apparent early in the work. We have determined which of the different bacteria occurred in predominating number in the sputums injected into guinea-pigs and mice and in the primary cultures from sputum injected into guinea-pigs, and also in exudates and blood of the animals that died as a result of the injections. In table 3 is given the percentage of incidence of the predominating organisms. It will be noted that the green-producing streptococcus was the predominating organism in the material injected in each group of experiments and, what is more significant, it was the predominating organism in a higher percentage of the animals after death, whereas the reverse was true of hemolytic streptococci and staphylococci. The relative importance of these three organisms in influenza might be said to be indicated roughly by the figures in the last line of table 3.

PROTOCOLS OF EXPERIMENTS FOLLOWING INJECTION OF
MATERIAL FROM INFLUENZA

Guinea-pig 846, weighing 420 gm., was injected intraperitoneally Dec. 28, 1918, with 2.5 c c of glucose-broth culture of the green-producing streptococcus from the blood of G. pig 828, which had been injected with the sputum from case 2,749. December 29 the animal was found dead. Marked hemorrhagic serofibrinous peritonitis, moderate distention and congestion of the lungs (11 c c), a large number of large and small subpleural hemorrhages, and beginning pleuritis were found. The pleura contained 3 c c of turbid, blood-tinged, chocolate-colored fluid. A moderate amount of bloody, frothy fluid escaped from the cut surface of the lungs. The uterus contained several hemorrhagic areas marking placental attachment. The cultures from the blood, pleural fluid, peritoneal fluid, and placental site showed many green-producing streptococci.

Guinea-pig 981, weighing 470 gm., was injected Jan. 16, 1919, intratracheally with 1.5 c c of the glucose-broth culture of the green-producing streptococcus in the second culture generation isolated from the blood in case 2,800. The white blood count before injection was 8,000; the temperature 102.2 F. January 17 the animal appeared less active than normal and the respirations were slightly increased. The leukocyte count was 2,000 and the temperature 103.2 January 18 the animal was more active, but the respirations were still slightly increased. The leukocyte count was 6,200, the temperature 102.8. January 19 the animal appeared quite well. The respirations were normal, the leukocyte count was 12,200, and the temperature 102.4. The animal made a complete recovery; when it was chloroformed January 24 it showed no lesions. The cultures from the blood and lung remained sterile.

Guinea-pig 995, weighing 470 gm., had injected into the trachea, Jan. 18, 1919, 1.5 c c of the glucose-broth culture of the green-producing streptococcus in the second culture generation isolated from the blood of case 2,800. The white blood count before injection was 9,200, the temperature 102.4. There were moderate symptoms of dyspnea immediately following injection. January 19 the animal appeared quite well but the respirations were definitely increased. The leukocyte count was 6,200, the temperature 103. January 20 the respirations were slightly increased, the leukocyte count was 14,400, the temperature 103. January 25 the animal appeared well. February 24 at 7:30 a. m. the animal appeared ill. The respirations were markedly increased and difficult. The animal when taken from the cage and placed on a table had a typical attack resembling anaphylactic shock with bronchial spasm. At noon the respirations were exceedingly rapid and the animal appeared to be very sick; at 4 p. m. it was found dead. The white blood count was 12,800. There was a large amount of bloody, turbid fluid in both pleural cavities; the right contained a moderate amount of adherent, partially organizing fibrin. The lungs were collapsed and the intermediate lobe was completely consolidated, grayish-red, and covered with a film of fibrin. There were several thickened areas in the mucous membrane of the uterus indicating a resorption of fetuses. The ovaries were normal. The heart muscle was grayish-red. Cultures from the blood and pleura showed green-producing streptococci.

Guinea-pig 1335, weighing 420 gm., was injected intratracheally, May 15, 1919, at 9:50 a. m. with 1.5 cc of glucose-acacia-broth culture of staphylococcus in the sixth subculture from case 2,623. At 10:15 a. m. respirations were rapid, difficult and irregular. There were repeated attacks bordering on bronchial spasm, expiration was forced and prolonged, and the animal was weak. At 10:30 a. m. the respirations were extremely difficult. The animal coughed violently at intervals making desperate efforts with each expiration, and during one of these violent efforts it ran about aimlessly with blood spurting from its nose and mouth; it fell on its side and died with its head in a pool of frothy blood. The lung was found greatly distended (20 cc) and hemorrhagic and edematous throughout. Sections showed marked distention of alveoli and destruction of the epithelium lining the alveoli and of the endothelium of the capillaries. In areas dissolution was so marked as to make it quite impossible to distinguish the alveolar boundaries.

Guinea-pig 956, weighing 280 gm., was injected intratracheally, Jan. 13, 1919, with 1.5 cc of glucose-brain-broth culture of the green-producing streptococcus from a single colony on a blood-agar plate inoculated with the swab from case 2,800. January 14 the animal was very ill; respirations were rapid and difficult. The fur was rough and the animal was restless and irritable. It died at noon. The lungs were markedly distended (15 cc). Both diaphragmatic lobes were dark and mottled. The cut surfaces everywhere were extremely moist and a large amount of bloody, frothy fluid exuded. The other lobes showed smaller areas of hemorrhagic edema. The alveoli were extremely distended, in places almost to the point of rupturing. The peribronchial glands were edematous. The trachea and bronchi were extremely hyperemic and contained a large amount of bloody, frothy fluid. There was a moderate amount of slightly turbid, blood-tinged fluid in the pleural and pericardial sacs. The mucous membrane of the nose was hyperemic. The suprarenals were swollen and there was cloudy swelling of the kidneys. The mucous membrane of the uterus was markedly hyperemic throughout and showed three hemorrhagic areas marking placental attachments. The vagina contained a moderate amount of bloody mucus. Cultures from the blood showed one colony of green-producing streptococci; from the lung and hemorrhagic areas of the mucous membranes of the uterus, large numbers of green-producing streptococci; from the spleen, kidney, liver, and suprarenals, no growth. In sections of the lung were noted marked dilatation of alveoli, marked desquamation of the epithelial lining of bronchi, and marked edema and hemorrhage in the alveoli with little cellular infiltration (fig. 13 b). The Gram stain showed enormous numbers of streptococci distributed particularly along the alveolar walls (fig. 14 c).

Guinea-pig 947, weighing 400 gm., had injected into the trachea, Jan. 10, 1919, 11 a. m., 1.5 c c glucose-brain-broth culture from the throat swab of case 2,800. At 6 p. m. the respirations were rapid and shallow; the voice was weak and the animal appeared sick. January 13 at 7:30 a. m. the animal was found dead. There was a large amount of hemorrhagic, dark colored fluid in the pleural cavities, containing practically no fibrin. The pleura was rough and covered with a thin fibrinous film, and the lung was compressed by the hemorrhagic fluid in the pleural cavities. The right diaphragmatic and intermediate lobes were extremely wet and edematous on the cut surface. A large amount of bloody, frothy fluid escaped. Portions of the diaphragmatic lobe barely floated in water. The mucous membranes of the bronchi, trachea, and nose were extremely hyperemic and covered with a bloody, frothy fluid. The uterus contained four hemorrhagic areas marking placental attachments. A moderate amount of bloody mucus was found in the uterus and vagina. The stomach was distended with gas rich in carbon dioxid, and showed marked postmortem digestion of the mucous membrane. The cultures from the blood showed a small number of colonies of Staphylococcus aureus and hemolytic streptococci; from the lung, pleura, pericardial fluid, and uterus, large numbers of hemolytic streptococci and staphylococci, and a few from the kidney, liver, and suprarenals. Sections of the lung showed extreme interstitial edema and hemorrhage with marked disintegration of the cells lining the alveoli. The gram stain showed enormous numbers of gram-positive diplococci in the pleura and subpleural spaces in the interstitial tissues and around the blood vessels (fig. 20 a and b).

Guinea-pig 948, weighing 300 gm., was injected intragastrically, Jan. 10, 1919, with 1.5 c c of the glucose-brain-broth culture from the throat of case 2,800. January 13 it appeared to be quite well. January 15 it appeared to be quite well, but was less active and sat humped up. January 19 it sat humped up with ruffled fur, with a dry crust about the nostrils, markedly increased respirations, labored and forced expirations and dilated chest. It had lost 40 gm. in weight. January 20 at 8 a. m. the breathing was rapid and difficult and the animal very much weaker. At noon when it was found dead, it weighed 250 gm. The thorax was distended with a large amount of chocolate-colored fluid (15 c c); there were marked pleuritis with loose fibrinous adhesions throughout and a thin layer covering the pleura. The peribronchial lymph glands were much enlarged and edematous; the lungs were collapsed, but hemorrhagic, and showed areas of bronchopneumonia with white necrotic spots in the intermediate lobe. The pancreas was edematous, the spleen enlarged, and the myocardium gray. No lesions in the stomach or intestinal tract were demonstrable. Cultures from the blood showed green-producing streptococci; those from the pleural fluid, green-producing streptococci and staphylococci.

Guinea-pig 1311, weighing 320 gm., was injected intratracheally, March 25, 1919, with 0.2 c c of the glucose-brain-broth culture from the throat swab from case 2,800 in the sixth subculture. March 26 and 28 the animal's respiration was increased but otherwise it appeared well. April 15 it was found dead and showed three circumscribed areas of necrosis with softening in the left diaphragmatic lobe. The pleura over each of these areas was bound down by organizing adhesions. One area over the diaphragmatic lobe showed localized hemorrhages and fibrinous deposit on the peritoneal side of the diaphragm, undoubtedly the source of the serofibrinous peritonitis. One area of consolidation in the right cardiac lobe occupying one third of its volume showed recent diffuse consolidation. The white necrotic areas on the cut surface were wedge-shaped and resembled infarcts; the urinary bladder contained a number of circumscribed hemorrhages in the mucosa; but no other lesions were noteworthy. Cultures from the blood, lung, peritoneal and pleural fluids showed green-producing streptococci.

Guinea-pig 1030, weighing 400 gm., was injected intratracheally, Jan. 22, 1919, with 1.5 c c of the lung emulsion from case 2835. The leukocyte count before injection was 10,200; twenty-four hours after injection it was 7,800, and the animal appeared quite well. February 3 the animal was chloroformed. It showed one large grayish-red area of consolidation posteriorly in the left diaphragmatic lobe and one area of consolidation which was dark red and edematous, and a localized necrotic, wedge-shaped, adherent area over the right diaphragmatic lobe.

The experiments cited in detail are representative of a much larger series. Examples of mild effects, mild early effects and severe late effects and marked progressive symptoms from the time of injection are given following injection of pure cultures of the green-producing streptococcus in the first to the sixth subculture, staphylococcus in the sixth subculture, and of a lung emulsion.

CONTROL EXPERIMENTS WITH CULTURES FROM THE THROATS OF NORMAL PERSONS DURING AND AFTER THE EPIDEMIC. THE DETECTION OF THE CARRIER STATE

The occurrence of voluminous lung, hemorrhagic edema, and bronchopneumonia associated with leukopenia following intratracheal injection of the influenza strains was a striking picture. It was thought that intratracheal injection of primary mass cultures from throats of normal persons might detect carriers of the influenza streptococcus. Two sets of experiments were done, one on persons in an institution during the prevalence in the disease in epidemic proportions, the other four months later when influenza had entirely subsided. In the former set, 12 guinea-pigs were injected with cultures from 4 patients. Seven of the guinea-pigs recovered and 5 died, a mortality of 42% (table 2). In 2 cases the animal injections were without apparent effects; in one, the 2 pigs injected died in three and four days, respectively, of bronchopneumonia without leukopenia. The lungs were only slightly enlarged (average volume 10 c c), and quite dry on the cut surface; the exudate was highly cellular. After death green-producing streptococci, or pneumococci, and staphylococci were isolated from the lung in large numbers. The streptococci were not agglutinated by the monovalent serum. The results in the fourth case were in sharp contrast. The 3 guinea-pigs and 1 mouse which were injected died. One pig and the mouse were injected subcutaneously, the other animals intratracheally. The 3 guinea-pigs showed a sharp drop in leukocytes. Death in all was due to green-producing streptococci (which were agglutinated by the monovalent serum) and staphylococci. The average leukocyte count before injection was 14,000, while twenty-four hours after injection it was 4,260, a loss of 64%. The two animals injected intratracheally showed voluminous hemorrhagic lungs.

Guinea-pig 1004, weighing 350 gm., was injected intratracheally Jan. 19, 1919, with 1.5 c c of the glucose broth culture from the throat of a normal person who had been exposed to influenza (case 2839). The leukocyte count was 13,000. January 20 the leukocyte count was 4,200, and there was marked shortness of breath and difficult breathing. January 21 at 4 p. m. the animal was found dead, with its head lying in a pool of hemorrhagic fluid. The white blood count was 2,600. The lung was distended, very heavy (14 c c and 12 gm.) and almost completely filled with a frothy hemorrhagic fluid. There was little evidence of consolidation. The peribronchial lymph glands were hemorrhagic and edematous. A thin fibrinous film covered the posterior aspect of the lung. Cultures from the blood, lung, suprarenals, and liver showed staphylococci and green-producing streptococci; those from the kidney and spleen were negative.

The experiments with cultures from normal persons months after the epidemic had subsided consisted of the intratracheal injection of 15 guinea-pigs with cultures from the throats of 15 persons. Of these animals, 12 recovered without developing noteworthy symptoms and 3 (20%) died (table 2). None of these animals showed the violent respiratory embarrassment noted in the animals following injection of the influenza strains. The lung picture after death was quite different than that following injection of the influenza strains. The animals died in one, two and five days, respectively, of green-producing streptococci or pneumococci in the two former, and of Bacillus mucosus in the third. The lungs averaged 8.5 c c in volume. The hemorrhages and consolidation were situated immediately around the bronchi and the consolidated areas were relatively dry on the cut surface, and the exudate highly cellular in character, as noted in the following experiment:

Guinea-pig 1364, weighing 280 gm., was injected intratracheally July 24, 1919, with 1.5 c c of the glucose brain-broth culture from the throat of a normal person (case 3515). July 25 the respirations were decidedly increased. At 4:30 p. m. it was found dead. The thorax was not distended. The pleural cavities were free from fluid; the lungs were only slightly distended (9 c c). There were areas in the diaphragmatic lobes of hemorrhage and beginning infiltration. The cultures from the blood were negative; cultures from the lung showed green-producing streptococci.

CONTROL EXPERIMENTS WITH CULTURES FROM THROATS AND SPUTUM OF PATIENTS WITH SIMPLE NASOPHARYNGITIS AND TRACHEITIS AND WITH CULTURES FROM THE NOSE OF NORMAL GUINEA-PIGS

In some cases there was a marked parallelism between the findings in the patient and in the animals injected (case 2798). Hence it was thought worth while to inject the sputum and cultures from patients with simple nasopharyngitis and tracheitis long after the epidemic had subsided and compare the results with those obtained following injection of the strains from influenza. The results are summarized in table 2. Thus, of 10 animals injected from cultures from 2 cases, 2 died (20%), both of bronchopneumonia. None showed marked respiratory embarrassment resembling anaphylaxis, and none died of hemorrhagic edema. Both of the patients showed leukocytosis, and leukocytosis was the rule in the animals injected.

In order still further to control the results of the experiments on intratracheal injections and to make sure that the bacteria of the upper respiratory tract might not be carried into the lung with the catheter, a series of guinea-pigs were injected with the cultures from freshly isolated strains of the green-producing streptococci normally present in the nose in some guinea-pigs.

The strains isolated from the nose of 2 guinea-pigs were each injected in the usual dose into the trachea of 2 guinea-pigs. The leukocyte count from the guinea-pig in which the culture was made was normal and remained so following injection of sterile broth. The 4 guinea-pigs injected were well the day after injection and remained so for a month thereafter. None of the animals showed leukopenia. All showed a slight rise in leukocyte count the day after injection, and only one a moderate reduction forty-eight hours after injection. The average leukocyte count before injection was 12,550, twenty-four hours after injection, 14,750, and forty-eight hours after injection, 10,200. It is thus apparent that the chance of carrying infection from the upper respiratory tract through the trachea is extremely slight, not even occurring when large doses of the normal flora of the upper respiratory tract are introduced.

CONTROL EXPERIMENTS WITH TYPE PNEUMOCOCCI FROM LOBAR PNEUMONIA

In order that a correct standard for comparison might be had in evaluating the results of the experiments in influenza, it was considered necessary not only to inject animals with type pneumococci, but also with strains having at least the same killing power, when injected intraperitoneally, dose for dose, as had the strains from influenza. The virulency of the strains were first determined for mice. Twelve strains * of the various types were injected intraperitoneally into 13 mice, the dose ranging from 0.8 to 1.0 c c of glucose-blood or glucose brain-broth culture. All died of peritonitis. The blood and peritoneal fluid in all showed large numbers of pneumococci, the latter often a few colonies of staphylococcus in addition. These 12 strains freshly isolated from the blood, and 2 other recently isolated strains, 14 in all, were then injected intraperitoneally and intratracheally into guinea-pigs. The doses in both were the same and varied from 0.3 to 3 c c of twenty-four-hour glucose brain broth cultures; the usual dose in these, as in the animals injected with the influenza strains, was 0.5 c c for each 100 gm. of body weight. The weight of the guinea-pigs ranged from 320 to 400 gm., the average being 330 gm. Intraperitoneal injections were made in 18 guinea-pigs with the 14 different strains of type pneumococci, 6 with 6 strains of type 1; 5 with 3 strains of type II; 6 with 4 strains of type III, and 1 with 1 strain of group IV. Eleven of the animals died on the first day and 7 on the second day after injection, a mortality of 100% (table 2). The blood and peritoneal exudate showed large or countless numbers of pneumococcus colonies in all these animals. The peritoneal exudate in most instances and the blood in some instances yielded in addition a small and variable number of staphylococcus colonies. The volume of the lungs ranged from 4 to 9 c c, averaging 7 c c. Noteworthy lesions in the lungs were absent in all. A few showed small hemorrhages. A beginning pleuritis was noted in 5.

* For the strains of pneumococci used in these experiments I am indebted to Dr. Rufus J. Cole of the Hospital of the Rockefeller Institute for Medical Research and Dr. Augustus Wadsworth of the New York State Board of Health.

Successful intratracheal injections were as follows: 7 guinea-pigs with 5 strains of type I; 4 with 3 strains of type II; 5 with 4 strains of type III, and 4 with 2 strains of group IV pneumococcus, a total of 14 strains and 20 animals (table 2). Respiratory embarrassment immediately after injection and the following day was relatively slight as compared with animals injected with the influenza strains. In 7 of those that recovered no noticeable increase in respiratory rate or illness could be detected the day after injection. Five of the others showed increased respiration and rise in temperature for a day or two, and then recovered. Two showed marked increased respiration for 4 days and when improving, on the fifth and sixth day, respectively, were chloroformed. The findings in the former are illustrated in the experiment in guinea-pig 1,450. The other showed a resolving pneumonia with a few pneumococci in the blood and lung exudate. The 6 animals that died (one each injected with types I, II and III, and 3 of group IV pneumococci) showed with one exception progressive increase in respiration rate until death. The one that did not, died eight days later with a resolving pneumonia. The respirations in the 3 that died within five days after injection were extremely rapid, the nostrils remained free from exudate, there was no bleeding from the nose, the animals were quiet, and the breathing was generally free and easy. The picture was thus in sharp contrast to that noted in guinea-pigs that died following intratracheal injection of the highly virulent influenza strains. The tendency to the production of leukopenia following injection of type pneumococci even in fatal infection was far less than that following injection of the influenza strains, occurring respectively in 11 and 57% of the animals injected. The lungs were moderately distended, but smaller than those observed following the injection of influenza strains. The consolidation usually involved whole lobes or was sharply outlined (fig. 4). The pleura overlying the consolidated area was opaque and rough, the consolidated areas, even in the stage of red hepatization, were less edematous than in the influenzal lungs, and the areas showing gray hepatization were uniformly dry and granular. Extensive gray hepatization was noted as early as forty-eight hours after injection. Sections in the early stages showed many red cells and moderate leukocyte infiltration in the alveoli. Later diffuse alveolar infiltration with leukocytes and fibrin occurred with a few red blood corpuscles and little edema. The bronchial and alveolar epithelium showed comparatively little damage (figs. 18a and 19b). The pneumococci were found diffusely distributed in large

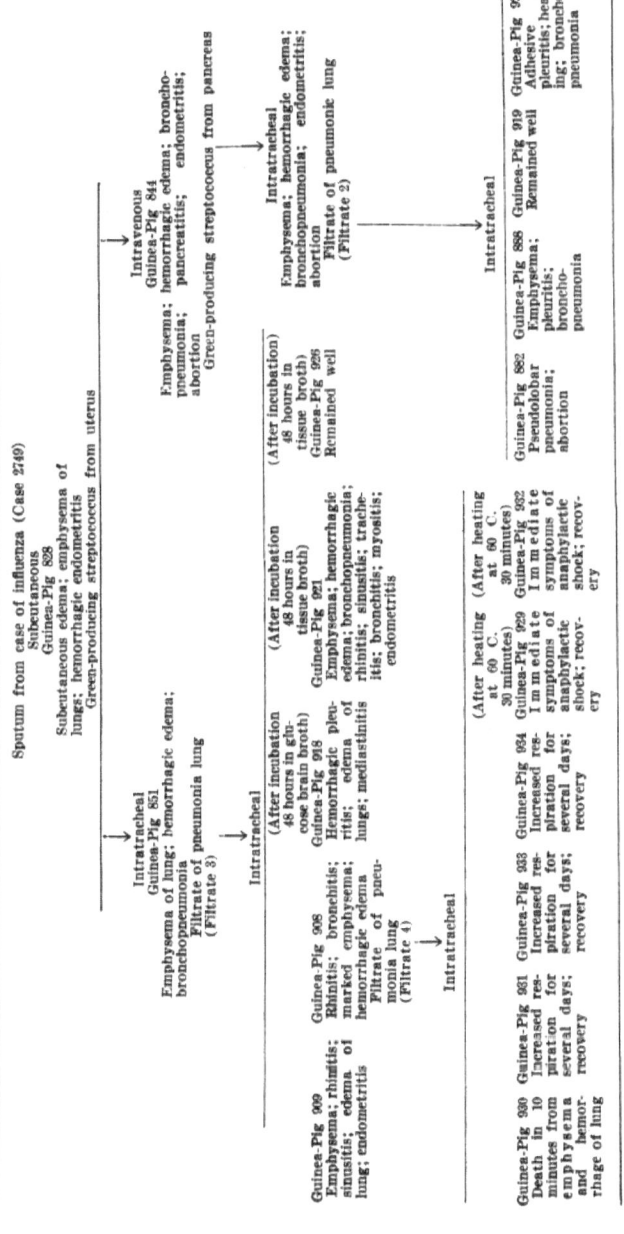

DERIVATION OF THREE FILTRATES AND THE RESULTS FOLLOWING THEIR INJECTION

numbers throughout the exudate and showed little tendency toward peripheral aggregation along the alveolar lining, and the perivascular and subpleural spaces (fig. 18b). There was no distinct difference in the exudate in animals injected with the different type strains. The findings in two experiments will suffice to illustrate:

Guinea-pig 1031, weighing 400 gm., was injected intratracheally, Jan. 22, 1919, with 1.5 c c of glucose-broth cultures of pneumococcus group IV after one (intraperitoneal) animal passage. The temperature before injection was 102.4 F., and the white blood count was 13,200. The following day the animal appeared quite well. The temperature was 99.6 and the white blood count was 18,600. January 24 the animal was found dead. The white blood count was 17,500. Most of the right lung was consolidated, uniformly grayish-red, firm in consistency, and quite dry on the cut surface. A number of smaller areas of consolidation were found in the left lung. The cut surface everywhere was fairly dry and nowhere could edematous fluid be made to drip from it. Emphysema was moderate. The total volume of the lungs was 10 c c. The cultures from the blood and lungs showed large numbers of green-producing pneumococci.

Guinea-pig 1448, weighing 380 gm., was injected intratracheally, Oct. 21, 1918, with 1.5 c c of glucose-blood-broth culture of pneumococcus type II (Strain 3625). October 22 the respirations were extremely rapid and the animal sat quietly. October 23 it was dead. A moderate amount of slightly turbid fluid was found in both pleural cavities. The lungs were moderately distended (14 c c) and weighed 10 gm. The right diaphragmatic lobe was quite uniformly gray and completely consolidated; it was dry and granular on the cut surface. A number of smaller areas of hemorrhage with decided consolidation were found chiefly around the bronchi in the left diaphragmatic and right cardiac lobes. There were marked myocardial degeneration and cloudy swelling of the kidneys, but the uterus and other organs were normal. Cultures from the blood yielded many pneumococcus colonies. Sections of the lung showed moderate distention of alveoli, absence of necrosis of alveolar epithelium and capillaries, and marked, highly cellular leukocytic infiltration of the alveoli in which large numbers of diplococci were distributed throughout the exudate with little tendency of the bacteria to be distributed along the alveolar epithelial lining (figs. 18 and 19 b).

PROTOCOLS OF CASES OF INFLUENZA AND INFLUENZAL PNEUMONIA AND ANIMAL EXPERIMENTS. SIMILARITY OF LOCALIZATION OF MICRO-ORGANISMS

Case 2607, a middle-aged woman developed pneumonia during an influenzal attack and died. The sputum obtained Nov. 21, 1918, was bloody; smears showed large numbers of gram-positive, lanceolate diplococci, gram-positive cocci, and small gram-negative bacilli of irregular size resembling influenza bacilli, and large numbers of gram-positive diplococci, at times in chains within epithelial cells. Blood-agar plates showed large numbers of colonies of green-producing streptococci and influenza bacilli. The sputum (0.3 c c) was injected intraperitoneally November 21, into Guinea-pig 737. November 22 at 8 a. m. the animal appeared to be ill, was irritable and short of breath. At noon it was worse. The respirations were greatly increased and it had repeated choking spells resembling anaphylactic shock. At 8 p. m. it was found dead, and was examined at once. A small amount of turbid fluid without fibrin was found in the peritoneal and pleural cavities. The lungs were distended (13 c c), hyperemic and edematous, and showed numerous small hemorrhages and a number of large subpleural hemorrhages posteriorly in the left diaphragmatic lobe (fig. 5). In cultures from the blood were a few green-producing streptococci; the hemorrhagic area in the lung and peritoneal fluid contained large numbers of green-producing streptococci in pure culture. No influenza bacilli were found in smears from the peritoneal fluid. Sections of the lung showed marked congestion of interalveolar capillaries, marked hemorrhage in the alveoli, and desquamation and necrosis of the alveolar epithelial cells in varying degree. Many alveoli and terminal bronchi were greatly dilated; others appeared to be collapsed. The larger bronchi were constricted and their lumen contained numerous red blood corpuscles and desquamated alveolar epithelium; the mucous membrane lay in great folds. The hemorrhagic areas were usually situated around bronchi and beneath the pleura. In the latter position they were often triangular in shape with the base toward the pleura. At no place was there marked leukocytic infiltration (fig. 10). Prolonged study of sections stained by Gram-Weigert and by the combination of Goodpasture and Weigert stains recommended by MacCallum showed an interesting distribution of the bacteria. None were found within capillaries and larger blood vessels. A few were found in the areas of hemorrhage in the alveoli, but by far the largest number were found, as shown in figure 11, just outside the capillary in the interstitial tissue of the alveolar wall (a), along the alveolar lining beneath the desquamated epithelium (b), in the epithelial cells showing poorly stained nuclei, but still in place lining the alveoli showing hemorrhage (c), and in the degenerated, desquamating alveolar epithelial cells (d).

The streptococcus from the peritoneal fluid in this guinea-pig in the third culture generation was injected intraperitoneally into another guinea-pig. It died in twenty-four hours with turbid hemorrhagic fluid in the peritoneal cavity and numerous hemorrhages in a large part of the secum, especially surrounding the lymph follicles, and hemorrhages in Peyer's patches, but with no lesions of the lung. Intraperitoneal injections of the sputum in 3 other normal guinea-pigs was followed by the death of all in from three to ten days. The animal that died in 3 days was found to have emphysema, hemorrhages and edema of the lungs. The others showed no lesions of the lung. Two guinea-pigs injected two weeks previously with the sputum from other cases of influenza recovered.

The points of particular interest in these experiments are the marked affinity of the streptococcus in the sputum for the epithelium of the alveoli of the lung (fig. 11), the noninvasive power of the influenza bacilli found in the sputum, the hemorrhages in the intestine in the second animal passage, and the acquired immunity in the two guinea-pigs previously injected with sputum from other cases of influenza.

Case 2769, Miss M. J., aged 38, came for examination on account of chronic loseness of bowels and loss of weight and strength. Her condition was found to be due to pancreatic insufficiency. The patient contracted influenza Dec. 16, 1918; developed symptoms and signs of bronchopneumonia December 22, and died December 28. The looseness of bowels was worse throughout the influenzal attack. At necropsy were found "a resolving 'lobar' pneumonia, seropurulent pleuritis (1,500 c c), of the right side, chronic parenchymatous and interstitial pancreatitis, and fatty degeneration of kidneys."

Cultures from the lung after death and pus from the right pleura showed many hemolytic streptococci and a few staphylococci. The primary culture in glucose broth from the lung was injected intratracheally into one guinea-pig and intraperitoneally into another. The guinea-pig (Guinea-pig 875) injected intratracheally died nineteen days after injection from hemorrhagic and purulent pleuritis, pericarditis and myocardial degeneration (fig. 7). The animal injected intraperitoneally died after twenty-four hours. It had diffuse peritonitis, extreme hyperemia of the large and small intestines, swollen lymph follicles throughout the intestinal tract, and numerous hemorrhages in the lower two thirds of the small intestine and in the cecum. The contents of the small intestine consisted chiefly of bloody mucus. The duodenum, stomach, and suprarenals were normal. The lungs were emphysematous (11 c c), and showed moderate edema and a number of small hemorrhages. The pleural cavity contained a small amount of hemorrhagic fluid. Cultures from the blood, peritoneal fluid, and intestinal contents showed hemolytic streptococci and staphylococci. The pleural exudate (1 c c) was injected directly into the trachea of a guinea-pig. It aborted four days later and died with marked leukopenia, increased respirations, voluminous lungs (17 c c), marked hemorrhagic pleuritis, hemorrhagic bronchopneumonia and lesions in the psoas muscles. Large numbers of green-producing streptococci were isolated from the lung, pleural fluid, and uterus but none from the spleen, liver, suprarenals and cervix. The culture from the peritoneal exudate was injected intravenously into a rabbit and one guinea-pig, and intratracheally into one guinea-pig. The rabbit died the day following injection with extreme distention of the abdomen due to a large amount of gas (rich in carbon dioxid) in the small intestines. The small and large intestines contained a large amount of mucus. The intestinal contents were liquid or semisolid throughout. The intestinal wall was opaque, but there were no hemorrhages. Six sharply circumscribed hemorrhages were found in the mucous membrane of the cardiac end of the stomach; in the medulla of the kidneys were a few embolic hemorrhagic areas. The myocardium was markedly degenerated. Cultures from the blood showed a large number of hemolytic streptococci and staphylococci. The guinea-pig injected intravenously died five days later. It showed two small areas of bronchopneumonia, swollen Peyer's patches and solitary lymph follicles, a large amount of mucus in the intestines, absence of food in the stomach, but a large amount of turbid mucus showing many gram-positive diplococci, edematous and hemorrhagic mesenteric lymph glands, marked hyperemia of the uterus, turbid mucus in both uterine horns, numerous small hemorrhages in the mucous membrane of the uterus and cecum, and focal lesions in the medulla of the kidney. Cultures from the blood showed one colony; cultures from the pneumonic areas, countless numbers, and from the mucus from the left horn of the uterus, a moderate number of staphylococcus colonies.

The guinea-pig injected intratracheally died six days later. It had voluminous lungs (15 c c), bronchopneumonia and edema of the right and left caudal lobes, hemorrhagic tracheobronchial lymph glands, purulent material in the nostrils, purulent bronchitis and tracheitis, a hemorrhagic fetus in the vagina and one still attached to the uterus; focal lesions in the medulla of the kidneys; and edematous mucous membranes of the pelvis of the kidneys. Cultures from the pneumonic lung and blood showed green-producing streptococci and staphylococci.

The striking features in the animal experiments in this case was the tendency to produce, in addition to the characteristic lung lesions and pleuritis in the first animal passage, lesions of the intestinal tract and medulla of the kidney in the second animal passage.

Case 2770, Mr. S. M., aged 33, was admitted to the isolation hospital Dec. 24, 1918, complaining of severe weakness, backache, aching all over, extreme nervousness and severe cough. These symptoms had begun two days previously. The leukocyte count the day of admission was 3,800. The temperature was 103 F., pulse 118, respirations 28. The patient grew progressively worse, the temperature ranging between 103 and 105. December 26 evidence of involvement of the lungs became apparent. Cyanosis and dyspnea increased as evidence of a rapid filling of the lungs appeared and the patient died December 28, forty-eight hours after the first signs of pneumonia had developed. Necropsy showed voluminous lungs, pseudolobar pneumonia associated with marked hemorrhagic edema involving all lobes, a large accumulation of bloody, turbid fluid in the left thorax (900 c c) and intense hemorrhagic bronchitis. In cultures made from the sputum December 26 were enormous numbers of green-producing streptococci and a few staphylococci; in the lung exudate and blood after death were many green-producing streptococci and staphylococci.

The primary culture in glucose broth from the blood of this patient was injected into the trachea of 3 guinea-pigs in doses of 0.1 c c, 1 c c and 2.5 c c, respectively. The one receiving only 0.1 c c had moderately increased respirations for several hours, then appeared quite well for four days, when the respirations again became rapid and the animal died six days after injection with a moderate amount of hemorrhagic turbid fluid in the pleural cavity, moderate distention of the lung (12 c c) with almost complete consolidation of the left anterior and cardiac lobes. The cut surface of the consolidated areas was mottled grayish-red and edematous between the areas of denser consolidations and necrosis. Cultures from the blood showed green-producing streptococci in pure culture; those from the lung and pleural fluid, green-producing streptococci and staphylococci. The leukocyte count was 17,000 before injection, 8,960 four hours after injection, and 5,200 the following day. The animal injected with 1 c c died in five days after having aborted. It showed acute diffuse peritonitis clearly secondary to infection in the uterus which passed through the left tube, voluminous lung (15 c c), hemorrhagic bronchopneumonia, pleuritis, and marked maxillary sinusitis, tracheitis, and bronchitis. The animal injected with 2.5 c c died in four and one-half hours. It had extreme difficulty in breathing and frequent paroxysms resembling anaphylactic shock; it was found with its head in a pool of hemorrhagic edema fluid. The lungs were voluminous (20 c c), hemorrhagic, and edematous throughout. The trachea, bronchi, and nostrils were filled with hemorrhagic frothy fluid.

The glucose-brain-broth culture of green-producing streptococcus derived from a single colony on the blood-agar plate from the blood in this case was injected into 3 guinea-pigs; all received 1 c c intratracheally. One of these had had an intraperitoneal injection of a primary culture from the sputum in another case of influenza 10 days previously. It showed no symptoms the day after injection and remained well subsequently. One of the others died the day after injection with leukopenia, voluminous lung (12 c c), marked hemorrhagic edema and bronchopneumonia, edematous peribronchial lymph glands, and a moderate amount of fluid in the pleural cavity. The third died in 3 days of hemorrhagic bronchopneumonia, tracheitis, and sinusitis. Both of these showed green-producing streptococci in the blood and green-producing streptococci and a few staphylococci in the lung and pleural fluid. The glucose-brain-broth culture injected into these 3 guinea-pigs was subcultured rapidly in duplicate from tube to tube of glucose-brain broth, and cultures made from one to three times a day. In the eleventh subcultures 2 guinea-pigs were injected intratracheally with 1 c c and 1.5 c c, respectively, of the two cultures.

Both were found dead the following day. The blood-agar plates of the culture injected showed a pure culture of staphylococci and smears showed the absence of streptococci. The lungs in both were hemorrhagic and edematous but were compressed (5 c c) by a huge accumulation of chocolate-colored fluid in the pleural cavities (20 c c in each). Both had hemorrhagic placental masses in the uterus; several were detached and being expelled (fig. 9). Sections of both showed large numbers of staphylococci throughout the lungs, especially beneath the pleura, and no streptococci. Cultures from the blood of both showed staphylococci; from the lung, pleural fluid, and hemorrhagic placental masses, large numbers of staphylococci and a few colonies of green-producing streptococci; and from the liver, kidney, and ovaries a small number of staphylococci. The symptoms in the guinea-pig (Guinea-pig 940) injected with 1.5 c c were noted for nine hours prior to death. Respiratory embarrassment at first consisted chiefly of difficulty in expiration; later breathing became easier but exceedingly rapid as from a filling thorax. The animal was examined immediately after death in order to note the condition of the uterus. Violent waves of uterine contraction continued for some minutes. One of the placental masses was partially detached; all were hemorrhagic. The hemorrhagic pleural fluid was immediately injected into the trachea of another guinea-pig, which showed moderately increased respirations immediately after injection, seemed well the following day and remained so for twenty-six days, when it was chloroformed. The pericardial sac was thickened and distended with bloody fluid. The peribronchial and mediastinal lymph glands were edematous and much enlarged. The pleura and lungs were normal. Cultures from the pericardial fluid and lymph glands showed staphylococci.

The points of special interest in the experiments in this case are the high virulency of the strain isolated from the blood, the tendency to produce the same type of lesions over a wide range of dosage, the immunity induced by a previous injection of a culture from influenzal sputum, the extreme contractions of the uterus, and the marked infectiousness of the culture, showing what seems must be considered as a mutation of green-producing streptococcus into staphylococcus.

Case 2787, a man, aged 59, had influenzal pneumonia and pleuritis from which he made a slow recovery. There was little expectoration. A diagnostic puncture of the chest was made Jan. 8, 1919. A small amount of turbid, bloody fluid was aspirated which showed countless numbers of colonies of hemolytic streptococci in pure culture. A suspension in salt solution of one-thirtieth and one-third of the primary growth on a blood-agar plate was injected into the trachea of 2 guinea-pigs, respectively. The former had increased respirations for several days and then recovered; the latter had increased respirations for several days and died two weeks later of abscess and gangrene of the right diaphragmatic lobe, pericarditis, and pleuritis. The pericardium was markedly thickened and distended with gelatinous organizing, fibrinous exudate. The pleural cavity contained a large amount of foul smelling pus communicating with the abscess (fig. 8). Cultures from the blood showed no growth; the pericardial fluid showed staphylococci, the pleural fluid, staphylococci and gram-negative bacilli.

Case 2798, Mr. E. C. B., aged 26, was admitted to the isolation hospital Jan. 7, 1919. He had been taken ill seven days before with cough, general malaise, sore throat, and chills, but he did not ache severely. The temperature on admission was 103 F., but it dropped to normal the following day. The leukocyte count January 8 was 11,400; January 10, 12,500, and January 11, 14,300. The patient had a moderately severe cough in which he raised mucopurulent sputum. No definite chest signs could be detected on physical examination, but the roentgen-ray examination on the day of admission showed slight bronchial infiltration in the left lung, and January 14 a small area of infiltration in the right middle lobe. The patient was discharged from the hospital January 14, after the temperature had been normal for 5 days, although the cough persisted. January 16, he was again admitted to the hospital complaining of a sharp, severe pain in the right lower chest aggravated by breathing, of malaise, and of feeling weak generally. At this time he had fever for five days; he developed outspoken signs of pleuritis over the right side of the chest, and pleural thickening over this area was manifested by roentgen examination January 26. The sputum obtained January 11 showed countless numbers of colonies of hemolytic streptococci, a few green colonies of streptococci, small indifferent colonies of influenza bacilli, and a number of staphylococci.

The culture in glucose brain broth from a single colony of hemolytic streptococcus (which yielded a pure culture of green-producing streptococci on blood-agar plates) was injected into the trachea of Guinea-pig 957, January 13. The leukocyte count was 16,000 and the temperature 102.4 F. The following day the animal seemed ill, respirations were rapid, the temperature was 97 and the leukocyte count was 19,000. On the second day the symptoms were about the same, the temperature was 103.6, and the leukocyte count was 16,500. January 16 the temperature was 102.8, the leukocyte count was 16,500. January 16 the temperature was 102.8, the leukocyte count was 17,000, the respirations were definitely increased, and the animal appeared sick. January 19 it was found dead. The pleural cavity was distended with a large amount of bloody, chocolate-colored fluid, partially walled off in pockets with fibrinous adhesions, and partially obliterated by fibrinous adhesions, and the visceral and parietal pleura and the pericardium were covered with a thick layer of fibrinous material (fig. 7). The lungs were moderately distended (14 c c), moist and edematous on the cut surface, but consolidation was limited to several small areas. Cultures from the blood, pleural fluid, and lung showed a large number of green-producing streptococci and some staphylococci; from the spleen and kidney, a number of green-producing streptococci, and from the liver and suprarenal, no growth.

The attack in this case of influenza was atypical; there was no reduction in leukocytes, and the attack occurred during a quiescent interval between two epidemic waves. The point of special interest is the fact that the findings in the animal injected with a culture from the sputum paralleled the findings in the patient quite accurately in that leukopenia did not occur; the lung lesions were slight, and the involvement of the pleura was the marked lesion.

Case 2809, M. D., a little girl, aged 3, was admitted to the isolation hospital Jan. 8, 1919, in a weak condition with a temperature of 103.4 F., pulse 152, respirations 32, moderate cyanosis, and a severe cough. She had been taken sick that day, and was running a typical course of influenza without apparent lung involvement. The temperature ranged between 101 and 102 degrees for four days, becoming normal on the fifth day. The throat was moderately red; the tonsils were normal, the tongue coated. The day after admission it was noted that the vulva was inflamed and that pus was discharging from the vagina. The condition yielded promptly to irrigations and douching with a weak solution of potassium permanganate. January 12 smears of the vaginal discharge showed a moderate number of leukocytes, many gram-positive, lanceolate diplococci, often in short chains, gram-negative bacilli, some resembling Bacillus coli and many smaller gram-negative bacilli resembling Bacillus influenzae. Blood-agar plates showed a large number of green-producing streptococci, a moderate number of colonies of colon bacilli, and many small colonies resembling Bacillus influenzae. The colonies of the latter were most numerous and the growth more luxuriant immediately surrounding the colonies of the streptococci. Smears of these small indifferent colonies showed gram-positive and gram-negative small bacilli or short-chained diplococci. A subculture on a blood-agar plate of a single colony of the green-producing streptococcus, including some of the small indifferent colonies, yielded pure growth of green colonies of streptococci; of four single colonies resembling Bacillus influenzae no growth was obtained, whereas subcultures from a group of these colonies yielded countless numbers of influenza bacillus-like colonies and a moderate number of green streptococcus colonies. Subcultures in two bottles of glucose-blood broth from the groups of isolated Bacillus influenzae colonies, well separated from green colonies of streptococci, yielded countless numbers of streptococci, blood-agar plates from these showing countless colonies of green-producing streptococci.

The primary culture in glucose brain broth from the vaginal swab was injected into the trachea of 2 guinea-pigs. Both pigs died within twenty-four hours of markedly dilated lungs filled with acute hemorrhagic edema fluid; both developed marked leukopenia, abortion with hemorrhage in the uterus, and both showed gram-positive diplococci in sections of the hemorrhagic edematous areas in the lung (fig. 17). A pure culture of the green-producing streptococcus in glucose brain broth in the second generation was injected into the trachea of 2 guinea-pigs. The female died within forty-eight hours with marked reduction in leukocytes, massive hemorrhagic bronchopneumonia, edematous mucous membrane of the uterus, cervix and vagina, hemorrhages in the cervix and upper portion of the vagina, and a large amount of turbid mucus in the vagina. Smears from mucus in the vault of the vagina showed a moderate number of gram-positive diplococci and a few large gram-negative bacilli. The male recovered and showed moderate reduction in leukocytes; he had fever for several days, but no other noteworthy symptoms.

The streptococcus isolated in this case, in addition to causing characteristic lesions of the lungs, showed marked affinity for the uterus and vagina; it was agglutinated specifically by the monovalent antistreptococcus serum.

Case 3171, Mr. P. H. L., aged 30, was taken with headache, severe aching all over and chilliness Feb. 26, 1919. He felt so sick that he was obliged to go to bed. After resting for a number of days he felt better, but March 2, after a hearty meal, he developed high fever, cough, and a headache with sweating. The following day cyanosis, rapid respirations, crepitant râles and bronchial breathing over the left lower lobe were noted. The next day numerous moist râles were heard over the right lower lobe, and the respirations were labored. The sputum became serous, bloody, and frothy March 5, and the patient died March 6. At necropsy marked bilateral hemorrhagic pneumonia of the greater portion of both lungs and marked hemorrhagic tracheo-broncho-bronchiolitis were found. Histologic examination of the lungs showed marked congestion of the alveoli which were filled with edematous exudate containing few cells.

Cultures from the mucopurulent material in the larynx, trachea, and bronchi showed numerous spreading, slightly hemolyzing streptococci, a moderate number of staphylococci, and hemolytic streptococci. Cultures from the pleural fluid showed a large number of green-producing streptococci and from the glucose broth inoculated with the blood, green-producing streptococci. The primary culture in glucose broth was injected into the trachea of male G. pig

1249. The respirations the following day were extremely rapid and labored. the animal appeared ill, and was found dead the next day. The lungs were huge, 26 c c, and extremely heavy, 21 gm. A large amount of bloody, edematous fluid ran from the cut surface. The whole left lung appeared uniformly consolidated, and most of the right lung showed irregular areas of consolidation, emphysema, and hemorrhagic edema (fig. 3). There were no other lesions. Cultures from the blood, lung, and spleen showed many large, moist, spreading, green colonies of streptococci.

The primary culture in glucose broth from bronchial exudate was injected intraperitoneally into a mouse and into the trachea of a female guinea-pig. The mouse died of peritonitis within twenty-four hours. The guinea-pig died of hemorrhagic bronchopneumonia, hemorrhagic pleuritis, and a hemorrhagic infection of three fetuses with abortion, in forty-eight hours. The cultures showed large numbers of colonies of typical hemolytic streptococci and a moderate number of staphylococci. The primary culture of the pleural fluid was injected into a male guinea-pig. It appeared ill the following day and sat humped up; its hair was rough, and the voice was hoarse. It gradually improved during the following four days and remained well.

The results in this case, in addition to the production of the characteristic lung and uterine lesions, are of interest because of the bacteriologic findings in the blood, pleural fluid and the lung exudate, and in showing changes in the character of these organisms as they were passed through animals, the green-producing streptococcus from the blood acquiring the property of producing large, spreading, moist, green colonies, and the spreading, slightly hemolyzing streptococcus from the bronchial exudate becoming a typical hemolytic streptococcus.

Case 3175, Mrs. C. S., aged 24, was operated on March 1, 1919, on account of recurring attacks of appendicitis which were considered sufficiently serious to warrant operation for the removal of the appendix even though she was four months pregnant. The patient did well for five days and then developed fever, cough, dyspnea, mucopurulent and bloody sputum, rapidly progressing pneumonia, and pleuritis of the right side. She aborted on the seventh day after the operation and died from acute pulmonary edema on the eighth. Necropsy was refused. The sputum obtained March 7 was purulent and chocolate colored. The blood-agar plate showed countless numbers of staphylococci.

The human fetus (male) was brought to the laboratory while fresh; the membranes had not ruptured. The trunk measured 10 cm. in length. There was marked edema in the anterior cervical region surrounding the trachea and in the left abdominal rectus muscle. The left pleural cavity was free from fluid; the right contained a large amount of turbid hemorrhagic fluid fully 5 c c. The pericardial sac contained a small amount of turbid fluid free from blood. Blood-agar plate cultures from the brain, intestinal contents, pericardial fluid, and edema fluid from the subcutaneous tissue remained sterile. Glucose brain-broth cultures of hemorrhagic fluid from the right pleural cavity, pericardial fluid, and subcutaneous edema fluid showed short-chained streptococci and staphylococci. Sections of brain, kidneys, suprarenals, liver, and spleen showed no noteworthy lesions and no bacteria. Sections of the right lung showed a moderate number of diplococci in the pleura and subpleura of the right side (fig. 22).

The sputum containing streptococci in addition to staphylococci was injected into the trachea of 3 female guinea-pigs. All died within twenty-four hours from hemorrhagic edema of the lung, and hemorrhagic pleuritis, and all aborted.

Two showed interstitial pulmonary emphysema, one in the form of pleural blebs only, the other in frothy fluid in the pleural cavity due to rupture of one of these blebs. Cultures from all yielded staphylococci and streptococci. In order to determine the infecting power of the staphylococcus, the culture in glucose blood broth from a single colony was injected into the trachea of another female guinea-pig. It died within twenty-four hours from hemorrhagic edema, hemorrhagic pleuritis, and abortion, and showed staphylococci in the blood and pleural fluid in pure culture. Sections of the lung of one of these pigs showed the characteristic hemorrhagic edema with slight cellular infiltration and large numbers of streptococci and staphylococci in the lung (fig. 21).

A large white and gray cat (cat 24), with advanced pregnancy, a leukocyte count of 11,600 and a temperature of 101.4 F., was injected in the trachea March 17, 1919, with 4 c c of glucose-blood-broth culture of streptococcus in the second culture from one of the guinea-pigs. March 18 the temperature was 101.4, the white count 6,600, and the animal appeared well. March 19 and 20 it appeared quite well but refused food, and the temperature was 102.2. March 21, 12 m., it was found in labor; one kitten was born. By 6 p. m. 4 kittens had been born; all were alive and appeared nearly full-time size. March 22 the cat and kittens appeared well, but the cat refused food; the kittens nursed. March 23, one kitten was found dead; the cat refused food and appeared sick. March 24, another kitten was found dead, and a third was sick. The cat was worse, refused food, the respirations had increased, and a vaginal discharge of bloody pus had developed. March 25 the third kitten was dead and the fourth was in a dying condition. The cat, which was so weak that she was just able to stand, and had a marked diarrhea and a temperature of 104, was chloroformed. The uterus showed large numbers of small submucous hemorrhages; the mucous membrane was swollen in places, necrotic, and covered with a thick layer of chocolate-colored pus. The liver showed marked fatty degeneration, the kidneys, acute nephritis. Smears from the uterine exudate contained many staphylococci and streptococci. In cultures from the uterus were countless numbers of colonies of staphylococci and green-producing streptococci and number of spreading gram-negative bacilli; from the blood, liver and spleen, a few colonies of staphylococci and streptococci; from the suprarenal and kidney, no growth. Sections of the uterus showed a thick layer of leukocytes covering the endometrium, containing enormous numbers of staphylococci and streptococci. Fetus 1 showed no lesions. Cultures from the blood showed large numbers of stphylococci and a few green streptococci. Fetus 2 was accidentally discarded by the animal keeper. Fetus 3 showed 5,800 leukocytes in the blood and a small amount of blood-tinged pleural fluid, staphylococci, and a few green streptococci in the blood and pleural fluid, together with a spreading gram-negative bacillus. Sections of the lung showed gram-positive diplococci in the subpleural space duplicating the findings in the human fetus (fig. 22). Fetus 4 showed no gross lesions, but the same organisms in blood and urine as in fetus 3.

The points of particular interest in this case are the invasion of the fetus with lesions of the pleura caused by the organisms found in the sputum, the production of marked lesions in the lung and pleura, including interstitial emphysema of the lung in guinea-pigs, the marked affinity for the placenta, the invasion with the production of pleural lesions of the fetuses in the cat, and the sensitiveness of the streptococcus to oxygen.

The findings in the patients and the results obtained in each case reported herewith in detail are quite accurately representative of the findings of the whole series studied. I have purposely included one case (case 2787) in which leukopenia was absent and in which the diagnosis of influenza was doubtful because the results in the animal injected paralleled so accurately the findings in the patient. The points noted which deserve special emphasis are the marked affinity of the streptococci for the epithelium of the lung, even after intraperitoneal injection (fig. 11), the occurrence of characteristic lesions of the lung and pleura, the frequent involvement of the uterus resulting in abortion, and the very great similarity of the results obtained in the animals and the findings in cases 2769, 2770, 2787, 2798, 2809 and 3175. The findings in the little girl who developed vaginitis during her influenzal attack leave little doubt that the vaginal discharge was the result of localization and infection by the streptococcus in the uterus and vagina. The localization of the streptococcus in the pleura of the fetus (fig. 22) of the pregnant patient (case 3175), and in the pleura of the fetuses in the pregnant cat injected into the trachea with the sputum of this case, when absent in other tissues, may be regarded as elective localization of bacteria of high order. On the basis of these findings a study of the tissues of fetuses and of the new-born said to have contracted influenza in utero should be undertaken, since the micro-organism found in the affected tissues under these conditions may be considered responsible for the production of the lesions, and thus add materially to our knowledge of the etiology of influenza.

EXPERIMENTS WITH FILTRATES OF LUNG EMULSIONS AND CULTURES

After it was noted that intratracheal application of the bacteria from patients with influenza had marked effect it was thought that this method of injection might prove valuable in studying the effects of filtrates of material from influenza. Exceedingly small forms of diplococci were frequently seen in smears of sputum, in throat swabs, and in cultures from influenza, especially in deep tubes of glucose brain broth. It was thought possible that the preformed toxic products in filtrates of cultures and lung emulsions might injure the respiratory epithelium and thus facilitate growth of the few organisms which might pass through the filter, and, since the lung appeared to be the point of predilection of these organisms, growth might occur when cultures were introduced in this manner even though control cultures on artificial mediums were negative. Moreover, valuable light might be thrown on the question of the presence or absence of a filtrable virus in this disease. I wish here to summarize the experiments done along this line. The filtrates studied were from sputum obtained, early in the course of the disease, from the lungs of dead animals, with the characteristic picture following injection of sputum or cultures from sputum, and from cultures from the sputum during life and from the blood and lung exudate after death of patients who had died from influenza.

Berkefeld N filters, Mandler filters, and dense unglazed porcelain filters were used. The filtrates from the lungs were obtained by making an approximately 10% emulsion of the pneumonic or hemorrhagic lung tissue in salt solution, centrifuging it fractionally, and filtering the opalescent fluid by the aid of a partial vacuum obtained with a water suction pump. The cultures of influenzal material in the tall tubes of broth were incubated twenty-four to seventy-two hours and filtered without centrifugation. The efficiency of the filters used was controlled with Bacillus prodigiosus, and they were found to remove these small organisms in every instance. Cultures from the filtrates were made on blood agar, and in deep tubes of glucose brain broth and in tissue broth. The brain, which weighed approximately 1.5 gm., was added to each tall tube of glucose broth before autoclaving; the tissue (rabbit kidney) was added in a sterile manner to meat infusion broth sterilized by the fractional method. The inoculations in these mediums were made with at least 0.5 c c of the filtrate. The tubes were incubated at 33 to 35 C. for a week before they were discarded. Altogether, 15 filtrates have been made and studied. The cultures on blood agar were negative in all. Those in broth remained free from growth in 13, while 2 (filtrates 6 and 7) yielded definite growths. In the former, filtration was slow; in the latter, rapid. In 4 of the broth cultures clouding was distinct, but smears and subcultures were negative.

The animal experiments consisted of intratracheal injection of the usual dose of the filtrate itself, of the "negative" cultures in the broth, and in some instances of the respective culture and lung emulsion as controls. Altogether, 42 guinea-pigs were injected intratracheally, 30 with the filtrate directly, and 12 with the "negative" cultures from filtrates. Of these, 13 died; 10 were anesthetized for examination, and 19 recovered. The immediate symptoms following injection of the filtrates were indistinguishable from those following injection of the cultures. Death from fatal infections occurred somewhat later following injection of the filtrates than following injection of the corresponding cultures or emulsions. The lesions were similar. Emphysema, hemorrhage and edema of the lung, with coalescing areas of lobular pneumonia and hemorrhagic pleuritis, were striking features. Microscopically dilated alveoli filled with blood and edema fluid with marked desquamation and destruction of the epithelium of the alveoli and bronchi with relatively slight leukocytic infiltration formed the dominant picture. Of the cultures from the 13 guinea-pigs that died, 8 showed green-producing streptococci as the predominating organism, 2 showed Bacillus bronchisepticus in addition, 1 Bacillus coli, and in 1 the cultures remained negative; cultures were not made from 1 guinea-pig. In the 2 that showed Bacillus bronchisepticus an old pneumonia, easily distinguished from the hemorrhagic lesions due to the injection, was present. Sections of the lungs showed gram-positive diplococci which were most numerous along the alveolar wall. The 10 anesthetized animals had the usual immediate symptoms, increased respirations for from two to three days. Two were anesthetized while the symptoms were severe and progressing. The findings in these were similar to those in the animals that died (guinea-pig 882, guinea-pig 885). The lungs of the rest were only slightly emphysematous; hemorrhagic edema with little infiltration in relatively small areas in the lung was noted in most of the animals. The cultures in these showed green-producing streptococci in 3, no growth in 6, and in 1 the cultures were contaminated accidentally. Symptoms in those that recovered were either absent the day after injection or consisted of increased respirations, lessened activity, and ruffled fur for several days.

Six animals were injected with heated filtrates; all showed the usual immediate symptoms of anaphylactic shock, somewhat less severe but otherwise comparable with the symptoms in animals injected with the corresponding unheated filtrate. They had no symptoms subsequently and all remained well.

Leukocyte counts were made in 26 animals injected with filtrates. In 17 a marked or decided drop in leukocytes occurred, in 2 a slight drop, while in 7 no noteworthy change occurred. None showed leukocytosis. The leukopenia was usually present twenty-four and forty-eight hours after injection, after which return to normal occurred in the animals that recovered; in those that died it usually persisted, and sometimes the count became progressively lower until death (guinea-pig 888). The drop was not usually as marked as that following injection of cultures.

Leukopenia occurred following injection of filtrates from sputum, from lung emulsions, and from broth cultures of freshly isolated strains. Heating to 60 C. for thirty minutes and to the boiling point for ten minutes was found not to destroy the substance causing a diminution in leukocytes, nor did heating destroy the property causing immediate symptoms of anaphylactic shock.

Two filtrates that produced marked effects in animals on intra-tracheal injection were injected subcutaneously into 3 persons in doses of 4 c c for one, and 5 c c for each of the other two. All developed only slight local reaction and none fever or constitutional reaction. One person's throat was swabbed with a mixture of 2 filtrates, one prepared from the lung, and the other from a culture from the blood of case 2800. No symptoms followed. These filtrates (5 c c) were also injected subcutaneously in each of two persons. No symptoms occurred other than a negligible local reaction.

The results following injection of 3 filtrates (filtrates 2, 3 and 4) in a series of animals, and the derivation of the strain from which they were prepared, are summarized in the tabulation. Two guinea-pigs (guinea-pigs 908 and 909) injected with the fresh filtrate and the 2 (guinea-pigs 918 and 921) injected with the "negative" culture in glucose brain broth developed the characteristic symptoms and findings; 1 (guinea-pig 926) injected with the fresh filtrate remained well. The filtrate from the pneumonic lung of one of these (guinea-pig 908) was injected intratracheally while fresh into 4 guinea-pigs (guinea-pigs 930, 931, 933 and 934), and after being heated to 60 C. for thirty minutes was injected in 2 guinea-pigs (guinea-pigs 929 and 932). All showed decided immediate symptoms and 1 died in ten minutes of anaphylactic shock. Three of the rest had increased respirations for several days and then recovered, while the other 2 showed no symptoms. The filtrate from the pneumonic lung of guinea-pig 874 was injected into the trachea of 4 guinea-pigs (guinea-pigs 882, 888, 919 and 923). Three developed symptoms and died. The usual findings were noted.

Green-producing streptococci in pure culture, or together with staphylococci, were isolated from the characteristic lesions in all that died. Injection of the corresponding cultures into other guinea-pigs was followed by very similar lesions (to be reported elsewhere). The parallelism was so striking that the mortality in the third animal passage (filtrate 3) was higher than in the fourth animal passage (filtrates 2 and 4). Sections of the lungs showed all the characteristic features peculiar to the influenza strains, including the localization of the streptococci. From the filtrate experiments it may be concluded that the green-producing streptococci from influenza in cultures and lung exudate may pass through filters through which Bacillus prodigiosus will not pass, and that they can multiply and grow when injected into the trachea of guinea-pigs, even though cultures remain negative.

Four protocols are given as illustrations:

Guinea-pig 921, weighing 260 gm., was injected intratracheally Jan. 6, 1919, with 1.5 c c of negative culture of the Berkefeld filtrate of the lung emulsion of Guinea-pig 851 (filtrate 3, see tabulation). January 7 the blood-agar plate from the nose made before injection showed a moderate number of colonies of Bacillus coli and staphylococci. January 8 the animal seemed ill and respirations were increased. January 9 and 10 there was marked increase in respirations and the animal seemed sick. January 11 it was found dead. The lungs were found moderately distended; their total volume was 9 c c. The diaphragmatic lobes were firm and heavy. The left lobe contained a whitish area of consolidation 1 by 0.5 cm.) along the margin surrounded by large areas of hemorrhage and edema. The cut surface of the lung was moist and a large amount of bloody fluid escaped. The peribronchial lymph glands were edematous. The uterus was small but showed a circumscribed area containing numerous punctate hemorrhages. On the flat muscles on the inner aspect of both thighs were numerous small whitish necrotic areas. The kidneys showed marked cloudy swelling. The left nostril and the corresponding sinus were filled with mucopus. The mucous membrane of the nose, trachea, and bronchi was edematous and congested. January 13 blood-agar plate cultures from the blood, the areas of consolidation, and edema fluid of the lung, the kidney, and mucus from the right and left horns of the uterus, contained large numbers of streptococci; emulsons of the muscles with lesions, contained 70 green colonies of streptococci; and the emulsions of the normal muscle, contained no streptococci.

Guinea-pig 908, weighing 350 gm., was injected intratracheally Jan. 4, 1919, with 1 c c of Berkefeld filtrate from Guinea-pig 851 (filtrate 3). The nostrils were dry at the time the cultures from the nose were made. January 5, at 11 a. m., the animal appeared to be quite well with slight increase in respiration. At 1 p. m. it suffered from a brief attack of shortness of breath and paroxysms of coughing; the voice was clear. At 5:30 p. m. the animal was hoarse and respirations were definitely increased. A violent attack of shortness of breath followed the making of a second culture from the nose. The blood-agar plate of secretion from the nose made before injection showed a large number of staphylococci and a few green-producing streptococci. January 6 a large number of staphylococci and green-producing streptococci were found in the cultures from the nose made the day after injection. At 9:45 a. m. the animal was short of breath. It had an attack resembling anaphylactic shock; the eyes were watery, the nostrils dry. At 3 p. m. the respirations were rapid and an expiratory grunt had developed. At 8:30 p. m. the animal was very weak; respirations were extremely rapid and difficult, and it often made violent efforts to get its breath. It died in one of these paroxysms. The lungs were found to be extremely distended; their volume was 17 c c and the weight was 14 gm. A large part of both lungs was consolidated. The cut surfaces everywhere were extremely moist; a large amount of bloody, frothy fluid escaped and the trachea and bronchi were filled with a similar fluid. An uninvolved portion of the lung was extremely emphysematous and the alveoli appeared to be at the rupturing point. There were no areas of old lung lesions. The mucous membrane of the nose, the trachea, and the bronchi was hyperemic. The peribronchial lymph glands were edematous. The mucous membrane of the uterus was hyperemic. January 7, blood-agar plate cultures from the blood, kidney, liver, brain, and mucous membrane from the right and left horns of the uterus were sterile; in cultures from the pneumonic lung countless numbers of green colonies of streptococci were found; and from the nose and the mucous membrane of the turbinate bones, countless green colonies of streptococci and a large numbers of staphylococci. Smears from the lung showed large numbers of gram-positive diplococci and those from the nose, gram positive diplococci and staphylococci. No organisms resembling the influenza bacillus were found.

Guinea-pig 888, weighing 490 gm., was injected intratracheally Jan. 3, 1919, with 1.5 c c of the porcelain filtrate of the lung of Guinea-pig 874 (filtrate 2, see tabulation). Before injection the leukocyte count was 10,500. The nostrils were dry when cultures were made. The animal coughed violently several times while being injected and had shortness of breath for 15 minutes following the injection. The temperature rose to 103.4 degrees. January 6, the condition of the animal was about the same although the shortness of breath had increased somewhat. The cultures from the nose showed large numbers of green-producing streptococci and moderate numbers of staphylococci. January 9 the animal was found very weak and short of breath. It acted strangely, constantly pushing its head into the side of the basket or under its mate until it was completely exhausted. At 9 a. m. its temperature was 94; the white count 4,300. At 11 a. m. it died during a violent effort at respiration. The lungs were found distended (14 c c); there was an extensive bronchopneumonia, a mild pleuritis, four hemorrhagic areas, markedly recent placental attachments, one in the right and three in the left horn of the uterus. There was a large amount of turbid mucus in the uterus. January 11 blood-agar plate cultures of the blood were negative; those of the lung showed countless numbers of colonies of streptococci and a few staphylococci.

Guinea-pig 882, weighing 300 gm., was injected intratracheally Jan. 2, 1919, at 10 p. m. with 2 c c of porcelain filtrate of the lung emulsion from Guinea-pig 874 (filtrate 2). Cultures from the nose contained large numbers of staphylococci and diphtheroid bacilli. January 3 at 7:30 a. m. the animal appeared quite well, and without definite shortness of breath. At 11 a. m. there was definite shortness of breath. Much mucus was noted in the left nostril. This was cultivated and was found to contain a large number of green colonies of streptococci and a moderate number of staphylococci. January 4 respiration was increased and the animal had grown thin, weighing 260 gm. January 5 it seemed ill; the nostrils were moist; the temperature was 103.6. It was etherized; the lung was found moderately distended and the left anterior lobe completely consolidated, uniformly grayish-red, and mottled on the cut surface. The consolidated areas were moist and surrounded by hemorrhagic edema. The uterus contained a hemorrhagic area, one in each horn, and bloody mucus in the fundus. In the right horn was found a chocolate-colored, hemorrhagic mass. January 7 blood-agar plate cultures of the blood showed a few green-producing streptococci; of the lung and nose, large numbers of green colonies of streptococci and a moderate number of Staphylococcus aureus; from edematous fluid of the lung, a moderate number of green colonies of streptococci; from the right horn of the uterus moderate numbers of green colonies of streptococci and one of staphylococci. Cultures from the liver and kidney were negative.

Guinea-pig 885, weighing 350 gm., was injected intratracheally Jan. 2, 1919, with 2 c c of Berkefeld filtrate with emulsion of the pneumonic lung of Guinea-pig 869. Cultures taken from the nose before injection showed staphylococci only. January 3 at 7:30 a. m. the animal appeared quite well; there was no apparent shortness of breath; at 11 a. m. the respirations were increased. Smears from the nose showed large numbers of diplococci, often in short chains. January 4 cultures from the nose made twelve hours after injection showed many staphylococci and green colonies of streptococci. The animal appeared sick, coughed and sneezed at intervals; respirations were rapid. January 5 shortness of breath had diminished. The animal was etherized. The lungs were moderately emphysematous (11 c c); one area of consolidation 1 by 0.7 cm. was found in the right diaphragmatic lobe. The pleura was dull over this area. The cut surface was markedly edematous and a large amount of bloody, frothy fluid escaped. A number of smaller areas of consolidation were found in the left diaphragmatic lobe. The peribronchial lymph glands were enlarged and edematous. There was mucopurulent material in the nostril. January 7, blood-agar plate cultures from the blood, liver, kidney and testicle were negative; those from the pneumonic lung showed large numbers of green colonies of streptococci, and those from the nose showed many staphylococci and green colonies of streptococci.

EXPERIMENTS INDICATING THE TRANSMISSION OF INFLUENZAL INFECTION BY CONTACT

The question of the possible transmission of infection by contact in the animals was also studied. Uninjected guinea-pigs and guinea-pigs injected with broth or salt solution were caged with animals inoculated intratracheally with cultures. All of the 8 uninjected pigs, and the 5 injected with salt solution remained well. In 5 of the former and 3 of the latter the nasal mucous membrane was injured with a sterile flexible wire coil when making cultures from the nose. Two of 10 guinea-pigs injected intratracheally as controls with glucose broth became ill with symptoms suggesting respiratory involvement. Both of these animals were caged with guinea-pigs injected with highly virulent cultures. One died in four days from hemorrhagic bronchopneumonia. Cultures from the blood and lung showed countless numbers of green-producing colonies of streptococci. The other died ten days after injection, with a large amount of a bloody fluid in the chest and marked bronchopneumonia. The blood contained green-producing streptococci and the pleural fluid, staphylococci. The green-producing streptococcus from both guinea-pigs was agglutinated specifically by the monovalent serum. It corresponded morphologically and culturally with the streptococci from influenza and neither strain fermented inulin. During the course of these experiments the supply of normal guinea-pigs was large and no epidemic of pneumonia occurred. Examination of those that died spontaneously was made as a further check on the experiments. Five were found with lesions in lungs. These lungs were different in appearance from those that followed injection of the strains from influenza. They were small, the pneumonia process, usually old, was most marked in the anterior lobes instead of the posterior lobes, and the more recent consolidations were ill defined, often resembling atelectatic areas. The cultures from these showed Bacillus bronchisepticus and two showed pneumococci. The latter were not agglutinated by pneumococcus type serums nor by the monovalent serum.

SYMPTOMS AND GROSS LESIONS FOLLOWING INTRATRACHEAL INJECTION OF INFLUENZAL MATERIAL

The more marked effects of intratracheal than of intraperitoneal injection were very apparent. The respiratory embarrassment on intratracheal injection, particularly in the infections that terminate fatally, was often marked immediately after injection and extreme the day following. The thorax was often in full expansion, the eyes had a glazed appearance, lacrimation was frequent, the mucous membranes were cyanotic, the breathing was difficult, rapid, irregular, and chiefly abdominal. The animals were restless and irritable, the fur ruffled. Expiratory efforts were often violent, and recurring coughing and choking spells resembling the bronchial spasm of acute anaphylaxis were common. The degree of respiratory embarrassment in the animals that died within twenty-four or forty-eight hours was found to vary considerably during the hours of observation. There were periods of some minutes when breathing, although rapid, was quite free and easy, and the animals often ate food or drank water. The quiescent intervals were followed by a return of marked difficulty in breathing, during which time, bloody, edematous fluid sometimes escaped from the nostrils. Finally the animals, while perfectly conscious, and bending every effort at breathing, would run about aimlessly with the head extended, often jump out of the basket in violent efforts to get breath, and die with symptoms of acute anaphylactic shock, and in addition with large amounts of hemorrhagic edema fluid escaping from the nostrils. The symptoms in these animals were clearly those of a prolonged anaphylaxis.

The lungs in the animals that died early were always voluminous, dark purplish red, and showed marked hemorrhage and edema with little or no true consolidation. This was true even in those in which the toxicity of the culture killed them in the course of a few hours (figs. 2 and 6), and even following intranasal insufflation. The dark, hemorrhagic and edematous areas often occupied almost the entire lung, but they were always more marked in the posterior lobes. The emphysema was often so extreme that the alveoli were distended to the rupturing point and in some instances rupture was indicated by the finding of subpleural, interstitial emphysema and by the escape of air into the pleural cavity and in the mediastinal and subcutaneous tissues about the chest. The cut surface was extremely wet and large amounts of hemorrhagic edema fluid escaped. The hemorrhagic, edematous areas were often wedge-shaped with the base toward the pleura, or peribronchial. The cyanosis in some of these animals became extreme. The blood was very dark and often remained liquid. In the animals that showed the symptoms described, and that died in two or three days, the lungs were also extremely voluminous and presented the picture of massive pseudolobar pneumonia. At times the consolidation involved almost the entire lung (fig. 3), but although most or all of certain lobes were involved the consolidation was not uniform or complete, but consisted of coalescing areas of lobular pneumonia varying in age and surrounded by areas of hemorrhagic edema. These lungs also contained large amounts of a thin, watery, bloody exudate, and were extremely wet on the cut surface; this was in sharp contrast to the areas of consolidation noted following intratracheal injection of type pneumococci. The smaller bronchi were often found plugged with a bloody exudate, and the mucous membrane of the trachea and larger bronchi was extremely red, and the lumen filled with a blood-tinged froth. These characteristic changes in the lung tended to occur also in the white rat and monkey. A small percentage of the guinea-pigs (about 10%), which showed soon after injection the symptoms of respiratory embarrassment just described, might live for some days with extremely rapid but not difficult breathing, and then die with compressed lungs from hemorrhagic fluid filling the thorax. In these the symptoms of anaphylaxis might be noted at intervals. Usually, however, death seemed to occur from want of air from a rapidly filling thorax. If death in these animals occurred late, the picture was that of hemorrhagic empyema. The fluid in the pleural cavities, whether death occurred early or late, was almost without exception tinged with blood and contained a relatively small amount of fibrin.

Some animals with not very marked symptoms recovered either in a few days or died at a later period. The symptoms of those that recovered usually consisted of a varying degree of increased respirations, of cyanosis of the mucous membrane with evidence of general illness in loss of action and weight, and in fever. The animals sat humped up and with ruffled hair. The drop in leukocytes lasted for from one to three days. When these animals were anesthetized for examination relatively little lung involvement was found, consisting of irregular areas of partial consolidation, often lobular and peribronchial with hemorrhage and edema, while some showed no lung involvement even when examined within four or five days after injection. The tracheobronchial lymph glands were almost constantly found enlarged and markedly edematous on the cut surface.

The animals that died from three to ten days or more after injection usually showed bronchopneumonia of varying extent associated with emphysema and hemorrhagic edema of various degrees of intensity. In some the pneumonia was lobar in distribution, but lobular in character. Some of the animals developed mucopurulent discharge from the nose associated with maxillary sinusitis and marked redness of the nasal mucous membrane. Occasionally after recovery seemed to be complete there was a return of respiratory embarrassment and death occurred from hemorrhagic edema associated with well defined areas of grayish bronchopneumonia. In not a few of these localized abscesses were noted in the areas showing consolidation.

Cultures from the blood of the animals that died within forty-eight hours were usually positive, but the number of colonies was relatively small, while in those that died later the cultures usually remained sterile. The cultures from the lung and pleural exudates were always positive in the animals that died soon after intratracheal injection, but were often negative in the animals anesthetized while recovering. The relative preponderance of the different strains isolated is shown in table 3. In some animals that died in from ten days to two weeks or more after injection, an entirely different picture supervened. In these the respirations became progressively slower as unconsciousness, great weakness, and a tendency to retraction of the head developed. In a few instances the animals appeared mentally deranged. The lungs were usually small, although occasionally there was moderate emphysema and lesions were slight or wholly absent. The brain and cord were soft, the cerebrospinal fluid was clear but increased in amount; the meninges were edematous and congested. Cultures from the brain and cord substance and spinal fluid were usually negative on blood-agar plates, but in some instances yielded green-producing streptococci in tall tubes of glucose brain broth. The blood in these was always sterile.

MICROSCOPIC ANATOMY OF THE LUNGS

The microscopic findings in the lungs of guinea-pigs varied greatly, depending on the method of injection and on how long after injection the animals survived. In those injected intraperitoneally or subcutaneously the lung findings were relatively slight and consisted of localized hemorrhage and edema with a minimal amount of leukocytic infiltration and desquamation of alveolar epithelium. The localization of the streptococci in the tissues about the capillaries and in the swollen and degenerating alveolar epithelial cells in their normal position or about the desquamated cells which showed nuclear degeneration was a striking picture (figs. 10 and 11). But the lungs of the animals injected intratracheally showed the changes that have come to be regarded as more or less characteristic of influenzal pneumonia. They showed marked distention of alveoli and of alveolar ducts with red blood cells, precipitated serum and a varying number of desquamated degenerating epithelial cells often resembling polymorphonuclear leukocytes, almost complete absence of leukocytes in the acute lesions (figs. 12, 16 and 17), and relatively few leukocytes, even in the more advanced stages of consolidation (figs. 13 and 15a). This picture was in sharp contrast to the consolidation due to type pneumococci (fig. 18a) and the consolidations noted occasionally following injection of the bacteria from normal throats. Besides the marked edema and hemorrhage, probably the most striking change noted in the lungs of these animals was the marked and widely disseminated areas showing necrosis of alveolar epithelial cells and interalveolar capillaries (fig. 19a), also a picture in sharp contrast to that noted following injection of type pneumococci (fig. 19b). The latter finding was strikingly similar to that first noted and so clearly described by LeCount in the case of influenzal pneumonia in man. In the experimental animal in which dosage, place of inoculation, and duration of experiment could be controlled, the cause of this necrosis and the resulting hemorrhage and edema has been found to be due to the localization and growth of the micro-organisms in these structures. The number of organisms was often so large that the outline of alveoli and alveolar ducts could readily be made out with the low power in sections stained by Gram-Weigert by means of the dark lines due to huge numbers of streptococci revealed under higher magnifications (figs. 14c, 15b and 16b). This, too, was in sharp contrast to the even distribution of type pneumococci throughout the highly cellular exudate filling the alveoli (fig. 18b) in experiments in lobar pneumonia in the guinea-pig.

The marked edema and dilatation in the perivascular lymph channels noted in many sections was likewise associated with the presence of enormous numbers of Gram-staining diplococci (fig. 20). Moreover, marked hemorrhagic pleuritis was invariably accompanied by the localization and growth of the micro-organisms in enormous numbers in the subpleural lymphatics (figs. 20, 21 and 22).

It has been possible to study the reparative process of the lungs in animals that were recovering from the effects of injections. The striking feature in the cellular reaction throughout was the relatively small part played by polymorphonuclear leukocytes and the large part played by the proliferated fixed tissue cells, probably endothelial leukocytes and the marked proliferation of epithelial cells.

Distinctive features in the gross and microscopic findings were lacking in the lungs of animals that died soon after injection of the various bacteria, green-producing streptococci, hemolytic streptococci, and staphylococci, except that the hemolytic streptococus tended to invade the pleura and produce hemorrhagic empyema more than the green-producing streptococcus. This is in accord with the findings in the lungs of persons dying from influenzal pneumonia, reported by Blanton and Irons. In the animals that lived for a longer period after injection of mixtures staphylococci were isolated in relatively large numbers, and the sections showed staphylococci in larger numbers or in pure form in the localized areas showing marked leukocytic infiltration, and in abscesses when streptococci were the predominating organisms in the larger intervening areas of hemorrhagic edema showing few leukocytes. The tendency of staphylococci to displace the streptococcal flora in the prolonged experiment even when pure cultures of the streptococci had been injected was often a striking feature (case 2787, fig. 8). These findings in general are in accord with those in human lungs described by Lord,[13] Weichselbaum,[23] Kuskow,[9] and others in previous epidemics of influenza, and by Le Count,[11, 12] MacCallum,[17] Bell,[2] Chickering and Park,[5] Lucke, Wight and Kime,[15] Opie,[18] Lubarsch,[14] Lyon,[16] and others during the recent epidemic.

Altogether, the virulency more than the species of organism injected determined whether hemorrhagic edema with slight leukocytic infiltration, or bronchopneumonia with marked leukocytic infiltration dominated the picture. As a rule, the leukocytic infiltration in the lung occurred more rapidly and to a greater degree in the animals that showed relatively slight leukopenia or even leukocytosis, and in those injected with cultures from patients with mild attacks who had little or no reduction or even a moderate increase in the leukocyte count than in animals injected with strains from cases showing marked leukopenia.

LESIONS OF THE FEMALE GENERATIVE ORGANS AND OF TISSUES OTHER THAN THOSE OF THE LUNG

By far the most important effects or lesions which have been noted outside of the respiratory tract were those of the female generative organs, especially the uterus, and those of the intestinal tract. A consideration of the latter is reserved for a separate paper.

The effect on the female generative organs in influenzal infection is so marked that many authors regard this as of diagnostic importance. The symptoms most commonly encountered are the occurrence of menstruation for the first time in young girls, of intermenstrual hemorrhages in women in whom the menstrual function has been established, its recurrence after the menopause, and the marked tendency to abortions associated with a high mortality rate in pregnant women.

We have injected, altogether, 98 female guinea-pigs, 76 intratracheally and 22 intraperitoneally or subcutaneously with bacteria from influenza. Of these, 61 died as the result of the injection (62%), and 37 either recovered or were anesthetized as recovery appeared likely, or after being caged with males for several months.

A study of the uterus and the other generative organs was made in 75 guinea-pigs, 57 injected into the trachea and 18 intraperitoneally or subcutaneously. Of the 75, 34 were undoubtedly pregnant at the time of injection as shown by examination after death. Only 6 of these showed normal uteri and normal placental masses when examined.

Four were anesthetized, and 2 died in one and eight days, respectively, from the effects of the injection. The cultures from the uterus in 5 were negative; 1 showed a few green-producing streptococci. In the remaining 28 pregnant guinea-pigs the uterus was either found empty with hemorrhagic areas marking the site of placental attachment or it contained one or more detached or attached hemorrhagic placental masses (fig. 9). Cultures from the hemorrhagic placental masses and bloody mucous in the uterus in these often showed exceedingly large numbers of the bacteria injected.

The uterus of the 27 guinea-pigs that died which were not pregnant showed a varying number of hemorrhagic areas in the endometrium. These were usually small in number and the individual hemorrhages relatively small, but in some instances, even in young guinea-pigs, the hemorrhages were more extensive and occurred over wide areas (fig. 9). They almost always occurred in the horns and rarely in the body of the uterus, cervix, or vagina. Lesions of the latter, however, were noted in the guinea-pigs injected with the streptococcus from the vaginal discharge in case 2809. Marked evidence of infection of the mucous membrane was usually limited to the areas marking placental attachment. In these and in the hemorrhagic placental masses, large numbers of the organisms injected were demonstrable in sections. There was a marked difference between the strains with respect to their power to invade the uterus. In some, all animals injected aborted; in others few or none. The affinity for the uterus was particularly marked in the cultures from the patient (case 3175) who aborted. Intratracheal injections of the sputum in a series of female guinea-pigs and a cat were followed by localization in the uterus and abortion in every animal injected.

The effects in the lung associated with marked bronchial spasm and emphysema, the finding in animals of violent contractions in the uterus immediately after death, and in some instances when anesthetized, and the absence of demonstrable infection either in the placental site or the mucous membrane of the uterus in some of the animals injected, are good reasons for the belief that the emptying of the uterus may be due in some instances to the violent contractions of the uterus from the formation and circulation of "anaphylatoxin" and may not always be the result of actual localization of the bacteria at the placental side.

Lesions of the ovary were relatively rare. In some instances, however, one or both were edematous, fully twice the normal size, and in sections evidence of degeneration of cells in the granular layer associated with edema and leukocytic infiltration in the graafian follicles were noted. Lesions in the interstitial tissues of the ovary were not found.

Cultures were made from the sections in the uterine horns in 75 guinea-pigs. In these the amount of material cultivated usually consisted of only one or two drops from the ends of a small pipet. Green-producing streptococci in varying numbers were isolated in pure culture or together with hemolytic streptococci and staphylococci in 28 animals, hemolytic streptococci in 10, and staphylococci in 25.

Altogether, 10 female guinea-pigs were injected with the control cultures, including those from normal throats, from cases of simple nasopharyngitis, and with type pneumococci from lobar pneumonia. Of these 10 were pregnant. Only 3 showed slight lesions of the uterus or placental masses and only 1 aborted. Cultures were made from the uterus in 10. One showed a few colonies of staphylococci; the rest remained sterile. It is thus apparent that the marked affinity for the uterus and the high incidence of abortions in the animals injected with the influenzal strains is not shared by the control strains. When we were dealing with controlled conditions the effects on the female generative organs in the guinea-pig paralleled in so far as is possible those observed in women.

In order to determine whether other effects on the female generative organs might not have occurred following injection of these strains, the female guinea-pigs that survived were mated with males and kept under observation for from two to three months. Only 2 became pregnant, 1 showing 1, the other 2 fetuses. The general health of all these animals appeared to be good. They gained in weight. There was no evidence of disease of the external generative organs either in the males or females and no gross lesions of ovaries, uterus, or vagina in the animals chloroformed to determine the presence or absence of pregnancy. It would appear, therefore, that infection with these microorganisms had a pronounced depressant effect on the female generative mechanism after a recovery in other respects seemed to be complete. On the basis of this experiment a diminution in the birth rate in human beings greater than can be accounted for by the death of women of the child-bearing age might be expected.

The kidneys often showed a marked degree of diffuse, cloudy swelling and less commonly, focal areas of infection situated most often in the medulla; in a few instances these areas seemed to have given rise to pyelitis. Hemorrhages in the mucous membrane of the bladder were rarely noted. The suprarenals were often much swollen and hemorrhagic on the cut surface.

Following intratracheal injection of a few strains, numerous lesions of the muscles occurred, and in a few animals single large, hemorrhagic, edematous, necrotic areas were noted in the abdominal rectus muscle. Lesions of the myocardium occurred not infrequently and consisted usually of a grayish white diffuse degeneration. The ventricles in most of these were of stony hardness and in firm systole.

Lesions of the stomach were rare and occurred almost exclusively in animals that died from overwhelming infection, and consisted almost wholly of small localized hemorrhages with or without superficial ulceration associated with marked distention of the stomach with gas rich in carbon dioxid and marked postmortem digestion of the stomach wall.

General peritonitis following intratracheal injection was noted in 12 guinea-pigs. This occurred usually only when marked pleuritis or empyema was present or when it was otherwise secondary to infection of the uterus and tubes.

EXPERIMENTS ON THE MECHANISM OF RESPIRATORY EMBARRASSMENT IN INFLUENZA

Many findings in influenzal pneumonia, and particularly those in guinea-pigs following injection of bacteria from influenza, suggest strongly that they may be due in part to the formation of "anaphylatoxin," and that the lung picture may be the result of a prolonged anaphylaxis, associated with bronchial spasm. The protective effects of epinephrin and atropin against fatal anaphylactic shock are thoroughly established. It was thought, therefore, that injections of these substances into guinea-pigs having symptoms resembling anaphylaxis might furnish experimental evidence of the nature of the respiratory embarrassment and the use of these substances in treatment.

The effects of subcutaneous injection of epinephrin were studied in 15 guinea-pigs. The dose ranged from 0.02 c c-0.05 c c of a 1:1,000 solution of epinephrin chlorid to each 100 gm. of body weight. Good effects were noted in all but 3 guinea-pigs which showed no improvement; respiratory embarrassment was found to be due either to filling of the pleura or to extensive consolidation of the lung. The improvement, although striking, was always temporary, lasting from one-half to five hours. In a few control experiments in which the same dose of culture was given, life appeared to be prolonged for from one to two days in the animals treated with epinephrin, but in no instances in which recovery took place could it be attributed to the effects of this drug. This would be expected because of the inexhaustible supply of anaphylatoxin causing bronchial spasm due to the multiplication of the bacteria. Protocols illustrate the results obtained.

Guinea-pig 750, weighing 350 gm., was injected intraperitoneally Nov. 25, 1918, at 5:30 p. m. with 0.3 c c of the sputum from case 2620. The white blood count before injection was 14,400. November 26 at 9 a. m. the animal appeared to be sick, the fur was rough, and the respirations were rapid and difficult. The chest appeared to be dilated, and breathing was accomplished chiefly by means of the diaphragm. There was an expiratory rattle in the throat, and the animal's repeated forced efforts at expiration resembled the symptoms of anaphylactic shock. The mucous membrane of the conjunctiva, mouth, and tongue was blue. The leukocyte count was 4,500. At 1 p. m. the condition was unchanged except that respiratory efforts were more labored. A small amount of fluid oozed from the mouth and there was intense cyanosis of the mucous membranes. At 2:30 p. m. the condition was about the same. At this time 0.2 c c of a 1:1,000 solution of epinephrin chlorid were injected subcutaneously. At 2:35 p. m. there was no apparent change in respiration. At 2:45 p. m. the respirations undoubtedly were less labored and the animal appeared to be improved. At 3 p. m. the respirations appeared to be quite normal and the animal appeared to be much improved. At 3:45 p. m. the animal seemed to be comfortable, ate food, and the respirations were only slightly above the normal; cyanosis was absent. At 5:30 p. m. the respiratory difficulty had returned to some extent and the animal had a violent attack resembling anaphylactic shock. November 27, at 8:20 a. m., it was found dead. It showed hemorrhagic serofibrinous peritonitis and moderate emphysema of the lungs (12 c c), and beginning bronchopneumonia associated with marked edema surrounding the consolidated areas. The blood was very dark and had not coagulated. Blood-agar plates of the blood showed a moderate number of green-producing streptococci; from the peritoneal fluid there was a large number in pure culture.

Guinea-pig 965, weighing 360 gm., was injected intratracheally Jan. 14, 1919, at 3 p. m. with 2 c c of the glucose-brain-broth culture of the vaginal swab of case 2809. At 7 p. m. the respirations were extremely rapid and chiefly abdominal, the chest was dilated, the hair ruffled; there was an expiratory grunt, and the animal was restless, appeared uncomfortable, coughed repeatedly, and scratched its nose at intervals; bloody, edematous fluid escaped from the nostrils. At 7:20 p. m. respiratory embarrassment was unchanged. At 7:30 p. m., 0.2 c c of a 1:1,000 solution of epinephrin chlorid were injected subcutaneously. At 7:45 p. m. the picture had completely changed. The respirations were free and easy; the animal walked about, and the discharge of bloody fluid from the nose had ceased. At 11:15 p. m. the respirations were growing more labored; the animal was weak and restless, and breathing was difficult;

there was an expiratory rattle, and the bloody discharge from the nose had returned. At 11:30 p. m. the animal had an attack of severe shortness of breath in which it made violent efforts to breathe, ran around its mate, jumped into the air in a last violent effort at breathing, fell on its side as bloody fluid spurted from the nose and mouth, and died. The lungs were voluminous (22 c c); practically the entire lung was hemorrhagic and filled with hemorrhagic edematous fluid. The peribronchial lymph glands were edematous. A small amount of bloody fluid was found in the pleural cavity and a large subcapsular hemorrhage in the lower pole of the left kidney. Sections of the lung showed marked dilatation of alveoli filled by hemorrhagic edematous fluid, with slight leukocytic infiltration, and large numbers of diplococci in the hemorrhagic areas (figs. 17 a and b).

RELATION OF MORTALITY IN GUINEA-PIGS TO VIRULENCY OF THE ORGANISM ISOLATED IN FATAL AND NONFATAL INFLUENZA IN PATIENTS

If the results obtained in the animals really indicate close etiologic relationship of these streptococci to the disease, the relative mortality in the animals should correspond roughly with that in the patients from whom the material for injection was obtained. During the course of the experiments, the impression was gained that the material from severe or fatal cases is more virulent, producing more severe respiratory embarrassment, more marked hemorrhagic edema, and a higher mortality rate than the material from patients with mild attacks who recovered. It was considered of value, therefore, to determine the mortality in the animals according to whether the material injected was from patients with influenza and influenzal pneumonia who recovered, or from patients with influenza and influenzal pneumonia who died. In table 4 is given the mortality according to the diagnosis made at the time the material injected into animals was obtained and according to whether the patient died or recovered.

The mortality in the animals injected (intratracheally and intraperitoneally) with material from patients with influenza in whom signs of lung involvement were slight or entirely absent at the time of the experiments and who recovered, was about the same (49%) as in patients with influenzal pneumonia who recovered (43%). The 3 persons who had influenza at the time of the experiments and who later died of influenzal pneumonia harbored streptococci which killed the 5 guinea-pigs injected. It should be noted that the mortality in the guinea-pigs injected with material from patients with influenzal pneumonia was 26% lower when the material was taken from patients who recovered than when taken from those who died. In the former it was 43% in 23 guinea-pigs injected with 23 strains; in the latter, 69% in 78 guinea-pigs injected with 39 strains. The average mortality following intratracheal injection of 67 strains in 109 guinea-pigs was

TABLE 4

MORTALITY IN GUINEA-PIGS ACCORDING TO PLACE OF INJECTION AND MATERIAL INJECTED, AND ACCORDING TO DIAGNOSIS AND ULTIMATE RESULT IN PATIENTS FROM WHOM MATERIAL WAS OBTAINED

Place of Injection and Material Injected	Diagnosis at Time of Animal Experiments and Ultimate Result	Number of Strains	Number of Animals			Percentage of Mortality
			Injected	Recovered	Died	
Trachea—sputum, primary culture, green-producing streptococci, hemolytic streptococci, staphylococci	Influenza—recovery	32	43	23	21	49
	Influenzal pneumonia—recovery	12	11	7	4	36
	Total	44	55	30	25	[45]
	Influenza—death	1	3	0	3	100
	Influenzal pneumonia—death	22	51	20	31	61
	Total	23	54	20	34	[63]
	Total all strains	67	109	50	59	54
Peritoneum—sputum, primary culture, green-producing streptococci, hemolytic streptococci, staphylococci	Influenza—recovery	36	42	21	21	50
	Influenzal pneumonia—recovery	11	12	6	6	50
	Total	47	54	27	27	[50]
	Influenza—death	2	2	0	2	100
	Influenzal pneumonia—death	17	27	4	23	85
	Total	19	29	4	25	[86]
	Total all strains	66	83	31	52	63
Trachea and peritoneum—sputum, primary culture, green-producing streptococci, hemolytic streptococci, staphylococci	Influenza—recovery	68	86	44	42	49
	Influenzal pneumonia—recovery	23	23	13	10	43
	Total	91	109	57	52	[48]
	Influenza—death	3	5	0	5	100
	Influenzal pneumonia—death	39	78	24	54	69
	Total	42	83	24	59	[71]
	Total all strains	133	192	81	111	58
Vein—primary culture, green-producing streptococci, hemolytic streptococci	Total all strains	9	19	5	14	74
	Grand total (111 cases)	142	211	86	125	59

54%. The average mortality in the 55 animals injected with 44 strains from patients who recovered was 45% in contrast to a mortality of 63% in the 54 guinea-pigs injected with 23 strains from patients who died. The results following intraperitoneal injection were similar.

The average mortality in 83 guinea-pigs injected with 66 strains was only 9% higher, 63%, than following intratracheal injection. The average mortality in 54 guinea-pigs injected with 47 strains from patients who recovered was 50%, in contrast to a mortality of 86% in the 29 guinea-pigs injected with 19 strains from patients who died. A summary of the results following these two methods of injection gives a total average mortality of 58% in 192 guinea-pigs injected with 133 strains from 111 cases, the average mortality in 109 guinea-pigs injected with 91 strains from patients who recovered being 48% in contrast to the mortality of 71% of the 83 guinea-pigs injected with 42 strains from patients who died. The average mortality following intravenous injection of 19 guinea-pigs with 9 strains was 74%. The grand total average mortality in 211 guinea-pigs injected with 142 strains, derived from 111 cases, was 59%.

It would seem from these facts that the virulency of the streptococci in patients who recover is less marked than in patients who die.

GENERAL DISCUSSION AND SUMMARY

The animal experiments that have been carried out heretofore with bacteria isolated quite constantly in influenza, both in 1889 and 1918, have consisted largely of virulency and toxicity tests in which only the usual methods of injection were used, and in which sufficient attention was not directed to the time and method of cultivation before injection. Statements have appeared concerning the high virulency of organisms of the streptococcus group [3, 7] and the ability of influenza bacilli to produce highly toxic products in cultures [19] and a tendency to produce lesions in the lung,[1, 8] but little has been accomplished in the way of reproducing the clinical and pathologic picture of epidemic influenza.

Intratracheal injection has been employed only occasionally in previous studies despite the fact that by this manner of injection of highly virulent pneumococci Lamar and Meltzer [10] have produced the typical picture of lobar pneumonia in the dog, Winternitz and Hirschfelder [24] in the rabbit, Cecil and Blake [4] in the monkey, and Wollstein and Meltzer [25] produced bronchopneumonia in the dog with bacteria isolated from bronchopneumonia in man.

The results of subcutaneous, intraperitoneal and intravenous injections, in my hands, show that the bacteria, particularly green-producing streptococci, isolated quite constantly in epidemic influenza possess high and peculiarly invasive powers. They have a marked tendency to produce leukopenia, to localize electively in the interstitial tissues and epithelial cells of the alveoli and smaller bronchi, and to produce hemorrhage and edema in the lungs, as symptoms of anaphylaxis and emphysema of the lung usually develop. Significant as these facts are, an accurate analysis of the effects of the bacteria and the precise rôle they play in influenza was possible only by the use of methods which simulated more closely the natural conditions, through the application of the bacteria to the normal uninjured epithelium of the lower respiratory tract by the method of intratracheal injection. The guinea-pig was considered the most suitable animal available for this study. Its resistance to streptococcal infection, although higher than that of man, its reaction to bacterial poisons and anaphylaxis are in general quite similar.

There has been much discussion, based chiefly on the results of cultures, with regard to the relative importance of the four main types of bacteria isolated in this disease, green-producing streptococci, including pneumococci, hemolytic streptococci, staphylococci and influenza bacilli. By a combined study of intraperitoneal injection in mice and guinea-pigs and intratracheal injection in guinea-pigs of sputum and lung exudates directly, and of the primary mixed culture of standard dosage a fair knowledge of the degree of the invasive power of these bacteria has been obtained. Invasion by the green-producing streptococcus in pure or almost pure form occurred in most instances even when the bacteria were not present in predominating numbers in the material injected. In some instances invasion by hemolytic streptococci occurred, but usually only when they were present alone or in predominating numbers, and more rarely by staphylococci, but only when they were present in predominating numbers in the material injected. Invasion by influenza bacilli following injection of sputum or lung exudate, which in some instances was proved to contain influenza bacilli, has not occurred in a single experiment. Similar results regarding the relative invasive power of these species have been obtained by injections of pure cultures of each, and again the independent invasive power of influenza bacilli was found to be slight. It should be emphasized that while it was necessary to use rather large doses for routine injections, owing to the relatively high and variable resistance of guinea-pigs and marked variations in invasive powers of the strains, small numbers of the more virulent streptococci sufficed to produce characteristic lesions. They followed intratracheal application of filtrates, intranasal insufflation of particularly virulent cultures and in a few instances through contact infection from guinea-pigs injected with especially virulent cultures.

The effects of intratracheal injection of mixtures of these organisms as they occurred in sputum and primary cultures and of pure cultures of recently isolated strains, varied within wide limits. The animals may be classified in four groups as follows:

Group 1. Animals that showed slight symptoms and then recovered.

Group 2. Animals that showed mild early symptoms and later suffered severe attacks.

Group 3. Animals that showed severe and progressive symptoms of marked lung involvement.

Group 4. Animals that showed extreme and rapidly fatal effects.

Group 1.—The symptoms of the animals in this group were relatively slight, consisting in the main of moderate illness, loss in weight, usually some fever, moderate leukopenia, and slight or moderately increased respirations for a number of days, followed by complete recovery. The animals were found to be immune to subsequent injections of heterologous strains. Those anesthetized for examination showed relatively slight or no lung involvement; the blood was sterile and the lungs were either sterile or contained a few of the organisms injected. These findings may be considered to parallel the clinical findings in patients with relatively mild influenza in whom little or no lung involvement can be demonstrated and in whom relative immunity is conferred as in the animals.

Group 2.—In the animals in this group the initial effects of the injection were more pronounced and lasted longer than those in the animals of group 1. Some of the animals, after apparent recovery, developed severe symptoms of respiratory involvement and died in from one to two days with anaphylactic symptoms, voluminous lungs, and hemorrhagic bronchopneumonia or, more rarely, from hemorrhagic pleuritis. In others the symptoms of respiratory embarrassment progressed more slowly; many of the animals developed rhinitis, and later died from purulent bronchitis and well-defined bronchopneumonia, often with small abscesses, and more rarely from abscess and gangrene, or from emphysema with or without bronchopneumonia. The cultures from the animals that died of relatively acute symptoms in the pneumonic attack usually showed green-producing streptococci, the pneumonic lung showing localized abscesses or abscess, usually staphylococci, or staphylococci and streptococci, and the empyemas usually hemolytic streptococci with or without staphylococci. The findings in this group may be regarded as representative of the findings in the group of patients with the more severe influenzal attacks who later develop influenzal pneumonia or, more rarely, well-defined coalescing bronchopneumonia with slight hemorrhagic edema, but with purulent bronchitis and localized abscesses or a single large abscess, or of empyema with or without bronchopneumonia.

Group 3.—In this group the initial symptoms were severe and usually progressed without intermission until death occurred in from two or three days from an increasing intense cyanosis and respiratory rate or from marked respiratory embarrassment from anaphylactoid symptoms during which in many instances, hemorrhagic edematous fluid escaped from the nose while the animals made violent efforts to breathe. The lungs were huge, in a few cases interstitial emphysema had occurred and extensive consolidation consisting of coalescing areas of pneumonia of different ages and intervening areas of hemorrhagic edema. The blood was dark and remained liquid for a long time. The postmortem and microscopic findings in this group were in every way like those described as typical of acute influenzal pneumonia in man.

Group 4.—In this group extreme dyspnea often occurred almost immediately after injection of highly virulent cultures and their filtrates. The symptoms were quite typical of acute anaphylaxis and many of the animals died while making violent efforts to breathe, as a bloody fluid ran from the nose and mouth. The lungs were huge, a dark purplish red, and hemorrhagic and edematous throughout. The symptoms and postmortem findings resembled very closely those noted in patients who died soon after being taken ill, usually in the initial attack of acute hemorrhagic edema of the lungs before sufficient time had elapsed for the development of extensive consolidation.

The distress from lack of oxygen, the intense cyanosis, and the extreme efforts at respiration of many animals in the latter two groups resembled the picture presented by patients dying from a rapidly filling lung who copiously expectorated a serous, bloody, frothy fluid, and who frequently sat up or left their beds in making violent efforts to breathe as death occurred.

The experiments with the filtrates show that under the proper conditions green-producing streptococci may become sufficiently small to pass through bacterial filters which prevent the passage of Bacillus prodigiosus, and that small numbers of the streptococci, when applied to the normal mucous membrane of the lower respiratory tract, are sufficient to produce the characteristic symptoms and pathologic changes in the lungs of guinea-pigs. Moreover, the results of the experiments with filtrates of cultures, pneumonic lungs, and sputum, and those on the mechanism of respiratory involvement show that the strains from influenza which have high invasive powers also have the power to produce anaphylatoxin in large amount, as measured by intratracheal injection. Many findings in influnza, such as the expanded, hyperresonant, relatively immobile thorax, cyanosis, the sharp leukopenia, the delayed coagulability of the blood, and the voluminous lung appear to be expressions of an anaphylactoid intoxication.

The results obtained following injection of guinea-pigs with influenzal material were so definite and so striking as to rule out quite effectively the possibility of spontaneous infection. However, this possibility was considered throughout the series of experiments. Only vigorous healthy looking pigs were used. No epidemic of pneumonia occurred among the reserve supply. The patchy areas of chronic bronchopneumonia, usually situated in the anterior lobes noted in guinea-pigs, at times were easily differentiated from the acute lesions due to the injections by their appearance and by the fact that cultures in the former condition nearly always showed Bacillus bronchisepticus: Control injections of salt solution and broth were without effect, and finally similar results followed intratracheal injections of influenzal material in other species (rat, rabbit, cat and monkey).

The effects following injection of the control strains of green-producing streptococci, hemolytic streptococci, staphylococci, and type pneumococci in like dosage were quite different. The immediate symptoms were less marked or absent, the mortality rate was much lower, leukopenia rarely occurred, leukocytosis was the rule, respirations while rapid in some instances, were usually free and easy, prolonged anaphylactoid symptoms did not occur, and hemorrhages from nostrils were not observed. The lungs were smaller, the exudate more cellular, the areas of consolidation occurred earlier and were more definitely outlined, and there was either no edema or relatively slight hemorrhagic edema at all times; marked necrosis of alveolar capillaries and epithelium were also absent. The contrast between the gross and microscopic picture of the lung following injections of highly virulent green-producing streptococci from influenza and of type pneumococci was particularly striking. In the former there was huge dilatation of the lung and alveoli, marked desquamation and degeneration of alveolar epithelium, necrosis of alveolar capillaries associated with peripherally placed streptococci in large numbers, and hemorrhage and edema everywhere with relatively slight leukocytic infiltration. In the case of type pneumococci the striking findings were moderate distention of the lung and alveoli with slight degeneration of epithelium and little change in interalveolar capillaries, but with marked diffuse, sharply demarkated, highly cellular exudate filling the alveoli, with the pneumococci diffusely distributed in the exudate, and with little edema.

The occurrence of marked lesions of the lungs, including well-marked pneumonia following injection of pure cultures of staphylococci and the presence of staphylococci in areas of softening in lungs injected with mixtures, and in large numbers in the sputum in some cases, but more particularly in the lung exudate after death, are in accord with the findings of Chickering and Park in Staphylococcus aureus pneumonia, and emphasize anew the importance of the staphylococcus as a cause of death and a factor in the production of lesions in the lung in epidemic influenza.

The theory that influenza and influenzal pneumonia are manifestations of the same infection varying only in degree is supported by these experiments. The bacteriology of the sputum and other exudates in influenza and of the early stages in influenzal pneumonia have been found to be identical. The infecting powers of the strains isolated in these two conditions, particularly of the green-producing streptococci, have been found to be very similar. The mortality in the guinea-pigs injected with strains from influenza is as high as in those injected with strains from patients with influenzal pneumonia who recovered. The mortality in the guinea-pigs was proportionately higher in those injected with material from patients who died than in those injected with material from patients who recovered. The leukocyte curves in the fatal and nonfatal infections in the guinea-pig ran parallel with the leukocyte curves in fatal and nonfatal infections in persos.

From a study of 266 cases of influenza and influenzal pneumonia in which accurate record of the exact onset of the attack was obtainable it was found that 145 patients either had no preceding influenzal attack or developed outspoken signs of pneumonia within three days from the onset of symptoms; 108 became ill with pneumonia after an interval of from four to nine days, and 13 only had an interval ranging from ten to twenty-one days. The number of patients who developed outspoken signs of lung involvement in the initial attack and without a quiescent interval is therefore large, and in general similar to that noted by others. By means of the more refined methods of examination, such as the roentgen ray, the incidence of lung findings in the primary influenzal attack has been greatly increased. Indeed, the manifestations of the disease and the bacteriologic findings in some instances have led good clinicians to regard the so-called complications as the disease itself,[6] and bacteriologists to look on the "secondary invaders" as the cause of sharp outbreaks.[7]

Through a painstaking study of the infecting powers of the streptococci in influenza and influenzal pneumonia throughout several epidemic waves, it has been possible to reproduce in animals, by various methods of injection, but particularly by intratracheal injection, the picture of influenza as seen in man. The symptoms both of influenza and influenzal pneumonia have been closely simulated in these animals as far as possible. Likewise, the gross and microscopic changes which have come to be regarded as quite characteristic of influenzal infection have been reproduced. The same varied picture that often supervenes in the latter stages of influenzal pneumonia in man, such as leukocytosis as evidence of pleural involvement and purulent infection, becomes manifest and the varied pathologic picture in the lung of patients who died late have been noted in guinea-pigs injected intratracheally with these strains. The tendency to involvement of the female generative organs, with a high mortality in pregnancy and a high incidence of abortion, of lesions of the heart, abscess in the rectus muscle, and interstitial emphysema have been noted in the experimental animal quite as they occur in man.

BIBLIOGRAPHY

1. Albert, H., and Kelman, S. R.: Pathogenicity of Bacillus influenzae for laboratory animals, Jour. Infect. Dis., 199, XXV, p. 433.
2. Bell, E. T.: The pathology of the lungs in pneumonia following influenza, Journal-Lancet, 1919, XXXIX, 3.
3. Blanton, W. B., and Irons, E. E.: A recent epidemic of acute respiratory infection at Camp Custer, Michigan, Jour. Am. Med. Assn., 1918, LXXI, 1988.
4. Cecil, R. L., and Blake, F. G.: Active immunity against experimental pneomococcus pneumonia, Jour. Am. Med. Assn., 1919, LXXIII, 715.
5. Chickering, H. T., and Park, J. H., Jr.: Staphylococcus aureus pneumonia, Jour. Am. Med. Assn., 1919, LXXII, 617.

6. Dunn, A. D.: Observations on an epidemic of bronchopneumonia in Omaha, Jour. Am. Med. Assn., 1918, LXXI, 2128.

7. Hirsch, E. F., and McKinney, M.: An epidemic of pneumococcus bronchopneumonia, Jour. Infect. Dis., 1919, XXIV, 594-617.

8. Huntoon, F. M., and Hannum, S.: The rôle of Bacillus influenzae in clinical influenza, Jour. Immunol., 1919, IV, 167-187.

9. Kuskow, N.: Zur pathologischen Anatomie der Grippe, Virchow's Arch., 1895 CXXXIX, 406-458.

10. Lamar, R. V., and Meltzer, S. J.: Experimental pneumonia by intrabronchial insufflation, Jour. Exper. Med., 1912, XV, 133-148.

11. LeCount, E. R.: The pathologic anatomy of influenzal bronchopneumonia, Jour. Am. Med. Assn., 1919, LXXII, 650-652.

12. LeCount, E. R.: Disseminated necrosis of the pulmonary capillaries in influenzal pneumonia, Jour. Am. Med. Assn., 1919, LXXII, 1519-1520.

13. Lord, F. T.: Influenza. In: Osler, Sir W., and McCrae, Sir T.: Modern Medicine, Philadelphia, Febiger, 1913, I, 534-549.

14. Lubarsch: Die anatomischen Befunde, von 14 tödtlich verlaufenden Fällen von Grippe, Berl. klin. Wchnschr., 1918, LV, 771. (Quoted in abstr. of foreign literature compiled by British Medical Research Committee, Jour. Am. Med. Assn., 1918, LXXI, 1573-1579.)

15. Lucke, B., Wright, T., and Kime, E.: Pathologic anatomy and bacteriology of influenza, Epidemic of autumn, 1918. Arch. Int. Med., 1919, XXIV, 154-237.

16. Lyon, M. W., Jr.: Gross pathology of epidemic influenza at Walter Reed General Hospital, Jour. Am. Med. Assn., 1919, LXXII, 924-929.

17. MacCallum, W. G.: Pathology of pneumonia following influenza, Jour. Am. Med. Assn., 1919, LXXII, 720-721.

18. Opie, E. L., Freeman, A. W., Blake, F. G., Small, J. C., Rivers, T. M.: Pneumonia following influenza (at Camp Pike, Arkansas), Jour. Am Med. Assn., 1919, LXXII, 556-565.

19. Parker, J. T.: The poisons of the influenza bacillus, Jour. Immunol., 1919, IV, 331-357.

20. Rosenow, E. C.: Prophylactic inoculation against respiratory infections during the present pandemic of influenza, Jour. Am. Med. Assn., 1919, LXXII, 31-34.

21. Rosenow, E. C.: Studies in influenza and pneumonia. II. The experimental production of symptoms and lesions simulating those of influenza with streptococci isolated during the present pandemic, Jour. Am. Med. Assn., 1919, LXXII, 1604-1608.

22. Rosenow, E. C.: Studies in influenza and pneumonia. III. The occurrence of a pandemic strain of streptococcus during the pandemic of influenza, Jour. Am. Med. Assn., 1919, LXXII, 1608-1609.

23. Weichselbaum, A.: Bakteriologische und pathologisch-anatomische Untersuchungen über die Influenza und ihre Komplikationen, Wien. med. Bl., 1890, XIII, 83-85.

24. Winternitz, M. C., and Hirschfelder, A. D.: Studies upon experimental pneumonia in rabbits, Jour. Exper. Med., 1913, XVII, 657-678.

25. Wollstein, M., and Meltzer, S. J.: Experimental bronchopneumonia by intrabronchial insufflation, Jour. Exper. Med., 1913, XVI, 126-138.

Plate I

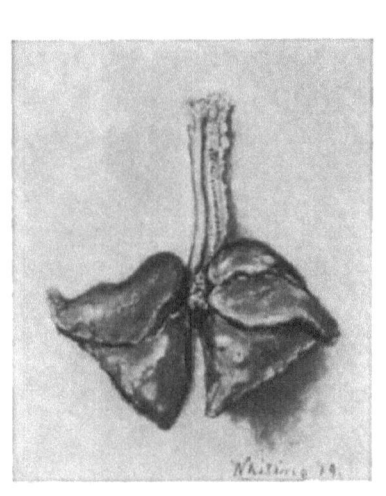

1

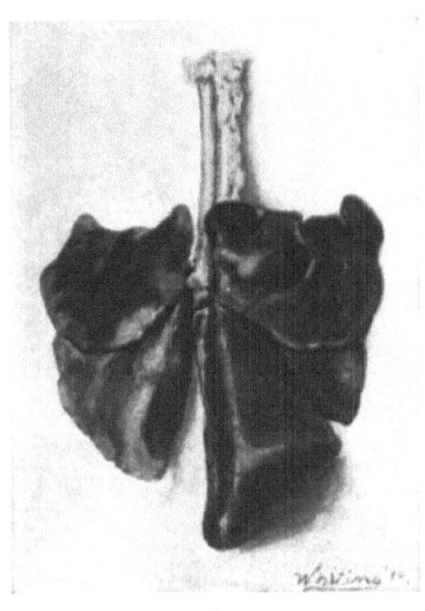

2

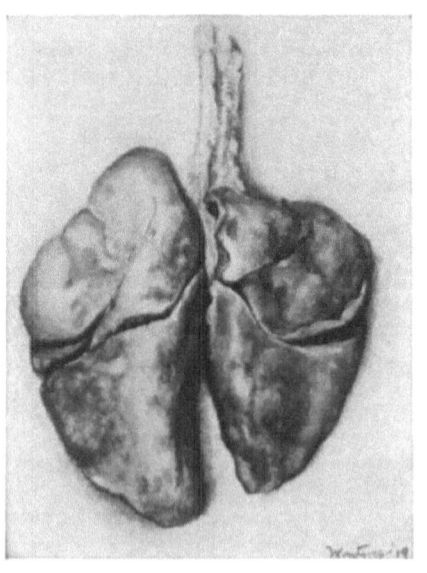

3

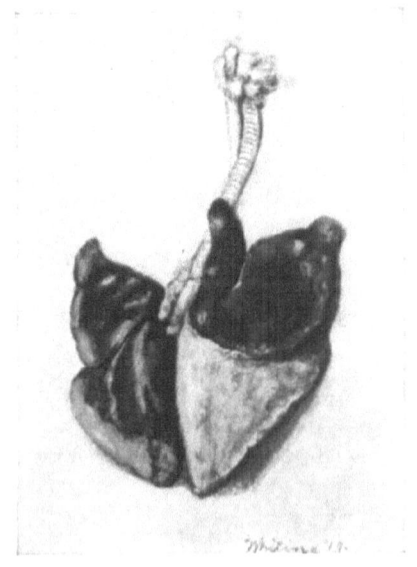

4

PLATE II

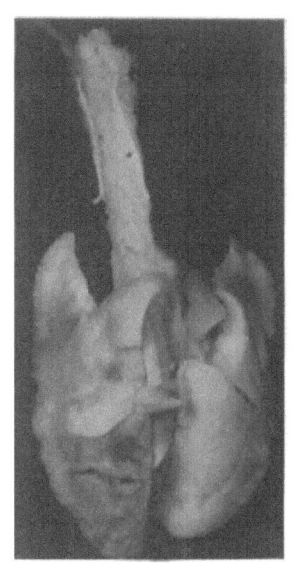

5

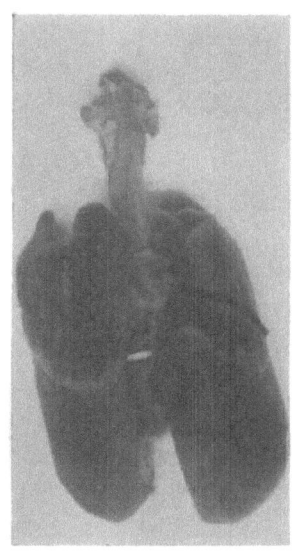

6

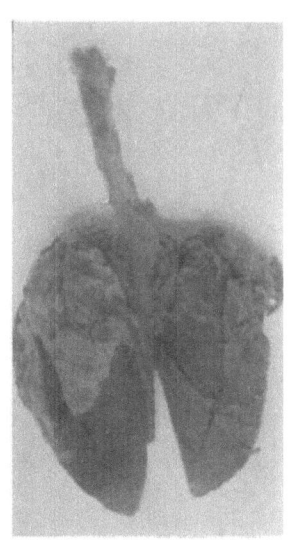

7

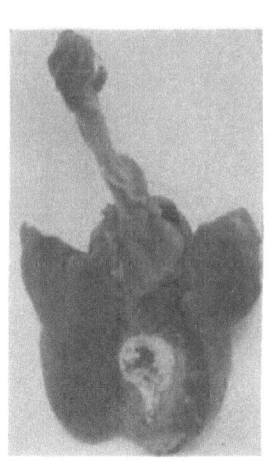

8

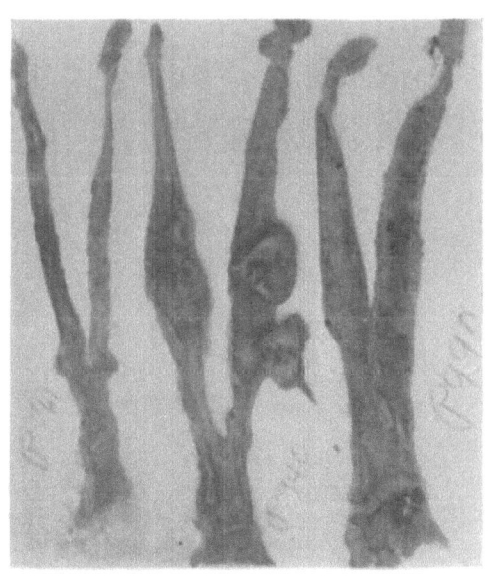

9

PLATE III

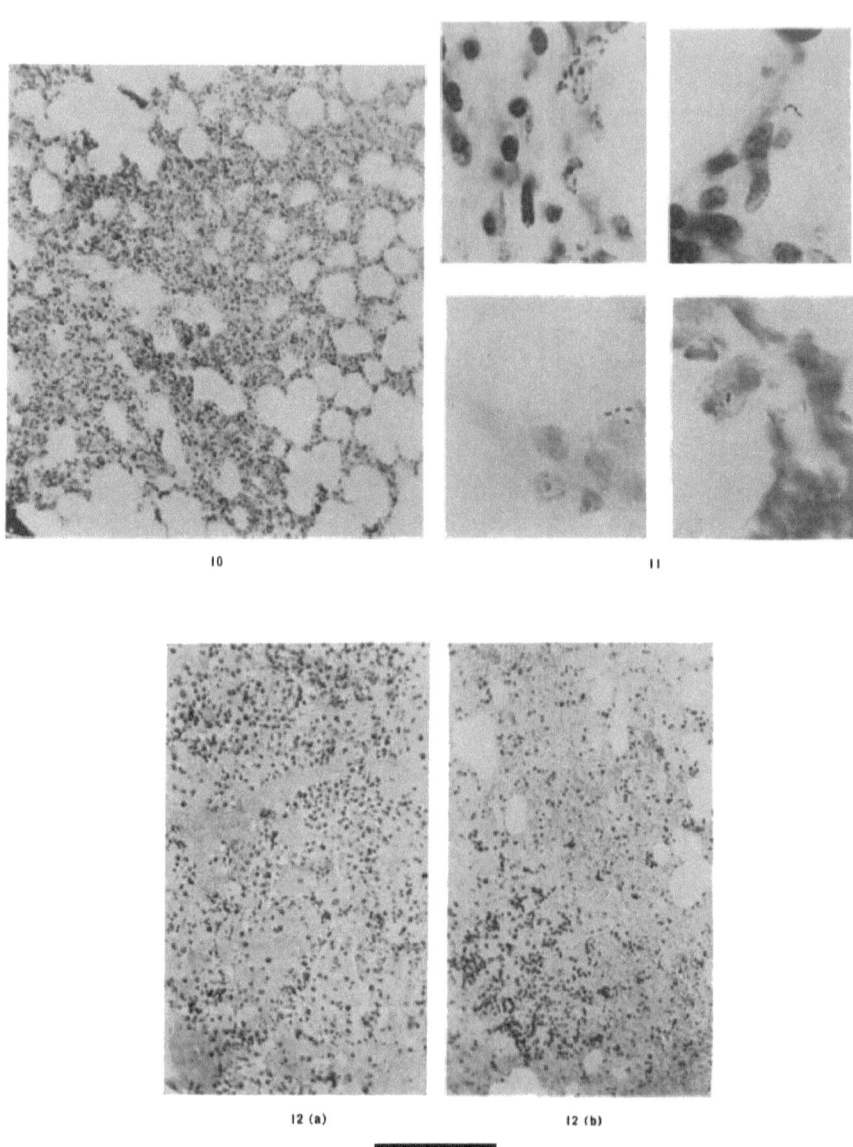

10

11

12 (a)   12 (b)

Plate IV

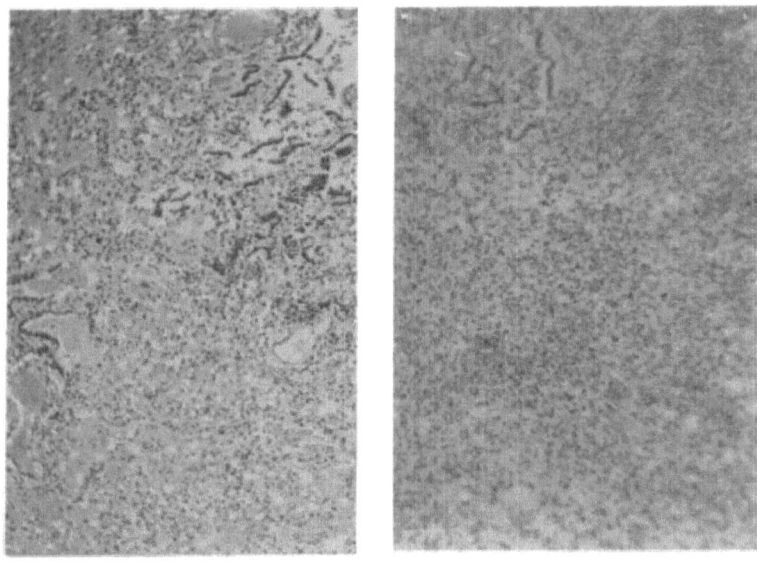

13

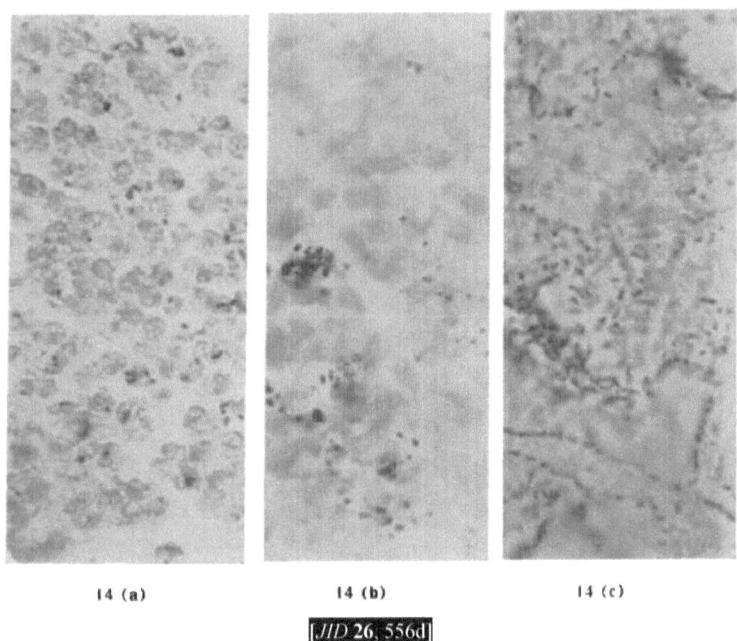

14 (a) 14 (b) 14 (c)

PLATE IV

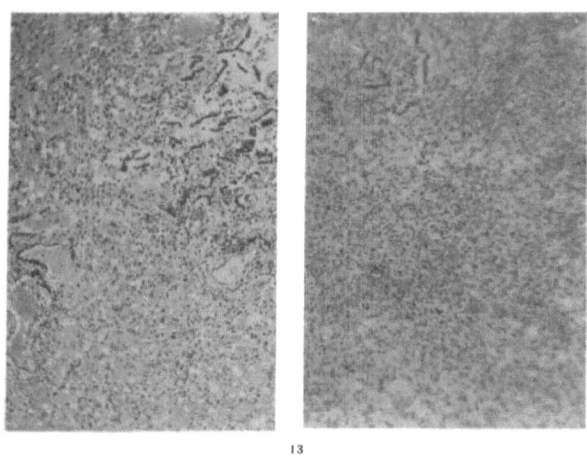

13

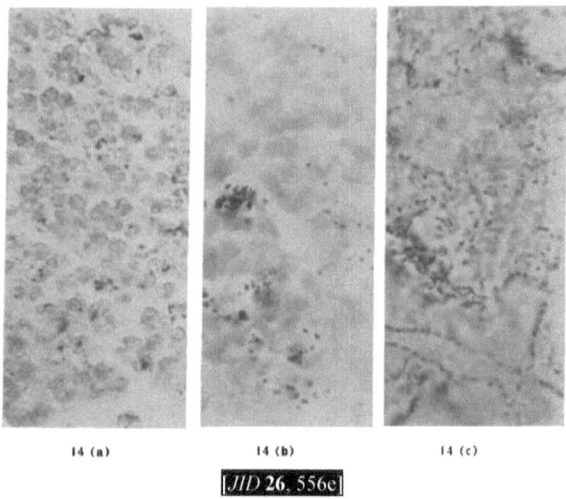

14 (a)   14 (b)   14 (c)

PLATE V

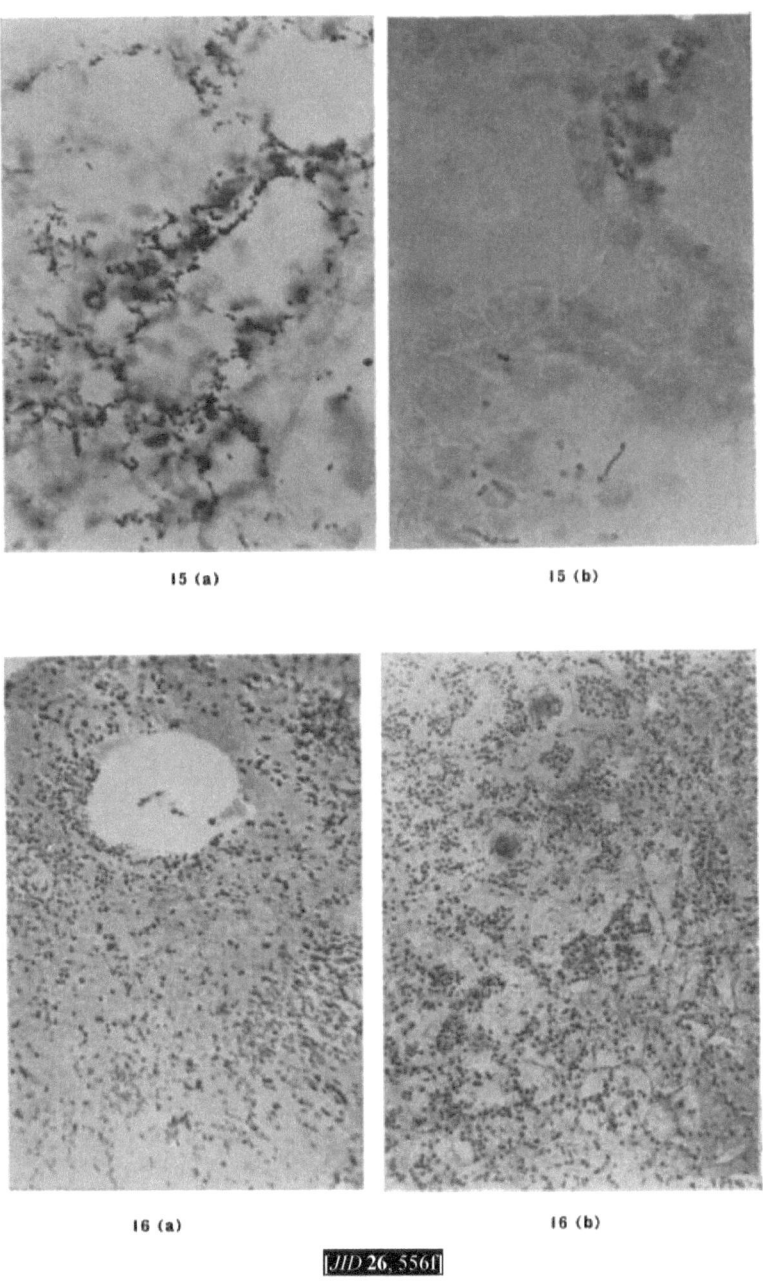

15 (a)   15 (b)

16 (a)   16 (b)

PLATE VI

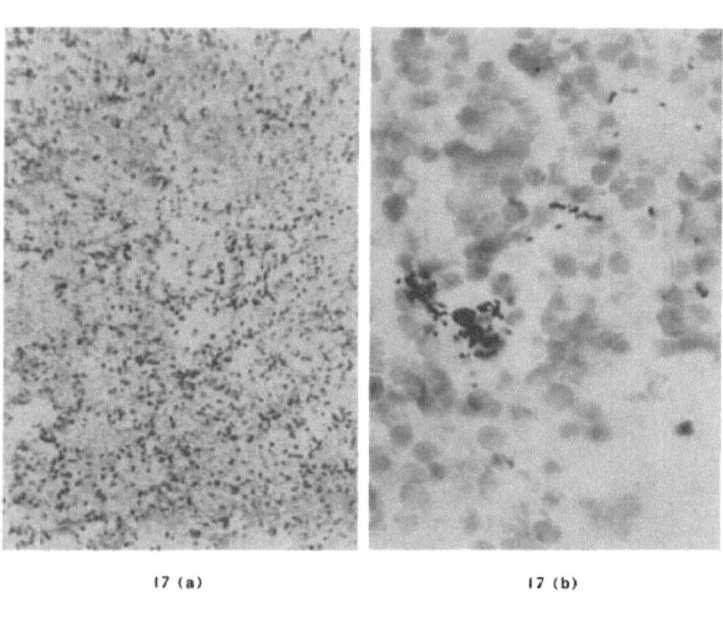

17 (a) 17 (b)

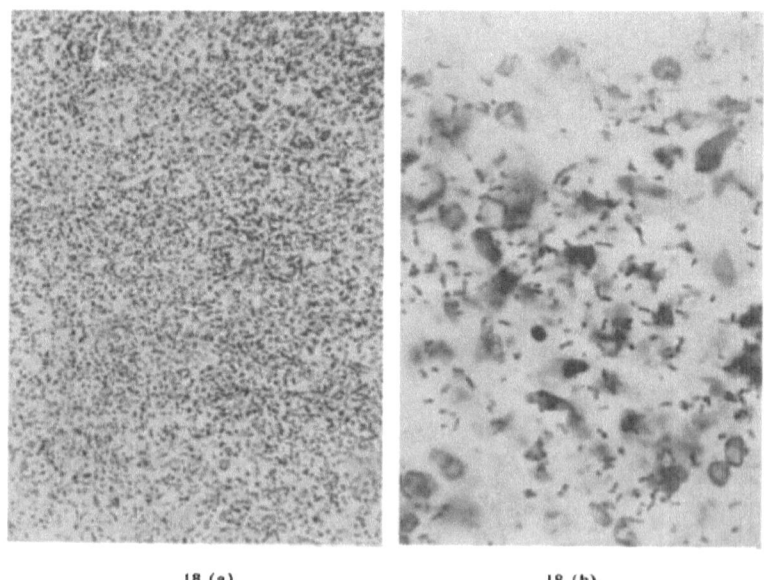

18 (a) 18 (b)

INFLUENZA/PNEUMONIA 1918-1919

Plate VII

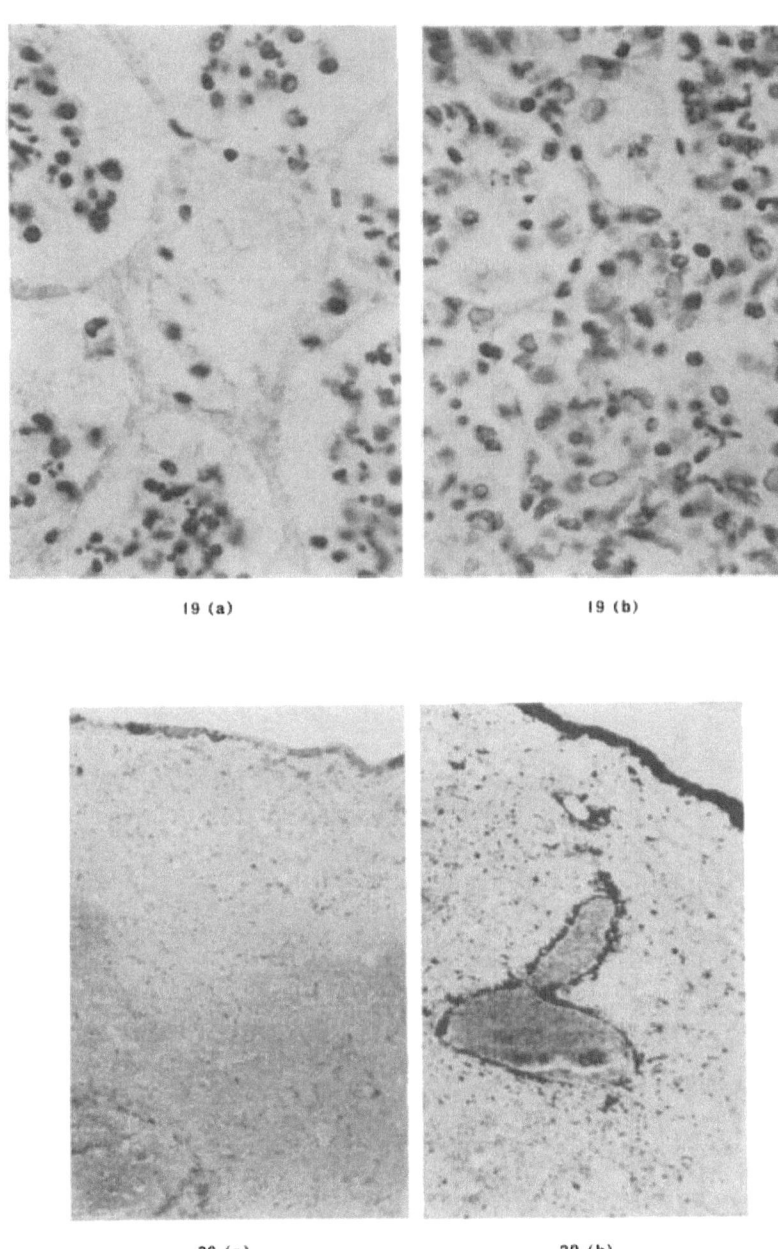

19 (a)   19 (b)

20 (a)   20 (b)

PLATE VIII

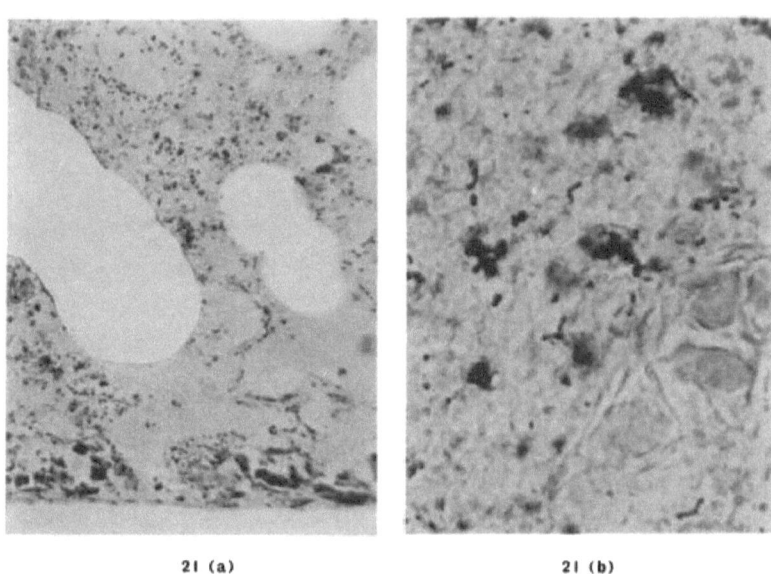

21 (a)   21 (b)

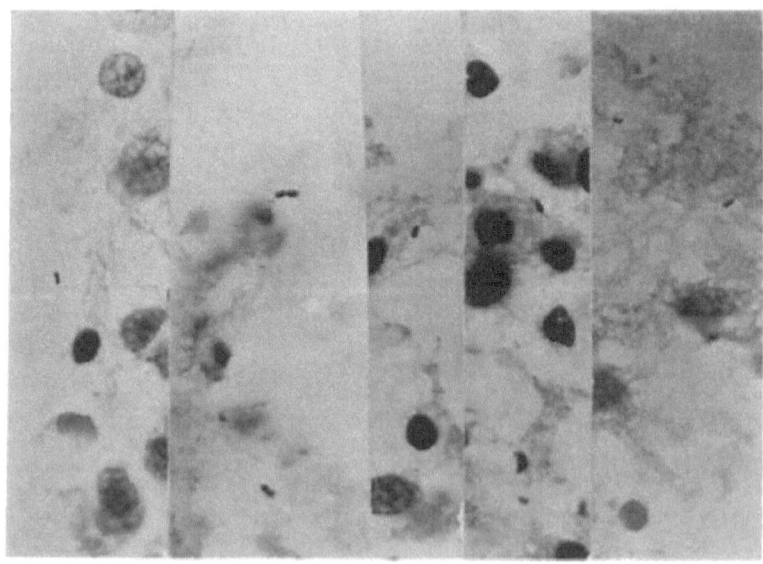

22

INFLUENZA/PNEUMONIA 1918-1919

EXPLANATION OF PLATES

PLATE 1

Fig. 1.—Lung of normal guinea-pig weighing 350 gm., killed with ether. Total volume of lung 5.5 c c, weight 3.5 gm. (× 1).

Fig. 2.—Lung of guinea-pig 1345, weighing 400 gm., showing acute hemorrhagic edema 2½ hours after intratracheal injection of a culture of green-producing streptococcus from influenza in the fourth culture generation. Total volume of lung 23 c c, weight 18 gm. (× 1).

Fig. 3.—Lung of guinea-pig 1249, weighing 380 gm., showing massive pseudolobar pneumonia 48 hours after intratracheal injecton of the primary culture of green-producing streptococcus from the blood of a fatal case of influenzal pneumonia (case 3171). Total volume of lung 26 c c, weight 21 gm. (× 1).

Fig. 4.—Lung of guinea-pig 1448, showing lobar pneumonia 48 hours after intratracheal injection of type II pneumococcus; total volume of lung 14 c c, weight 12 gm. (× 1).

PLATE 2

Fig. 5.—Lung of guinea-pig 737 that died 24 hours after intraperitoneal injection of sputum from case 2607. Note the large size (12 c c) compared with the lung shown in figure 1, and the hemorrhage and edema over the posterior aspect (× 1¼).

Fig. 6.—Lung of guinea-pig 1335 injected intratracheally with culture from sputum (case 2623) 40 minutes before death occurred with symptoms of acute anaphylaxis. Total volume of lung 20 c c. Note the extreme hemorrhage and edema (× 1).

Fig. 7.—Lung of guinea-pig 957 injected 6 days previously with hemolytic streptococci from case 2798. Note the marked thickening of the pleura (× 1).

Fig. 8.—Lung of guinea-pig 944, injected two weeks previously with hemolytic streptococci from case 2787, showing a large gangrenous abscess, numerous small abscesses in the cut surface of the right diaphragmatic lobe and marked pericarditis (× 1).

Fig. 9.—Photograph of uteri of three guinea-pigs, laid open presenting anterior view, illustrating the type of lesions noted in this organ following injection of influenzal material. Note the hemorrhages in the mucous membrane of the left horn of the uterus of guinea-pig 861 and both horns of guinea-pig 990, and their absence in the cervix and vagina, the hemorrhagic fetal masses and the localized edema, and infiltration of the endometrium marking placental attachments in guinea-pig 940 (× 1).

PLATE 3

Fig. 10.—Section of the lung of guinea-pig 737, injected intraperitoneally with the sputum of case 2607. Note the marked dilatation of alveoli, congestion of the capllaries, and the alveolar and interstitial edema and hemorrhage. Hematoxylin and eosin (× 100).

Fig. 11.—Sections of the lung of guinea-pig 737, shown in figures 5 and 10; (a) diplococci beneath the epithelial cells in the alveolar wall and just outside of a capillary; (b) chain of diplococci in alveolar wall where epithelial cells have desquamated; (c) diplococci in an epithelial cell in its normal position, but showing disintegration of the nucleus in the wall of an alveolus with hemorrhage; (d) diplococci in desquamating epithelial cell. Gram-Weigert (× 1000).

Fig. 12.—(a) Section of lung of case 2800 showing marked hemorrhagic edema; (b) lung of guinea-pig shown in figure 2 with dilatation of alveoli, marked hemorrhagic edema, and dissolution of parenchymatous cells. Hematoxylin and eosin (× 100).

PLATE 4

Fig. 13.—Section of lungs showing (a) hemorrhagic edema with relatively slight cellular infiltration and marked destruction and desquamation of the bronchial epithelium in case 2800, and (b) in guinea-pig 956 twenty-four hours after intratracheal injection of the culture of green-producing streptococcus from a single colony from the throat in this case. Hematoxylin and eosin (× 100).

Fig. 14.—(a) Diplococci in the lung of case 2800 shown in figures 12 and 13; (b) diplococci in the lung of guinea-pig shown in figure 12; (c) diplococci distributed along the alveolar lining of the alveoli in the lung shown in figure 13b.

PLATE 5

Fig. 15.—Lung of guinea-pig shown in figure 3; marked hemorrhagic edema, dilatation of the alveoli, desquamation and disintegration of the alveolar epithelium, necrosis of capillary epithelium with relatively slight leukocytic infiltration, and many diplococci lining the alveolar walls; (a) hematoxylin and eosin (× 100); (b) Gram-Weigert (× 800).

Fig. 16.—Lung of monkey 228 injected intratracheally with the emulsion of the hemorrhagic mucous membrane of the stomach in case 2979. Note the hemorrhagic edema, desquamation of the epithelial cells of the alveoli and ductus alveolaris, and the diplococci chiefly along the alveolar lining; (a) hematoxylin and eosin (× 100); (b) Gram-Weigert (× 1000).

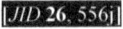

PLATE 6

Fig. 17.—Section of the lung of guinea-pig 965 injected intratracheally with a culture from the vaginal swab in case 2809. Note the dilatation of the alveoli, the marked edema and hemorrhage, the relatively slight cellular infiltration, and the large number of diplococci in the hemorrhagic and edematous areas; (a) hematoxylin and eosin ($\times$ 1000); (b) Gram-Weigert ($\times$ 1000).

Fig. 18.—Section of consolidated right diaphragmatic lobe of lung shown in figure 4. Note the marked and uniform cellular, chiefly leukocytic infiltration, relatively slight edema, and the even distribution throughout the alveolar exudate of the pneumococci; (a) hematoxylin and eosin ($\times$ 100); (b) Gram-Weigert ($\times$ 1000).

PLATE 7

Fig. 19.—(a) High power photomicrograph of the lung of guinea-pig 1249 (figures 3 and 15) showing marked dilatation of alveoli, necrosis of capillary endothelium, desquamation and degeneration of the alveolar epithelium, and slight leukocytic iinfiltration. Hematoxylin and eosin ($\times$ 500). (b) Section of consolidated lobe of lung of guinea-pig 1448 injected with type II pneumococcus. Note the lesser dilatation of alveoli, the marked leukocytic infiltration, absence of necrosis of endothelial cells lining the alveolar capillaries, and the lesser damage to alveolar epithelium. Hematoxylin and eosin ($\times$ 500).

Fig. 20.—Section of lung of guinea-pig 947 injected intratracheally with the primary culture of the throat swab from Case 2800, which died 24 hours after injection with compressed lung from hemorrhagic fluid in the pleural cavities. Note the marked hemorrhage and edema and the poorly staining cells throughout, and the dark areas beneath the pleura and around the large blood vessels. Hematoxylin and eosin ($\times$ 50).

PLATE 8

Fig. 21.—(a) Section of lung of guinea-pig 1262, injected into the trachea with the sputum of case 3175. There was a moderate amount of turbid hemorrhagic fluid in the pleural sac and a corresponding tendency of the bacteria to localize in the subpleural lymphatics as shown in the dark areas. Note the marked dilatation of the alveolar ducts and the alveoli, and the edema, hemorrhage, and desquamation of cells with relatively slight cellular infiltration throughout. Hematoxylin and eosin ($\times$ 100). (b) Diplococci and cocci in hemorrhagic, edematous areas. Gram-Weigert ($\times$ 1000).

Fig. 22.—Photomicrograph of diplococci in the edematous and hemorrhagic subpleural space of the pleura of the fetus in case 3175. Gram-Weigert ($\times$ 1000).

STUDIES IN INFLUENZA AND PNEUMONIA

STUDY VIII. EXPERIMENTS ON THE ETIOLOGY OF "GASTRO-INTESTINAL" INFLUENZA

E. C. ROSENOW

Division of Experimental Bacteriology, The Mayo Foundation, Rochester, Minnesota.

Symptoms of gastro-enteritis, alone or in association with respiratory involvement, have occurred with such regularity during the course of epidemics of influenza and the accompanying prostration has been so pronounced, that a gastro-intestinal type of this disease has come to be quite generally recognized. Kuskow cites cases of his own and of others in which lesions of the gastro-intestinal tract were found, varying from simple enteritis with the swelling of Peyer's patches and hyperplasia of mesenteric lymph glands to severe ulcerative and hemorrhagic gastro-enteritis. Bacteriologic studies, however, are quite lacking; no one has demonstrated bacteria in the lesions, and many regard the severe cases as due to enteritidis-like organisms. The investigations of Sherwood, Downs, and McNaught do not support the latter view since this type of organism was isolated in cases of influenza without symptoms referable to the gastro-intestinal tract and in those with symptoms. I shall report herewith the results of a study of a series of cases of gastro-enteritis, including one fatal case, which occurred during the first two waves of the epidemic of 1918.

The incidence of gastro-enteritis during the first wave was quite high; it was more common in children, but occurred also in adults. The symptoms varied greatly, but prostration and high fever were the striking features. In some instances the symptoms referable to the gastro-intestinal tract occurred without accompanying respiratory involvement; in most instances more than one member of a given family were affected. Cultures from the stools, usually from only one specimen taken at the height of the attack, were made in 15 cases during the first wave. Flakes of bloody mucus were fished out and washed in salt solution and plating on blood-agar made. Varying numbers of green-producing streptococci resembling those from the sputum in influenza were isolated in 9 instances and hemolytic streptococci were isolated in 2. Influenza bacilli were not isolated. Smears from flakes of bloody mucus often showed a large number of gram-positive diplococci resembling those from the sputum. Owing to stress of other work no animal experiments were made at this time. During the second wave opportunity presented itself for the study of one fatal case and one other case in the same family. The findings in detail are:

CASE 2979,—A boy aged 3, a patient of Dr. C. T. Granger, after having had symptoms of a slight sore throat for several days, suddenly became ill Feb. 3, 1919, with vomiting, diarrhea, high fever and delirium. The stools showed blood on the first day; this continued and he passed almost pure blood and mucus at times. He grew gradually weaker, vomited blood February 9 and died the following day. Dr. Peters brought the internal viscera to me for examination. The lungs revealed marked hypostatic congestion, moderate edema, but no outspoken areas of consolidation. The stomach contained a moderate amount of dark red, partially clotted, blood. The mucous membrane was covered with chocolate colored blood mixed with mucus. This was removed and numerous small hemorrhages with beginning ulceration, more numerous in the pyloric end, were found. The duodenum was normal. The mucous membrane of the ileum was extensively hyperemic throughout and was covered with mucopurulent bloody material; numerous punctate hemorrhages and in places beginning ulceration were found. The mesenteric lymph glands were edematous and hemorrhagic. The kidneys showed marked cloudy swelling; the spleen and heart were normal. Blood-agar plate cultures of an emulsion of the hemorrhagic mucous membrane of the stomach contained fully 5,000 rather moist, green colonies of bacteria resembling pneumococci and 5 colonies of staphylococci. The emulsion of the mesenteric lymph glands contained 260 colonies of green-producing streptococci, 4 of staphylococci, and a number of colonies of Bacillus coli. Emulsions of the washed intestinal wall revealed 120 colonies of green-producing streptococci, 50 colonies of staphylococci, and 30 colonies of Bacillus coli. Cultures of the spleen were negative. In sections made through the hemorrhagic areas in the ileum were found wedge shaped and diffuse areas of hemorrhage in the mucosa, with only moderate infiltration and edema, and in some instances with superficial ulceration of the mucosa (fig. 1). A large number of gram-positive diplococci were found throughout the hemorrhagic areas, but were most numerous near or on the surface of the ulcerated area (fig. 2a). The hemorrhagic areas in the stomach showed a similar picture; they contained a large number of gram-positive diplococci. In either case few or no diplococci were demonstrable in the tissues without lesions.

Feb. 12, 1919, the primary culture in dextrose-brain broth of the emulsion of a mesenteric lymph gland was injected, under ether, through a laparotomy incision into the duodenum of one guinea-pig. The leukocyte count was 25,000 before injection. The animal was found dead the following day. Examination revealed 7,200 leukocytes, fibrinous and clotted blood deposit about the point of puncture of the duodenum, a normal intestine above this point, and an extremely hyperemic intestine below. The lumen of the intestine contained a large amount of mucus mixed with chocolate colored blood. The mesenteric lymph glands were edematous. The mucous membrane of the stomach, the uterus, and the cecum was hyperemic and contained a few hemorrhages. The primary culture in glucose-brain broth of the stomach emulsion of the patient was injected in doses varying from 0.1 to 1.5 c c, intratracheally into one monkey and 5 guinea-pigs, and intravenously into one rabbit. The guinea-pig that was given 0.5 cc and the one given 1 cc died in twenty-four hours. Both had hemorrhagic edema of the lungs and hemorrhagic pleuritis; óne had marked lesions of the intestine and stomach, the other slight lesions. The other 3 animals were chloroformed for examination the third day. All had bronchopneumonia, one had a large amount of turbid fluid in the pleural cavity, and 2 had lesions of the intestinal tract; cultures from the lung of one of these were agglutinated specifically by the monovalent antistreptococcus serum. One of the guinea-pigs had leukopenia, 1 leukocytosis, and in 2 there was no change in the leukocyte count. The monkey died in twenty-four hours. Examination revealed hemorrhagic edema of the intermediate lobe, marked

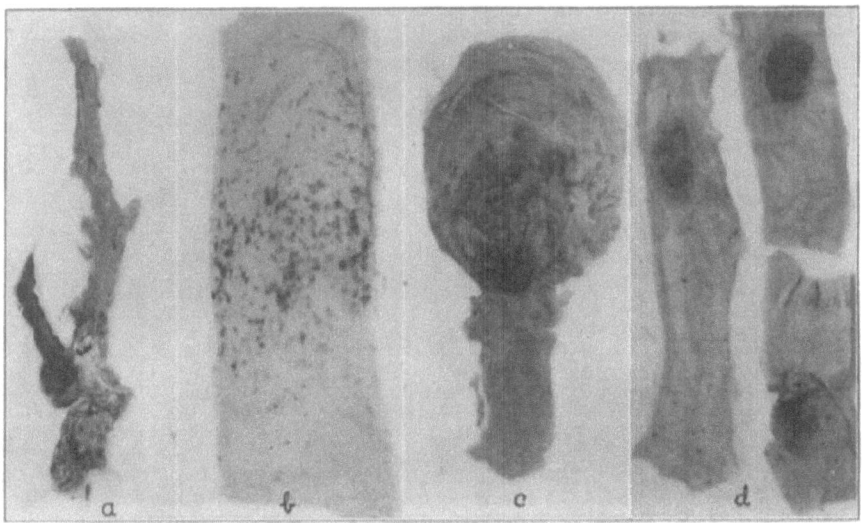

Fig. 1.—Photographs of lesions of the pancreas, intestine, stomach, and Peyer's patches following injection of green-producing streptococcus from influenza. × I.

a. Pancreas of guinea-pig forty-eight hours after intravenous injection of a strain after one animal passage. Note the edema, hemorrhage, and fat necrosis; × I.

b. Ilium of rabbit twenty-four hours after intravenous injection of a strain in the third animal passage. Note the numerous circumscribed hemorrhages in the mucous membrane; × I.

c. Edema and extensive hemorrhages in the stomach of a guinea-pig fifteen days after intratracheal injection of a strain in the third subculture; × 0.5.

d. Swelling and hemorrhages of Peyer's patches and the mucous membrane of the duodenum in the ileum and duodenum of rabbit forty-eight hours after intravenous injection of a strain in the fourth animal passage.

distention of the stomach with gas rich in carbon dioxid, edematous and hemorrhagic Peyer's patches and mesenteric lymph glands, and hyperemia and edema of the mucous membrane of the small intestine, especially in the ileum, where it was covered with mucus containing flakes of blood. The leukocyte count dropped from 35,000 before injection to 7,200 after death. The blood contained a moderate number of green-producing streptococci and staphylococci; the upper intestinal contents, a moderate number of staphylococci and green-producing streptococci; the lower intestinal contents, colon bacilli only. Cultures from two mesenteric lymph glands, the kidney, and the peritoneum were negative. Sections of the lower ileum contained subperitoneal hemorrhages and areas of hemorrhage in the mucous membrane showing desquamation of epithelium but no distinct ulceration. A large number of gram-positive diplococci were found in the hemorrhagic areas of the mucous membrane (fig. 3), a smaller number in the subserous hemorrhages, but none in the adjoining normal tissue. The rabbit injected intravenously with the primary

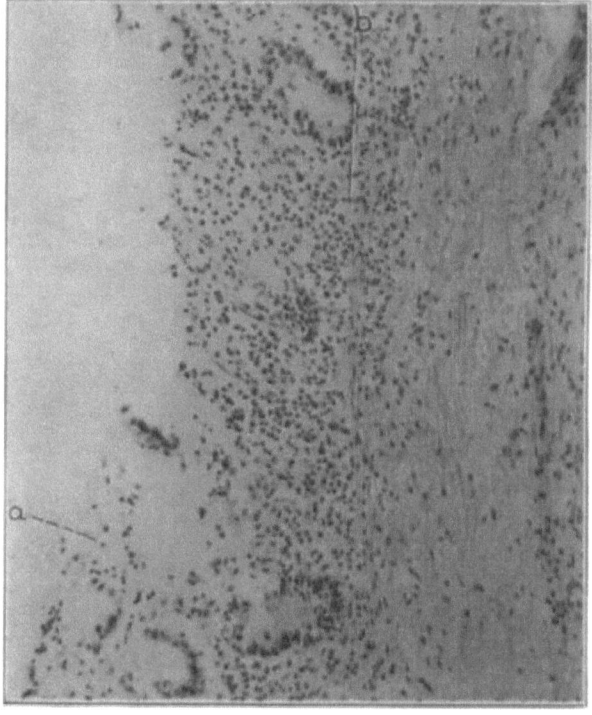

Fig. 2.—Photomicrograph of section of ileum in case 2979. Note the loss of tissue, infiltration by erythrocytes and leukocytes; hematoxylin and eosin, × 100.

culture from the stomach emulsion developed diarrhea and died three days later. Examination revealed two areas of bronchopneumonia posteriorly in the diaphragmatic lobes, hyperemia of the small intestine, swollen Peyer's patches and lymph follicles, much mucus in the intestine, edematous mesenteric glands, embolic lesions in the medulla of the kidney, and a few lesions in the myocardium and skeletal muscles. Cultures from the blood were negative and those from the pneumonic areas in the lung contained green-producing streptococci and staphylococci.

CASE 2981.—A baby girl aged fifteen months, sister of the patient whose case (case 2979) is first recorded, became ill Jan. 9, 1919, with vomiting, high fever (104 F.), and diarrhea six days after her brother had been taken sick. January 11, the child was apathetic, and fussy; the fever and diarrhea continued, and the leukocyte count was 5,400. The skin was dry and without rash, and there was no throat infection; the abdomen was scaphoid; and the stool consisted largely of blood-tinged mucus resembling pus. The diarrhea continued for five days, after which the child gradually recovered. Cultures were made from the tonsils, and from four samples of bloody mucus in the stool. The cultures from the tonsils showed the usual streptococcal flora. The blood-agar plates of the bloody mucus contained countless numbers of Bacillus coli, a few staphylococci, and rather moist, green-producing colonies of streptococci. Three guinea-pigs were injected, one intrarectally, one intratracheally with a salt solution suspension of the bloody mucus, and one with the pure culture of green-producing streptococcus in the second generation. The guinea-pig injected intrarectally appeared well

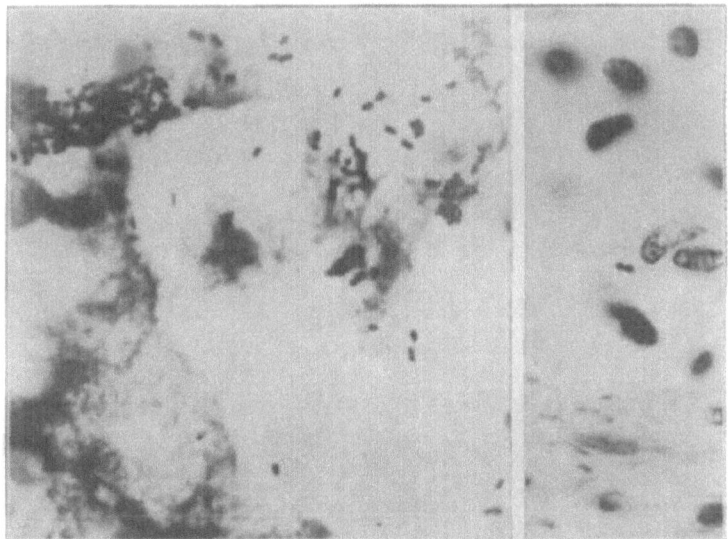

Fig. 3.—Diplococci in ulcerating area shown in figure 2 at a and b.

the following day when it was chloroformed. In the cecum were a large number of small hemorrhages and swollen lymphoid follicles; in the stomach, large circumscribed areas containing small punctate hemorrhages surrounding the cardiac orifice; and in the duodenum a few hemorrhages in the mucous membrane just beyond the pyloric ring. Cultures from the blood, adrenal. spleen, kidney, and liver were negative; staphylococci and green-producing streptococci were produced from the mesenteric and perigastric lymph glands, and from the lung. Sections of the hemorrhagic areas in the duodenum showed marked extravasations of red blood corpuscles, especially in the submucosa in which a large number of diplococci were found. In the guinea-pig injected intratracheally with a suspension the leukocyte count dropped 66 per cent. the following day. The temperature increased 2 degrees, and respirations increased slightly. The animal appeared well four days later when it was chloroformed. The transverse colon and cecum were found to be extremely hyperemic; the intestinal contents contained an abnormal amount of mucus, but otherwise showed no lesions; there was a large subcapsular hemorrhage in the lower pole of the left kidney, consolidation of the upper one-third of the right diaphragmatic lobe, and marked congestion and mucopurulent material in the mucous membrane of the trachea and nose. Cultures from the blood and the uterus were negative; the mucous membrane of the nose and trachea contained a large number of green-producing streptococci and staphylococci. In the guinea-pig injected with the pure culture of the green-producing streptococcus a diminution of 33 per cent. in leukocyte count and a slight increase in respiration occurred the day following the injection. Two days after the injection, when the animal appeared quite well, it was chloroformed. Examination revealed uniform grayish areas of consolidation of the right diaphragmatic lobe, a few hemorrhages in the mucous membrane of the stomach

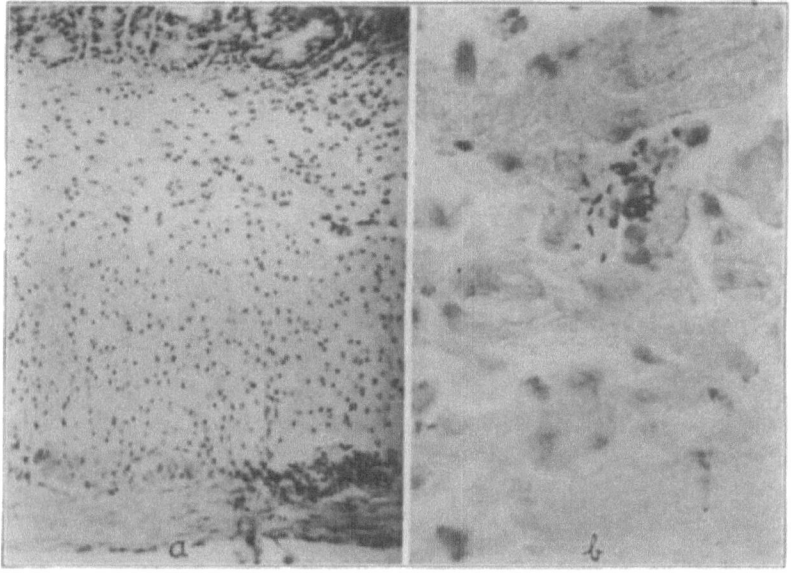

Fig. 4.—Section of the ileum of a guinea-pig injected intrarectally with a suspension of hemorrhagic mucus from the stool in case 2981. Hemorrhage and infiltration and thrombosis of vessel in subperitoneum by leukocytes and by swollen degenerating, desquamated endothelium; gram-positive diplococci in the area of infiltration in the submucosa. a., Hematoxylin and eosin, × 100; b. Gram-Weigert, × 1000.

along the lesser curvature and cardiac end, but no lesions of the intestine. The cultures from the lung contained a moderate number of colonies of staphylococci and green-producing streptococci.

Many green-producing streptococci were isolated from the lesions in the intestines of the patient with the fatal gastro-intestinal infection (case 2979), and from stools in the sister of this patient whose attack was milder and who recovered (case 2981). These attacks occurred at a time when influenza was epidemic in the surrounding community. The organism was present in large numbers in the lesions of the intestines and stomach, and absent in the normal tissues. Injection of the freshly isolated strains from these 2 patients into 14 animals produced well marked lesions in the gastro-intestinal tract, in 12 in which the organism was demonstrable in large number; the lesions were similar to those noted in the patients. In view of these facts there can be no reasonable doubt that this organism was the cause of the gastro-enteritis in these patients. Lesions of the gastro-intestinal tract following injection of streptococci isolated in influenza were noted only occasionally, but they occurred more often after

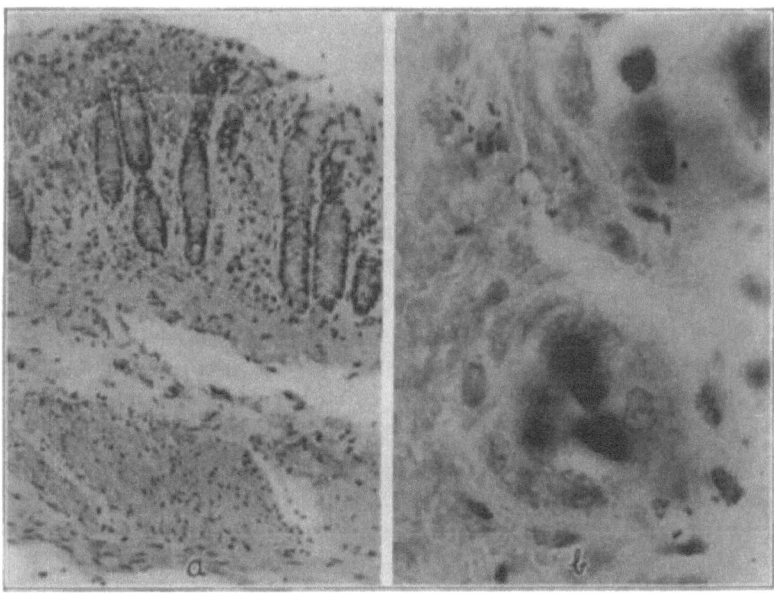

Fig. 5.—Section of transverse colon of a rabbit injected intragastrically with a strain in the fourth animal passage; marked infiltration by red blood corpuscles throughout the mucosa; gram-positive diplococci in the interstitial tissue between the acini. a, Hematoxylin and eosin × 100; b, Gram-Weigert, × 1000.

one or more animal passages. Thus from a series of 176 animals (guinea-pigs, rats, and dogs) injected in various ways with strains from influenza, outspoken hemorrhages of the stomach were noted in 9, hemorrhages or other lesions of the intestines in 12, and hemorrhagic pancreatitis in 5. Cholecystitis did not occur in a single case. The hemorrhages followed injection of the strains as isolated from influenza in 6 instances; the others occurred in animals injected with strains after from one to four animal passages. The lesions of the stomach consisted usually of multiple punctate hemorrhages varying in size, but whether small or large they usually involved considerable areas (fig. 4). Marked edema, and at times necrosis with beginning ulceration of tissue was often associated with the hemorrhages. Post-mortem digestion was often marked. Sections and cultures made in some instances showed that the lesions were the result of localization of streptococci and not due wholly to general toxic effects. Moreover, in nearly all instances the hemorrhage in the stomach occurred only when the virulence was high and when streptococci were isolated from the blood after death. Besides the swelling, hemorrhage, and the edema of Peyer's patches, lymphoid follicles, and mesenteric lymph glands, the most common lesions of the intestinal tract consisted of small but usually numerous hemorrhages of the mucous membrane or submucosa. The hemorrhages were more common in the small intestine but occurred also in the cecum, transverse colon (fig. 4 b), and in one instance in the appendix of a rabbit. The mucous membrane in the area showing hemorrhages was usually covered with a blood tinged mucus. Large amounts of mucus and fluid contents in the intestine were noted in some instances in which the mucous membrane was hyperemic. Peyer's patches and the lymphoid follicles were swollen, but no hemorrhages could be made out. Only a few animals developed outspoken diarrhea. Sections of the intestines through the hemorrhagic areas showed most of the hemorrhages to be in the mucous membrane. The areas were often wedge shaped, with the base toward the lumen, but they extended well into the deeper layers and mucosa, and in some instances into the submucosa. Superficial erosions were noted in some instances, but marked ulcerations were not found. In either case gram-positive diplococci were easily demonstrable throughout the areas, but not in the normal tissues. The diplococci were most numerous near the surface of the hemorrhage, as if the bacteria had been excreted into the lumen of the intestine, but at times they were found in large numbers in the deeper layers of the mucosa. Leukocytic infiltration was quite marked in some instances, and wholly lacking in others. Marked damage to the endothelium of the blood vessels was noted in many sections in, or adjacent to, the areas of hemorrhage and infiltration. In some cases this was evidenced by swelling of the endothelium and irregular staining of the nuclei; in others by the occurrence of masses of desquamated, swollen endothelial cells, with fragmented nuclei, partly or completely plugging the lumina of fair sized vessels. This finding was similar to that of Kuskow in lesions in the intestines in influenza in man. The lesions were particularly common in the vessels in the subperitoneum. More rarely the vessels were filled with leukocytes in which only a few endothelial cells could be found (fig. 4 a). Cultures from the upper intestinal contents, rich in mucus, and of emulsions of washed pieces of hemorrhages from the mucous membrane often yielded a large number of the green-producing streptococci, cultures from the lower respiratory tract usually only colon bacilli. Localization in the intestinal tract rarely occurred following the injection of the hemolytic streptococcus isolated in influenza, but in two instances in which hemorrhages were found, hemolytic streptococci were isolated in large numbers and diplococci were demonstrated in the lesions.

If lesions developed in the pancreas, they were usually severe, and always most marked in the head. They consisted of marked edema, diffuse and circumscribed hemorrhages usually associated with fat necrosis (fig. 4). Sections showed marked separation and degeneration of parenchymatous cells, edema, hemorrhage, and moderate infiltration of interstitial tissue. Some of the capillaries and larger vessels were partially or completely plugged with desquamated and degenerating endothelial cells. Gram stains revealed many diplococci in the thrombosed vessels and throughout the hemorrhagic and edematous areas, but the organisms were not demonstrable in the lumina of vessels and in the tissues, which were unchanged.

The islands of Langerhans were changed little or not at all, and were quite free from bacteria. The lesions noted following the injection after animal passages of strains from cases in which there was no gastro-enteritis, were due to localization of streptococci and not wholly to general toxic effects. They were similar to those noted following injection of the two strains from the cases of gastro-intestinal influenza, similar to those found in persons during the pandemic of 1889 to 1890, and the pandemic of 1918-1919 (Kuskow, Lucke, Wight and Kime). They occurred following intravenous, intraperitoneal, and intratracheal injection, and after introduction into the stomach, duodenum, and lower bowel.

Localization in the gastro-intestinal tract was found to be due largely to peculiar qualities in the streptococci. It occurred in nearly all animals injected with strains from the patients who had similar lesions. It occurred even in different species after injection of some strains isolated from cases of respiratory influenza after one or more animal passages. Thus a strain that produced pancreatitis in a guinea-pig in the second passage produced this condition in the guinea-pig, rat and dog on intravenous injection in the third passage, a property which had disappeared in the fourth passage. The strain from case 2979 was agglutinated specifically by the monovalent antistreptococcus serum from influenza.

The experiments made as a basis of this study suggest that there is a true gastro-intestinal type of influenza and that green-producing streptococci similar to those isolated from the respiratory type of the disease but which tend to localize in the gastro-intestinal tract, are the chief cause. It is not to be concluded, however, that all symptoms in influenza referable to the gastro-intestinal tract are due to localization of bacteria in its mucous membrane. In experiments reported elsewhere [3] it has been shown that the symptoms and findings in influenza are due in part to an anaphylactoid reaction; the severe vomiting and diarrhea noted at the outset of some cases may be an expression of this mechanism.

BIBLIOGRAPHY

[1] Kuskow, N.: Zur pathologischen Anatomie der Grippe, Virchows Arch. f. path. Anat. u. Physiol., 1895, cxxxix, 406-458.

[2] Lucke, B., Wight, T., and Kime, E.: Pathologic Anatomy and Bacteriology of Influenza, Epidemic of Autumn, 1918, Arch. Int. Med., 1919, xxiv, 154-237.

[3] Rosenow, E. C.: Studies in Influenza and Pneumonia. VII. A Study of the Effects Following the Injection of Bacteria Found in Influenza in Normal Throats, in Simple Naso-Pharyngitis, and in Lobar Pneumonia. (This issue, p. 504.)

[4] Sherwood, N. P., Downs, C. M. and McNaught, J. B.: Nonlactose Fermenting Organisms from the Feces of Influenza Patients. Jour. Infect. Dis., 1920, xxvi, 16-22.

STUDIES IN INFLUENZA AND PNEUMONIA

IX. CHANGES IN THE GREEN-PRODUCING STREPTOCOCCUS INDUCED BY SUCCESSIVE ANIMAL PASSAGE AND THEIR SIGNIFICANCE IN EPIDEMIC INFLUENZA

E. C. ROSENOW

Division of Experimental Bacteriology, The Mayo Foundation, Rochester, Minnesota.

In a previous paper [3] it has been shown that the green-producing streptococcus isolated quite constantly in influenza and early in influenzal pneumonia has peculiar and high invasive powers not possessed by the Streptococcus viridans or pneumococci normally present in the upper respiratory tract. By the intratracheal injection of this organism the findings which have come to be regarded as more or less characteristic of influenza have been reproduced. The severity of reaction, the degree of leukopenia, and the mortality in the animals were roughly proportional to the severity of the symptoms, the degree of leukopenia, and the mortality in the patients from whom the strains were isolated. In this paper I shall report the results obtained in the animals following successive animal passage of this strain, the changes induced in the bacteria, and correlate the findings with those noted in patients at different stages of epidemic waves of influenza.

The changes wrought in the green-producing streptococci by successive intratracheal injections as measured by the leukocyte count and mortality are summarized in table 1. It was found that the leukocyte count made twenty-four hours after injection was quite representative of the total reduction in leukocytes, and hence it is used as a standard for comparison. The average count before injection and twenty-four hours after injection, the percentage of reduction in leukocytes, the percentage of animals developing leukopenia, leukocytosis, or no change in the number of leukocytes, respectively, and the mortality percentage were determined for each series of animals. The reduction in leukocytes, and the percentage of animals showing leukopenia run roughly parallel with the mortality rate; the greater the former two, the greater the latter. The average percentage reduction in leukocytes in the first animal passage was 51, in the second 66, in the third 50, and in the fourth 38. The mortality percentage was

57, 100, 57, and 38, respectively. There were a progressive diminution in the percentage of animals showing leukopenia from 92 to 47, an increase in the animals showing leukocytosis, and no change in leukocytes in from 4 to 25 from the first to the fourth animal passage.

I shall now consider the changes wrought in these strains as evidenced by the character of pulmonary and other lesions in guinea-pigs and by the mortality rate following successive intratracheal application.

The technic employed throughout these experiments was uniform. The dose was 0.5 c c of a twenty-four hour dextrose-brain broth, or

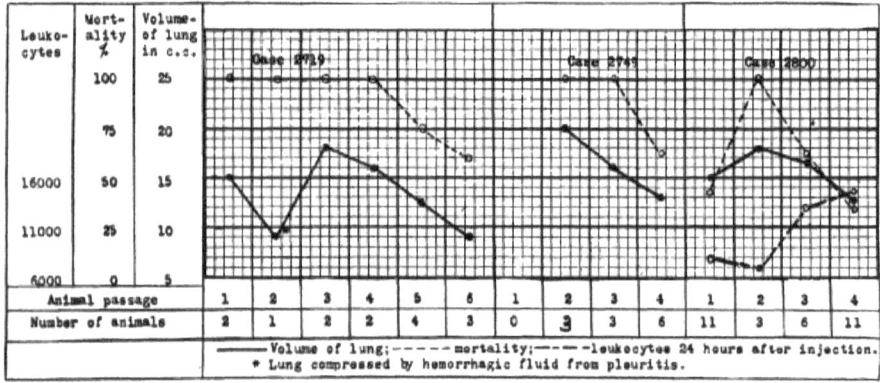

Chart 1.—Volume of lung, mortality and leukocyte count in experimental influenzal pneumonia in guinea-pigs following successive intratracheal injections.

dextrose-blood-broth culture. In order to prove viability and identity of the bacteria injected a plating was made of all cultures which were injected.

The results summarized in chart 1 were obtained from a study of the cases of typical influenza or influenzal pneumonia, and owing to the importance of the findings it is best to consider them separately in some detail.

CASE 2719.—A woman, aged 41, was admitted to the Isolation Hospital Dec. 12, 1918, with a temperature of 103.3, pulse 96, and respiration 31. The patient had been taken sick one week before with headache, backache, aching of the limbs, and fever; this lasted for three or four days, then was less severe until the day before her admission. Examination showed decided cyanosis, moderate dyspnea, scattered râles and areas of dulness, and bronchovesicular breathing over the right lung. Two days later fine râles were heard over both lower lobes and distinct dullness over most of the right lung. December 16, the patient was worse and the right lower lobe was found to be completely consolidated. December 18 the patient became delirious and constantly tried to get out of bed, and at intervals she was markedly cyanotic. In the evening cyanosis grew worse as the respirations became labored and very rapid, and death occurred four hours later.

The white blood count the day after admission was 7,400; no counts were made after that. The sputum December 19 was bloody and

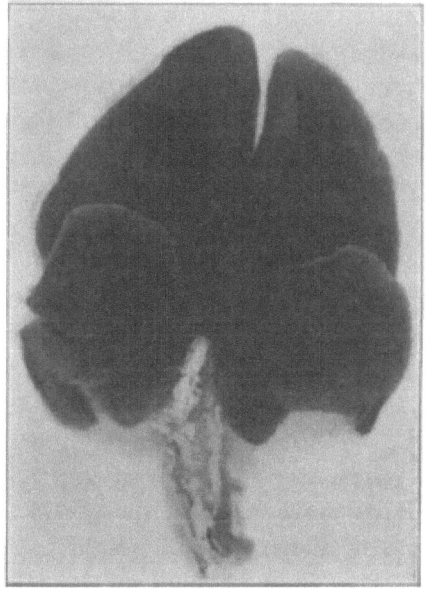

Fig. 1.—Photograph of lung of guinea-pig 853 twenty-four hours after intratracheal injection of green-producing streptococcus from case 2719 in the third animal passage; × 1.

frothy, and the culture showed a large number of characteristic green-producing streptococci and many staphylococci.

The main findings at necropsy were: Lobar pneumonia of the right upper lobe in the gray hepatization stage; bronchopneumonia of the right lower lobe; hemorrhagic edema and edema of the left lower lobe; hypostatic congestion; and emphysema of the left upper lobe. Sections of the lung showed marked congestion, a filling of the alveoli with degenerating red cells, giant cells, degenerating necrotic alveolar epithelial cells in large numbers, and a relatively small number of leukocytes.

The culture from the lung exudate after death contained almost pure growth of the green-producing streptococcus. The washing from a small part of a blood-agar plate was injected intraperitoneally into a guinea-pig; it died in twenty-four hours from peritonitis. The moderately emphysematous lung contained localized hemorrhages and edema. Large numbers of the characteristic streptococcus were found in cultures from the blood and peritoneal fluid. The strain from this animal was used in the successive injection of 20 guinea-pigs; 14 intratracheally and 6 intraperitoneally. The average volume of the lungs and the mortality on successive intratracheal injections are summarized in chart 1. In this series the peritoneal exudate of the first animal was injected directly into the trachea of one guinea-pig (second passage). The culture in dextrose-brain broth from a single colony on a blood-agar plate from the lung of this animal was injected into 2 guinea-pigs (third passage). In the fourth, fifth and sixth passages the primary culture in dextrose-brain broth of the lung of the preceding animal was injected intratracheally.

In order to make sure that the diminution in virulence was not due to cultivation on artificial mediums the emulsion of the lung of one of the sixth passage series was injected directly into the trachea of one guinea-pig. The duration of the successive experiments in animal passages (chart 1) in the animals that furnished the strains for succeeding injections, was one, three, one, one, one, and four days, respectively, or eleven days; the duration of cultivation on artificial mediums between the animal passages was six days, the total seventeen days. Blood-agar plate cultures were made of the exudates of the lung and pleura, the blood, and of the material injected to control the results obtained. No marked change in morphology occurred, but the colonies which at first were quite moist and spreading became smaller and less moist after successive animal passages. None of the strains fermented inulin, nor were they bile soluble. The agglutinating power of the various immune serums, including the monovalent serum, was tested over this strain on isolation, and after one, two, three and four animal passages. It was agglutinated specifically by the monovalent serum for the influenza streptococcus in each of these, but in the fourth passage the strain was less highly differentiated for it was partly agglutinated by type I and type II pneumococcus serums and by antihemolytic streptococcus serum, but to a lesser extent than in the influenza serum. The best measure of the changes which the micro-organism had undergone was found to be its effect on the animals. During the seventeen days of growth differences were noted in the character of the lesions of the lung, and in the mortality.

During the first three animal passages the effects were striking. Intraperitoneal injections were rapidly fatal and the tendency to localize and produce lesions in the lung was marked. The intratracheal injections in the second and third passages were followed by extreme lesions of the lung, consisting of marked exudation of dark hemorrhagic fluid into the alveoli or pleura, and increase in the size of the lung (fig. 1),

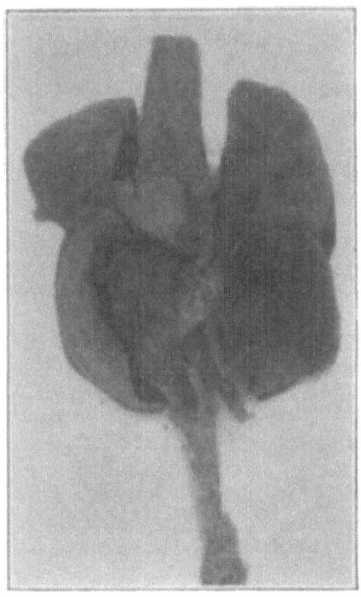

Fig. 2.—Lung of guinea-pig 869 thirty hours after intratracheal injection of the same strain in the fifth animal passage. Note the consolidation of the right diaphragmatic lobe and part of the left diaphragmatic lobe; × 1.

associated with marked degeneration of alveolar epithelium and endothelium (figs. 4 a, 5 a, and 8 a) with relatively slight cellular infiltration and aggregation of large numbers of streptococci along the alveolar lining (figs. 4 b and 5 b). In the fourth passage both guinea-pigs showed relatively less hemorrhagic edema and more leukocytic infiltration. In the fifth passage the difference was striking. In all 4 guinea-pigs well marked areas of consolidation, mostly of lobar distribution, occurred. In 2 this was extremely marked twenty-four (fig. 1) and thirty hours after injection (fig. 2). The consistency of the involved areas was quite firm, the cut surface quite dry, and grayish red, instead of hemorrhagic and edematous as noted in the earlier passages; sections showed marked leukocytic infiltration and relatively slight hemorrhagic edema, and the bacteria were no longer found chiefly along the alveolar lining, but more diffusely distributed throughout the exudate (figs. 6 a and b). In the sixth passage the picture of true pneumonia with no hemorrhagic edema was noted in all of the guinea-pigs injected (fig. 3). Sections showed marked leukocytic infiltration, little hemorrhagic edema, little necrosis of alveolar lining (fig. 8 b) and micro-organisms

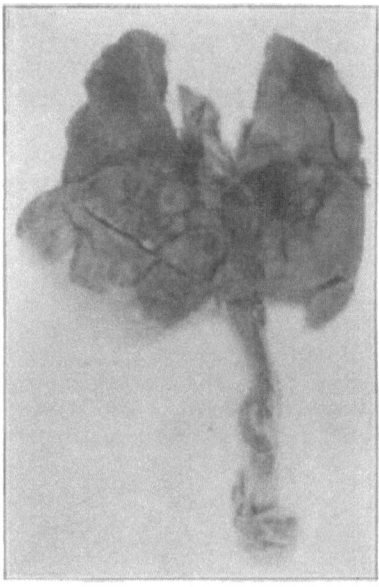

Fig. 3.—Lung of guinea-pig 886 four days after intratracheal injection of the strain in the sixth animal passage. Note the complete grayish consolidation of the left and part of the right diaphragmatic lobe; × 1.

diffusely distributed throughout the exudate (fig. 7). The guinea-pig injected with the lung emulsion from the sixth animal passage developed slightly increased respirations, fever for a few days, and moderate leukocytosis; it then recovered. No pulmonary or other lesions were found when it was chloroformed on the twelfth day. As the gross and microscopic picture of the lung changed from that of a violent destructive reaction with little evidence of response on the part of the host to a less violent reaction in which marked exudation of leukocytes occurred, the volume of the lung and mortality rate decreased. The following experiments are illustrative:

Guinea-pig 820, weighing 370 gm., was injected intratracheally Dec. 23, 1918, with 0.15 c c of a suspension of the peritoneal exudate of a guinea-pig injected intraperitoneally with the sputum from case 2719. December 24 the animal appeared ill. It was short of breath, uncomfortable, made repeated violent efforts at respiration, and coughed violently at intervals. December 26 it was found dead. The pleural cavity contained a moderate amount of bloody turbid fluid. The lungs were only moderately distended (9 c c), and covered with a thin fibrinous film. The left diaphragmatic lobe was large and almost completely consolidated. The areas of consolidation were irregular, and mottled red and gray. Areas of irregular size showing hemorrhagic edema and partial consolidation were found in all the other lobes. The peribronchial lymph glands were edematous and hemorrhagic. The pleural fluid showed many green-producing streptococci; the blood, five colonies of green-producing streptococci; and the pneumonic lung, a large number of green-producing streptococci and a moderate number of staphylococci. In sections of the lung patchy areas of marked leukocytic infiltration were surrounded by areas in which the terminal bronchi were enlarged, the epithelium was desquamated, and the alveoli were greatly distended and completely filled with coagulated serum in which a variable number of red blood corpuscles and relatively few leukocytes were found (fig. 4 a). Exudate in sections stained by the Gram stain showed a large number of diplococci and streptococci which usually were peripherally placed in the alveoli (fig. 4 b). The subpleural and the perivascular lymph channels in areas were completely plugged and distended with gram-positive diplococci and streptococci. In the areas of marked leukocytic infiltration a rather large number of staphylococci were found, whereas in the areas showing hemorrhagic edema, few or none could be demonstrated. Under high power marked nuclear fragmentation and degeneration of epithelial cells and marked necrosis of endothelial cells of the capillaries in the alveoli were observed (fig. 8 a).

Guinea-pig 853, weighing 440 gm., was injected intratracheally Dec. 28, 1918, with 0.5 c c of the dextrose-brain broth culture of the strain isolated from the blood of guinea-pig 820. The animal coughed up immediately a large part of the material injected. December 29 it was found dead. The trachea, larynx, and bronchi were filled with a bloody, frothy fluid. Approximately 5 c c of turbid chocolate colored fluid were found in the pleural cavity. The lungs were voluminous (18 c c), hemorrhagic throughout, and very heavy (fig. 1). The stomach was partially digested and a number of circumscribed areas in the horns of the uterus were congested and swollen. The uterus and vagina contained bloody mucus and the uterine horns a number of submucous hemorrhages. Cultures from the lung, pleural fluid, tracheal mucus, blood, and mucus from the left horn of the uterus showed a large number of the green-producing streptococci. Sections of the lung showed marked dilatation of alveoli and terminal bronchi, extreme congestion of the capillaries and veins, and marked constriction of the larger bronchi which were filled with coagulated serum and blood. There was marked desquamation of the alveolar epithelium and necrosis of the endothelium of the interalveolar capillaries (fig. 5 a). Some areas were slightly infiltrated with leukocytes. The Gram stain showed enormous numbers of diplococci and streptococci. These were especially numerous along the alveolar walls surrounding the bronchi and blood vessels (fig. 5 b). The number of gram-positive diplococci was so large that the outline of the alveoli could be made out readily under the low power of the microscope.

Guinea-pig 869, weighing 330 gm., was injected intratracheally Dec. 31, 1918, with 1 cc of the dextrose-brain broth culture of strain 2719 in the fifth animal passage. January 1 at 1 p. m. the animal was extremely short of breath, it had an expiratory grunt, its hair was ruffled, it was just able to walk, it sat humped up, breathing with all its might, the thorax appeared distended, and the respirations were chiefly abdominal. At 9 p. m. the animal was found dead, the body still warm. The lungs were moderately distended (15 cc); the right lung was almost completely consolidated; the areas of consolidation were quite uniform in consistency and grayish-red. The pleural cavity contained 2 cc of turbid, bloody fluid; the mediastinal lymph glands were edematous and surrounded by bubbles of gas in the mediastinal tissue. One fetus was aborted into the vagina. The area showing its attachment in the left horn of the uterus was hemorrhagic and edematous, and in the right horn was a loosely attached hemorrhagic fetal mass. Other parts of the mucous membrane of the uterus were markedly congested and showed small punctate hemorrhages. Cultures from the blood, liver, spleen, and adrenal were negative; those from the pleural fluid, lung, and the mucous membrane of the uterus and hemorrhagic placenta, showed a large number of green-producing streptococci in pure form. Cultures from the mucous membrane of the nose showed green-producing streptococci and some staphylococci; from the kidney, a few green-producing streptococci. Sections of the consolidated right diaphragmatic lobe presented a very different picture from those in the preceding animals. The alveoli were moderately distended; the epithelial lining only slightly desquamated; the nuclei of these cells and endothelial cells of the capillaries stained normally. The alveoli were filled with a highly cellular exudate consisting largely of polymorphonuclear leukocytes and a relatively small amount of coagulated serum and red blood corpuscles (fig. 6 a). Gram-positive diplococci and streptococci were found in large numbers distributed throughout the alveolar exudate (fig. 6 b).

Guinea-pig 886, weighing 320 gm., was injected intratracheally Jan. 2, 1919, with 1.5 cc of the dextrose-brain-broth culture from the lung of guinea-pig 869. The nostrils, before injection, were dry and clean; cultures from the right nostril showed a large number of indifferent colonies resembling staphylococci. January 3 at 7:30 a. m. the animal appeared quite well, although respirations were definitely increased. At 11 a. m. it appeared well; the respirations were still increased, and cultures from the nose showed a large number of green-producing streptococci and a moderate number of staphylococci. January 4 the nose was wet with a mucopurulent discharge; the weight loss was 50 gm., the respirations were somewhat rapid, and coughing occurred at intervals. January 6, 10 a. m., there was marked crusting about the nostrils almost to the point of causing obstruction, and on removal of the crust, several drops of mucopurulent secretion escaped from the nostril. At 6 p. m. the animal was found dead. The lungs were only slightly distended (9 cc). The left diaphragmatic lobe was completely consolidated and mottled grayish-red; the right diaphragmatic lobe and irregular areas in the right cardiac and apical lobes showed grayish consolidations surrounding the bronchi (fig. 3). The left nostril was plugged with a bloody, mucopurulent material. The right maxillary sinus was filled with bloody pus; the mucous membrane of the nose, trachea, and bronchi was extremely hyperemic. Cultures from the blood were negative. Cultures from the pleura, consolidated areas of the lung, and pus from the nose showed a large number of green-producing streptococci and some staphylococci. Sections of the lung showed slight dilatation of the alveoli, marked cellular leukocytic exudate of quite uniform distribution filling the alveoli completely, with little or no admixture of coagulated serum and blood (fig. 7 a). The epithelial cells lining the terminal bronchi and alveoli, and the endothelial cells of the inter-alveolar capillaries stained quite normally (fig. 8 b). The bacteria were diffusely distributed in large numbers in the alveolar exudate (fig. 7 b).

CASE 2749.—A man, aged 29, a nurse, developed headache, sore throat, severe aching all over, dry cough, and temperature.of 100.2, Dec. 16, 1918. The following day his temperature ranged from 102.6 to 103. The headache continued, there were marked backache, soreness through the chest, and a severe cough. December 18 the patient felt weak, perspired, and was chilly at intervals; the ache in the back, soreness in the chest, and the cough were worse. The temperature ranged from 100.6 to 101.8. The cough and soreness in the

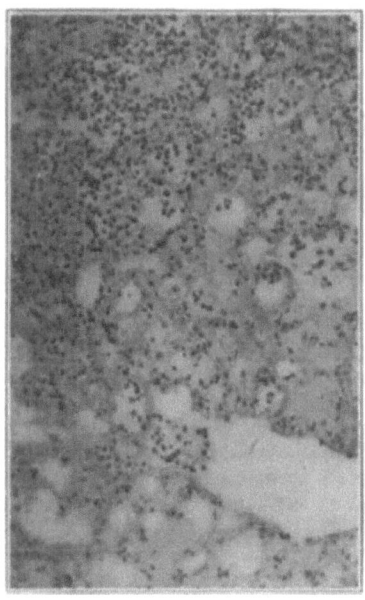
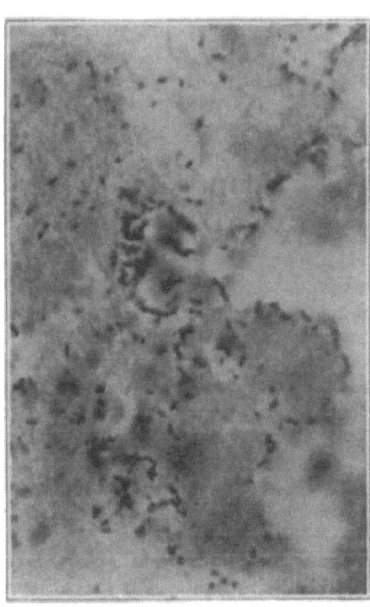

A   B

Fig. 4.—Photomicrograph of sections of lung of guinea-pig injected with the green-producing streptococcus from case 2719 after one animal passage. Note the marked edema, hemorrhage, dilatation of terminal bronchi and alveoli, necrosis of cells in alveolar walls and the relatively slight leukocytic infiltration in a, and the distribution of the bacteria along the alveolar wall in b. a. Hematoxylin and eosin; × 100. b. Gram-Weigert; × 500.

chest continued for a week; the nose bled December 22, and a large amount of mucopurulent blood-tinged sputum was raised December 23. This sputum was cultured and injected into animals. The temperature became normal December 23 and the patient made a good but slow recovery. Blood-agar plate cultures from the sputum showed almost pure culture of moist, spreading, green-producing streptococci, a few staphylococci, no hemolytic streptococci, nor influenza bacilli. The sputum, 0.2 c c was injected subcutaneously into a guinea-pig; it died three days later of subcutaneous cellulitis, beginning bronchopneumonia, and hemorrhagic endometritis. Cultures from the blood, lung, and bloody mucus from the uterus, contained a large number of the characteristic green-producing streptococcus colonies. The culture from the uterus was used to inject 7 guinea-pigs, 4 intravenously, and 3 intratracheally, and 2 rats, one subcutaneously, the other intratracheally. All died as a result of the injection. All 4 animals injected intravenously showed moderate emphysema and evidence of localization in the lung, indicated by localized areas of hemorrhage and edema with or without beginning consolidation. The 2 females showed lesions of the mucous membrane of the uterus and both aborted. Two showed, in addition, localization in muscles and myocardium, one acute peritonitis, and one marked hemorrhagic pancreatitis. Cultures from all yielded the organism injected, together with a few staphylococci, and in one a few colonies of hemolytic streptococci developed from the lung and uterus. All 3 guinea-pigs and the rat injected intratracheally died from emphysema of the lungs filled with hemorrhagic bloody fluid, or with bronchopneumonia in various stages of development. The average volume of the lung in the guinea-pigs was 20 cc (chart 1). The rat and 2 of the guinea-pugs showed decided involvment of the pleura in addition to the lung involvement. The only female injected aborted; one of the others showed peritonitis and one hemorrhage and edema of the head of the pancreas. The characteristic streptococcus was isolated from all. The rat injected subcutaneously died in three days from subcutaneous cellulitis, emphysema, and slight hemorrhages of the lung. The green-producing streptococcus was found in the edema fluid and in the bloody mucus in the uterine horns.

The primary culture in dextrose broth from the pancreas, which showed marked swelling and inflammation, was injected intravenously into 2 guinea-pigs and 2 dogs; intratracheally into a guinea-pig and a rat; intraperitoneally into a mouse, and subcutaneously into a rat. All the animals except the dogs died. Both guinea-pigs injected intravenously developed well marked areas of localized bronchopneumonia, and one developed acute hemorrhagic pancreatitis and myocardial degeneration. The dogs were etherized on the fifth day. Lung lesions were absent, but there were lesions in the mucous membrane of the uterus; the one animal that had aborted showed pancreatitis. The green-producing streptococcus was isolated from the mucous membrane of the uterus in both dogs, from the blood of both guinea-pigs, and from the pancreas of the dog showing pancreatitis. The guinea-pig and rat that were injected intratracheally developed marked rhinitis and tracheitis, emphysema of the lung with hemorrhagic edema, and bronchopneumonia. The guinea-pig had endometritis and aborted. The rat injected subcutaneously and the mouse intraperitoneally developed, beside cellulitis and peritonitis, respectively, definite lesions of lung and pleura, from which the organism was isolated.

The primary culture from the hemorrhagic lung of one of the guinea-pigs injected intratracheally in the second animal passage was injected intratracheally into 2 guinea-pigs. Both developed massive bronchopneumonia and purulent bronchitis, and both yielded the organisms in pure cultures. The filtrate from this lung was injected directly intratracheally into 2 guinea-pigs, and after incubation in dextrose-brain broth into 4 guinea-pigs. One of the latter remained well, all the others developed well marked lesions of the lung, quite similar to those in the animals injected with the corresponding culture. The 2 females had endometritis, 3 had rhinitis, sinusitis, tracheitis, and bronchitis, and 1 each had myositis and mediastinitis. Cultures from the lesions and the blood in these yielded the characteristic organism. The details of these and other filtrate experiments have been given elsewhere.

Cultures from 3 of the animals injected with this strain in the third passage were injected intratracheally into 5 guinea-pigs. All developed moderate emphysema and bronchopneumonia of lobar type, 2 developed high grade myocardial degeneration, and 2 marked rhinitis and bronchitis. Two of the females had endometritis. The primary culture in dextrose-brain broth from the pneumonic lung of 2 of the guinea-pigs, third animal passage series, was injected intratracheally into 4 guinea-pigs, and cultures from the uterine horns of the dog that had aborted were injected into 2 guinea-pigs. One of the former and one of the latter recovered after several days of illness. The others died from two to four days after injection. All showed well marked exudative pneumonia, 2 definitely lobar in type with relatively slight hem-

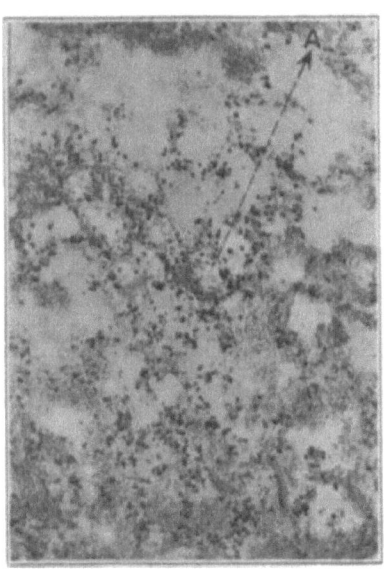
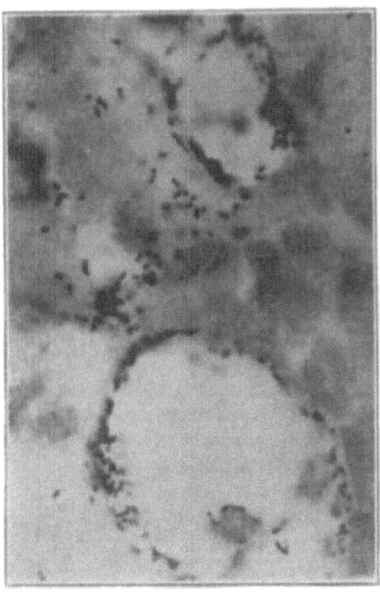

A B

Fig. 5.—Sections of lung of guinea-pig shown in figure 1. Note the marked hemorrhage and edema, the absence of leukocytic infiltration and the marked necrosis of alveolar walls in a, and the peripherally placed streptococci in b. a. Hematoxylin and eosin, × 100. b. Gram-Weigert, × 500.

orrhagic edema, and only moderate emphysema (chart 1). Two of the 3 females had endometritis and myocardial degeneration and 2 had well marked rhinitis, and tracheitis; 1 had hemorrhages in the rectus muscle. The green-producing streptococcus was isolated from all. The filtrate from the lung of 2 of the guinea-pigs (third animal passage series) was injected into the trachea of 12 guinea-pigs. The 2 that were injected with the heated filtrate recovered after severe immediate symptoms of anaphylactic shock, 1 injected with the unheated filtrate died in ten minutes from anaphylactic shock, 6 of the others recovered after severe immediate symptoms, and 3 died. All showed bronchopneumonia; 2 showed marked lesions of the pleura, and 1 aborted. The green-producing streptococcus was isolated from the lesions, and from the uterus of the one that aborted. The curves giving the volume of the lung and the mortality rate (chart 1) represent roughly the effects from the successive injections of this strain. The difference in the symptoms and types of lesions of the lung in the early and in the later animal passages was striking. In the former respiratory embarrassment, hemorrhage, and edema with relatively slight exudation of leukocytes in the lung dominated the picture; in the latter, respiratory embarrassment was less marked; exudative pneumonia, and a relatively slight edema with a greater tendency to involve the upper respiratory tract as well as the pleura, dominated the picture. The greater tendency of leukocytic infiltration was noted even in animals that lived the same length of time. The results on intravenous injection of the organism in the second and third passages, besides showing a tendency to localize in the lung and uterus, showed a marked affinity for the muscle, myocardium, and pancreas; pancreatitis occurred in three species of animals (guinea-pig, dog and rabbit). The lesions in the muscles were focal and hemorrhagic, often occurring in clusters, and often surrounded by edema and hemorrhage. Streptococci were found in large numbers in these lesions and in the pancreas, showing pancreatitis. Altogether 19 animals (guinea-pigs, rats, and mice) were injected with this strain intratracheally, intravenously, intraperitoneally, and subcutaneously, in the first, second, and third animal passages. All succumbed to the effects of the injection. Two of the 6 injected in the fourth passage recovered.

CASE 2800.—A woman, aged 24, was admitted to the isolation hospital Jan. 9, 1919, in a very weak condition with a temperature of 104, pulse 120, and respiration 34. The patient had been taken sick six days before with aching of limbs, headache, backache, chills and fever. She complained of pain over the entire chest, and coughed a great deal. The day after admission, her respirations were shallow and labored, she was pale and cyanotic, and the pulse was extremely rapid. A diffuse bronchopneumonia of the right base and bronchial breathing in the area opposite the angle of the scapula on the left side were found. January 12 her condition was very much the same; the chest was in full expansion and respirations were almost wholly diaphragmatic. The symptoms persisted, she grew worse as cyanosis increased and died January 14. The leukocyte count was persistently low, ranging between 1,900 and 3,700.

The chief findings at necropsy were: Bilateral pseudolobar pneumonia; hemorrhagic edema; left hemo-hydro-thorax, 500 c c; and mild acute nephritis. Sections of the lung showed dilatation of alveoli, marked congestion, and alveolar exudate rich in red blood corpuscles, edema fluid, little fibrin, and only a moderate number of leukocytes.

A culture from a throat swab January 12 showed a large number of moist, spreading colonies of green-producing streptococci, many colonies of Staphylococcus aureus, and moist hemolyzing streptococci. Cultures from the blood after death contained green-producing streptococci, hemolyzing streptocci, and staphylococci; and from cultures from the pleural fluid hemolyzing streptococci and staphyloccocci. The history and findings in this case are clearly those of influenza in which well marked lung lesions developed as the symptoms persisted.

The bacteria isolated from the sputum, blood, and lung exudate were a mixture of the organisms most constantly present in influenza. Aside from hemolysis the morphology and type of colony of the green-producing streptococci and hemolyzing streptococci were identical. It was thought worth while to study the effects, including the leukocyte counts, of the injection of mass cultures containing a mixture of these strains, and of pure cultures in a large series of animals in order to note the changes which might occur in the lesions produced following successive animal passage. The effect of intratracheal injections of cultures of the green-producing and hemolytic streptococci or mixtures that occurred in the primary dextrose-brain broth from the blood, and sputum, throat, and lung exudates were very similar. Emphysema of marked grade and hemorrhagic edema with localized areas of peribronchial consolidation of varying size and age dominated the picture. Leukopenia was equally marked regardless of whether the strain was hemolytic or green-producing. The results obtained following successive intratracheal injections of the green-producing streptococci are summarized in

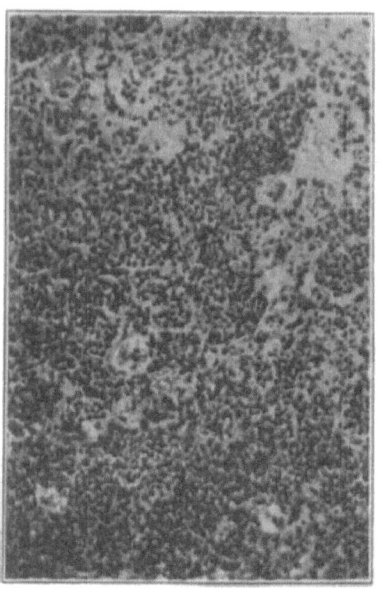 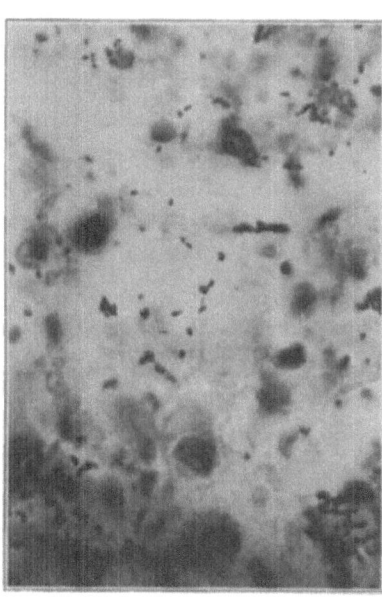

A B

Fig. 6.—Sections of lung shown in figure 2. Note the marked leukocytic infiltration and the slight edema and hemorrhage, and the diffuse distribution of the streptococci in the exudate. a. Hematoxylin and eosin, × 100. b. Gram-Weigert, × 500.

chart 1. In this series of animals the strains used for subsequent injections were first plated on blood-agar. From this subcultures of green-producing streptococci were made in dextrose-brain broth and injected.

It will be noted that during the first and second animal passages, as the volume of lung (severity of reaction) increased, the mortality increased, the drop in leukocytes occurred, and as the volume of lung diminished during the third and fourth passages the mortality and the drop in leukocytes became less marked. The difference in the character of lesions in the lungs was similar to the difference noted between cases 2719 and 2749.

It has been pointed out elsewhere that the green-producing streptococci may acquire typical hemolyzing power (beta type hemolysis), and that the hemolyzing streptococci may acquire the power of producing typical green colonies (alpha type hemolysis). Moreover, a green-producing flora in patients is often displaced by a hemolytic flora and this in turn by a green-producing flora, especially in patients who recover. It was thought worth while to pass the hemolytic streptococcus through a series of guinea-pigs in the same manner as the green-producing streptococcus had been passed, and to observe whether or not the type of lesion produced changed, and whether the streptococcus changed. The primary culture in dextrose-brain broth of the throat swab was injected into the trachea of 6 guinea-pigs and a rat. Two of the guinea-pigs and the rat recovered. Four of the guinea-pigs died from typical lung lesions with or without pleural involvement, and all showed hemolytic streptococci in pure culture, or together with a few staphylococci.

Guinea-pig 947, weighing 400 gm., was injected intratracheally Jan. 12, 1919, 11 a.m., with 1.5 c c dextrose-brain broth culture of the throat swab. A blood-agar plate of the culture injected showed green-producing, hemolytic streptococci, and a few staphylococci. At 6 p.m. the respirations were rapid, the voice was weak, and the animal appeared ill. January 13, 7:30 a.m., the animal was found dead. A large amount of hemolyzed, dark chocolate colored fluid was found in the pleural cavity. The right diaphragmatic and intermediate lobes were large, extremely hemorrhagic and edematous on the cut surface. Both uterine horns contained a moderate amount of blood tinged mucus, and the mucous membrane was hemorrhagic in areas. Cultures from the blood and from the lung and pleural fluid showed a large number of hemolytic streptococci, a smaller number of staphylococci, but no green-producing streptococci; those from the mucus in the left horn of the uterus showed 150 colonies of staphylococci, 9 colonies of hemolytic streptococci, and 21 colonies of green-producing streptococci. The primary culture of the pleural fluid of this animal which yielded hemolytic streptococci and a few staphylococci was then injected into the trachea of another guinea-pig; it died within six hours. The leukocyte count dropped from 15,000 before injection to 3,100 after death. The lungs were huge in size (18 c c) hemorrhagic and edematous throughout, and the pleura contained about 1 c c of hemorrhagic fluid. Cultures from the blood, pleural fluid, and lung exudate showed many moist, spreading colonies of hemolytic streptococci, while those from the liver and kidney showed a few. The dextrose-broth culture from the blood of this guinea-pig was injected into the trachea of 5 guinea-pigs. One recovered and 4 died of hemorrhagic edema and bronchopneumonia, from one to four days after injection; two died with hemorrhagic pleuritis and 2 without. All showed predominating or pure cultures of green-producing streptococci. The findings in the animal whose strain was passed to the next series were similar to those in the others.

Guinea-pig 1043, weighing 480 gm., was injected intratracheally Jan. 23, 1919, with 2 c c of the glucose-broth culture from the blood of the guinea-pig that died six hours after injection. The leukocyte count was 16,800. January 24, 10 a.m., the respiration was extremely rapid, the leukocyte count was 2,200; at 9 p.m. respiration was extremely rapid, the animal was weaker, it made repeated violent efforts at breathing, resembling anaphylactic shock, and had an expiratory grunt. January 25 it was found dead. The pleural cavity contained a moderate amount of bloody chocolate colored fluid. The left diaphragmatic lobe was covered with a fibrinous film. The lung was greatly distended (18 c c) and heavy (17 gm.). A large part of the left lung was consolidated, consisting of coalescing areas of bronchopneumonia, which in places on the cut surface had become grayish and quite dry. Several

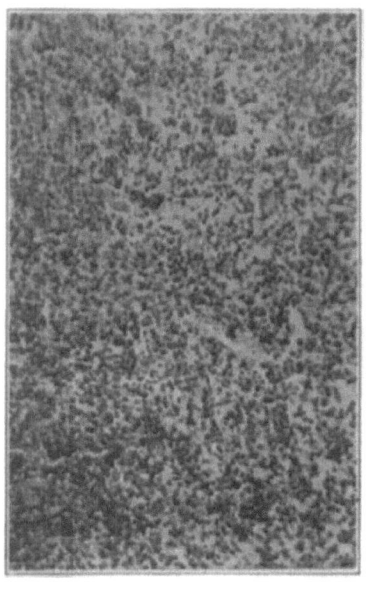
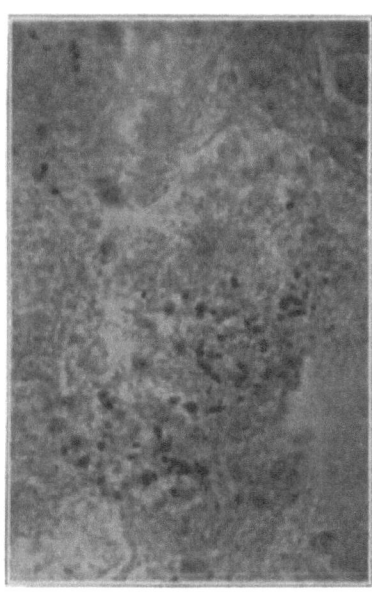

A   B

Fig. 7.—Section of lung shown in figure 3. Findings similar to those in figure 6. a. Hematoxylin and eosin, × 100. b. Gram-Weigert, × 500.

similar but smaller areas were found in the right diaphragmatic lobe. Generally the mucous membranes of the nose and trachea were extremely hyperemic and the trachea was filled with a hemorrhagic frothy fluid. A large area (2 by 1.5 cm.) of hemorrage and edema was found in the right rectus muscle of the adominal wall. The involved muscle was friable and ruptured on slight stretching. The leukocyte count of the blood from the heart was 4,400. The myocardium was yellowish gray, the ventricles were in firm contraction, and the auricles dilated. Cultures from the blood, pleural fluid, and lung showed a large number of green-producing streptococci in pure culture, and the liver, adrenal, kidney, brain, and spleen, showed a few. The culture in dextrose broth from the blood after one plating was injected into the trachea of 3 guinea-pigs; 1 of these died of bronchopneumonia in forty-eight hours,

1 recovered, and 1 was chloroformed three days after injection. The third had a moderate amount of bloody fluid in the right pleural cavity, a large wedge-shaped area of grayish consolidation of the right diaphragmatic lobe, and slight emphysema of the lung. The uterus was opaque and contained a moderate amount of mucus. The leukocyte count before injection was 9,400; twenty-four hours after injection 10,400; forty-eight hours after injection 7,200; and after death 8,000. Cultures from the blood were negative; those from the consolidated lung showed large numbers of staphylococci and green-producing streptococci, and the pleural fluid and uterus showed a few green-producing streptococci and staphylococci. This, then, is an example in which a hemolytic streptococcus remained as such throughout two animal passages, but in 4 animals in the third passage it appeared to lose the hemolytic power and to produce green colonies, a property which it retained through the next animal passage. Fifty-three guinea-pigs were injected with cultures of green-producing and hemolytic streptococci isolated from this case and after animal passage. Twenty-three were injected in the first passage, 14 (60%) died; 9 were injected in the second passage, 8 (90%) died; 9 were injected in the third passage, 7 (78%) died; and 14 were injected in the fourth passage, 6 (43%) died.

The average mortality resulting from the animal passage after intratracheal injection of the strains from the 3 cases reported herewith was 57 per cent. of 22 animals injected in the first animal passage, 90 per cent. of 10 animals in the second, 87 per cent. of 16 animals in the third; and 55 per cent. of 22 animals in the fourth. The total mortality, irrespective of the place of injection, ranged as follows: 60 per cent. of the 30 animals injected in the first animal passage, 94 per cent. of the 17 animals in the second, 90 per cent. of the 21 animals in the third, and 52 per cent. of the 19 animals in the fourth passage.

A study of the 3 cases shows clearly that the lesions in the lung in the first few passages resemble very closely those noted in the lungs of the 2 patients who died. They are characterized by marked emphysema, extreme hemorrhage and edema of the lungs (fig. 1), marked evidence of destruction and desquamation of epithelial lining (figs. 3 and 4 a), absence of staining or fragmentation of nuclei of endothelial cells, of capillaries of alveoli (Fig. 8 a), and aggregation of streptococci along the alveolar lining (figs. 3 b and 4 b). Moreover, the relative lack of response, on the part of the host, is evidenced by the slight leukocytic exudation in the lung and the marked reduction of leukocytes in the blood. The symptoms of respiratory embarrassment are often extreme, the mortality rate is high, and death occurs early. After a number of animal passages the picture becomes quite different. The respiratory embarrassment is less violent, the reduction in leukocytes less marked, and the exudation of leukocytes in the lung is the dominant picture (figs. 6 a and 7 a) as hemorrhage and edema become less prominent. The lungs are not so voluminous (figs. 2 and 3). Degeneration and desquamation of the epithelial cells and necrosis of the capillaries are slight (fig. 8 b) and the bacteria are diffusely distributed throughout the exudate instead of along the alveolar lining (figs. 6 b and 7 b). The difference in amount of leukocytic infiltration depends not on the duration of the experiment, but varies with the number of animal passages. The diminution of virulency of these strains from

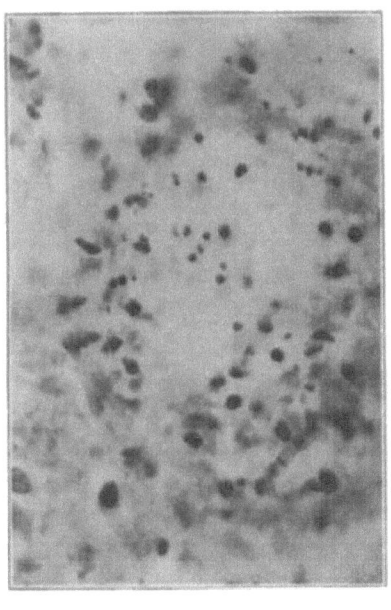 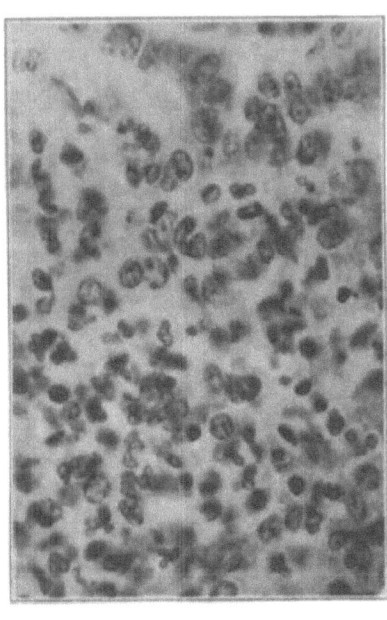

A B

Fig. 8.—High-power magnification of sections of lungs shown in figures 4 and 7, illustrating type of lesions obtained during the first few and higher numbers of animal passages. a. Note the marked fragmentation of nuclei of alveolar epithelium and capillaries, the marked hemorrhage and edema, and the almost complete absence of leukocytic infiltration. b. Note the marked leukocytic infiltration and the relatively slight necrosis of cells of alveolar walls. Hematoxylin and eosin, × 500.

cases of influenza as a result of successive intratracheal injections is contrary to the result following successive intraperitoneal injection of strains of the pneumostreptococcus group. The latter method was tested to determine whether the green-producing streptococcus from influenza is peculiar in this respect.

In chart 2 is given a summary of the results of successive intraperitoneal and intratracheal injections of a series of strains of green-producing streptococci from influenza. In the forced experiment on intraperitoneal injection the virulency of the green-producing streptococci increases as that of streptococci and pneumococci from other sources. But when the former micro-organisms are applied successively to the normal mucous membrane of the lower respiratory tract their invasive power increases only during one or two animal passages; it then becomes progressively less during three or four subsequent passages. Most of the strains that were passed through animals were cultivated on artificial mediums for one generation and in one strain

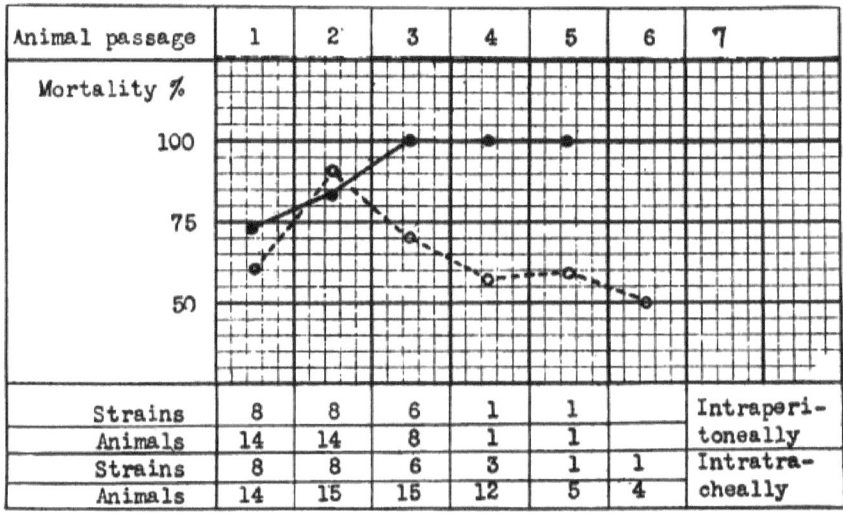

Chart 2.—Mortality in guinea-pigs following successive intraperitoneal and intratracheal injections of streptococci from influenza. The straight line denotes intraperitoneal injection; the broken line denotes intratracheal injection.

(case 2800), for two generations between each passage. In order to make sure that the diminution in invasive power on successive intratracheal application was due to effects exerted on the micro-organism by the body cells or fluids and not due to the culture mediums, control experiments were carried out; emulsions of the consolidated lung were injected directly from animal to animal. The results were similar. The diminution in infecting power was even more rapid than when intervening cultures were injected. This result, contrary to what might be expected, considering what usually happens after direct successive intraperitoneal injections, is in keeping with what has been observed repeatedly when emulsions of lung and pleural fluid from man and from animals are injected directly into the trachea and compared with the results following the injection of the corresponding cultures. The severity of reaction and the mortality following injections of the cultures were greater even when the number of viable bacteria was no larger than that in the exudate. The cells or fluids in the exudate seemed to rob the bacteria of their bite, as it were, a property which they often regained during the growth in suitable artificial mediums. Moreover, in harmony with this idea is the fact that the mortality was higher following the injection of sputum during life than following the injection of the bloody lung exudate after death. During the course of the experiments on intratracheal injection it was also noted that cultures of the green-producing streptococci from the blood and pleural exudate after death in cases of long standing were not so virulent as those from the sputum or throat. Thus in 22 guinea-pigs injected intratracheally with the strains cultured from the sputum of one patient the mortality was 64 per cent., whereas in a series injected with the strains cultured from the blood the mortality was 33 per cent.

Hirsch and McKinney found that the pneumococci at the height of the epidemic at Camp Grant were far more virulent when injected intraperitoneally or intravenously in animals than those isolated as the epidemic was subsiding, and, moreover, the strains isolated from the blood at the height of the epidemic were less virulent than those from the sputum.

EXPERIMENTS SUGGESTING THE OCCURRENCE OF MUTATION IN VIVO

It has been shown elsewhere that marked changes occurred in the bacterial flora in the later stages of influenzal infection, that similar changes often occurred in vitro, and that the new strains or variants were not only virulent on injection in animals, but also tended to produce leukopenia. Following intratracheal injection the changes in the lung closely simulated those of influenzal infection.

Owing to the instability of the streptococci from influenza noted at the onset of this work, we have taken particular pains to observe whether the changes noted in patients and in vitro might occur in the body of the experimental animal. A striking example of the mutation of a hemolytic streptococcus into a green-producing streptococcus simultaneously in a series of guinea-pigs has been detailed in the experiments recorded in case 2800. The lesions produced by the intratracheal injection method resembled closely those observed following injection of the green-producing streptococcus from influenza.

On the other hand, the green-producing streptococcus often appeared to become a hemolytic streptococcus. Thus in case 2749 one of four guinea-pigs injected intravenously with a pure culture of green-producing streptococcus from the blood of a guinea-pig injected subcutaneously with the sputum, showed a moderate number of hemolytic streptococci and Staphylococcus aureus in the pleural fluid, hemorrhagic areas in the lung, hemorrhagic mucus in the uterine horns, and in the pancreas. The pancreas showed a moderate number of green-producing streptococci. The green-producing streptococcus from 2 animals in the second-passage series were injected in various ways into 7 guinea-pigs, 2 rats, 2 dogs, and a mouse. The organism injected was isolated in pure form from all the guinea-pigs, one rat, and one dog. One rat injected subcutaneously yielded a large number of the green-producing streptococci from the blood and subcutaneous tissues, and from the latter a moderate number of Staphylococcus aureus also. The mouse injected intraperitoneally died in forty-eight hours from hemorrhagic peritonitis and pleuritis. The blood and pleural fluid yielded a moderate number of green-producing streptococci, slightly hemolytic streptococci, and Staphylococcus aureus. The one dog which aborted following intravenous injection had a large number of moist spreading hemolytic streptococci, and a moderate number of staphylococci in the bloody mucus of both uterine horns, and the blood yielded a few colonies of green-producing streptococci. The culture in dextrose-brain broth of the hemolytic streptococcus from the uterus, and the green-producing streptococcus from the blood were injected intratracheally into one guinea-pig each. The first animal showed leukopenia for forty-eight hours, then leukocytosis, and died on the third day with distended lungs (17 c c) showing marked exudative pneumonia of pseudolobar type (14 gm.). The lung and pleura yielded green-producing streptococci. The second animal showed a progressive and marked leukopenia and died with similar lung findings the day of injection. Cultures from the blood and kidney showed a few colonies of green-producing streptococci in pure form, while the pneumonic lung and mucus in the right horn of the uterus showed the green-producing streptococci and Staphylococcus aureus.

The results in case 2851 are similar to those observed in others. The patient developed an attack of influenza of ordinary severity, but on the sixth day became suddenly worse and died on the eighth day from acute hemorrhagic edema and bronchopneumonia. The sputum on the second day was mucoid and contained a large number of the green-producing streptococci, a few slightly hemolyzing streptococci, and a few staphylococci. On the seventh day the sputum was blood-tinged but purulent, and showed Staphylococcus aureus in pure form in large number. Permission for necropsy could not be obtained, but a syringe-full of bloody fluid was withdrawn from the left pleural cavity. The blood-agar plate inoculated with this fluid contained a large number of Staphylococcus aureus and a few moist slightly hemolyzing colonies of streptococci. The culture in dextrose-brain broth from a single well isolated colony of the slightly hemolytic streptococcus from the pleural fluid was injected into the tracheas of 3 guinea-pigs. Pure growth of slightly hemolyzing colonies of streptococci was obtained from the blood-agar plate of the culture injected. In all 3 guinea-pigs there was a reduction in leukocytes in from twenty-four to forty-eight hours after injection; the average count before injection was 12,900, twenty-four hours after injection 7,600, and forty-eight hours after injection 8,260. The animals seemed quite well three days after injection, when they were chloroformed. All had bronchopneumonia, and the one female had endometritis with hemorrhagic mucus in both uterine horns. None had pleuritis. In 2 the cultures from the blood were sterile; cultures from the blood of the female contained a few colonies of streptococci. Cultures from the pneumonic lung of all yielded a pure culture of Staphylococcus aureus. The hemorrhagic mucus in the uterine horns yielded Staphylococcus aureus and a few colonies of green-producing streptococci. Cultures from the adrenal, kidney, spleen and liver were sterile.

The culture in dextrose-brain broth from a single well isolated colony of Staphylococcus aureus which showed no streptococci in smears and only staphylococcus colonies on plating was injected intra-tracheally into a guinea-pig; it died in twenty-four hours from hemorrhagic edema of the lung. The pleural cavity was filled with hemorrhagic fluid, and the visceral pleura was covered with a thin fibrinous film. The leukocyte count of 12,400 before injection dropped to 3,400. Blood-agar-plate cultures from the blood, pleural fluid, lung, kidney and liver showed Staphylococcus aureus in large numbers, those from the adrenal and spleen a few. A few colonies of moist spreading green-producing streptococci in addition to Staphylococcus aureus were isolated from the pleural fluid and lung. A culture in a tall tube of dextrose broth from a single well isolated green-producing colony of the streptococcus from the pleural fluid was made and injected intratracheally into 2 guinea-pigs and intraperitoneally into 1. The latter showed a drop in leukocytes of from 19,000 to 7,600 twenty-four hours after injection, and then recovered. One of the former, a female, died in two days from hemorrhagic edema of the lung, bronchopneumonia, a large amount of hemorrhagic fluid in the pleural cavity, and hemorrhagic endometritis. Cultures from the blood, uterus, lung and pleural fluid revealed a large number of moist spreading green-producing streptococci, and a few Staphylococcus aureus; those from the adrenal, spleen, liver, and brain contained a smaller number of both. The leukocyte count dropped from 6,600 before injection to 2,000 twenty-four hours after injection. No count was made after death. The other pig injected intratracheally had a drop of from 14,200 to 10,000 leukocytes, and increased respiration for a few days; it then seemingly recovered, but died seventeen days after the injection. Serofibrinous pleuritis and peritonitis were found. There were no lesions of the lung. Cultures from the blood remained sterile, while those from the peritoneal exudate contained many colonies of Staphylococcus aureus in pure form. The blood-agar plate made at the time the culture was injected into these animals showed a pure growth of a green-producing streptococcus, and after the same tube was incubated for fifteen days a blood-agar plate showed a moderate number of rather dry green-producing and slightly hemolyzing colonies of streptococci and a large number of colonies of staphylococci.

A dextrose-brain broth culture from a single green-producing colony from the blood of the female guinea-pig that died from hemorrhagic edema and pleuritis was injected into the trachea of one guinea-pig. The leukocyte count dropped from 15,800 to 4,000 in twenty-four hours, respiration was increased moderately for a few days, and the animal then recovered. The strain was lost.

This case is an example of a predominant green-producing streptococcal flora noted early in influenza being replaced by Staphylococcus aureus. Hemorrhagic pleural fluid after death showed a preponderance of the Staphylococcus aureus and a few slightly hemolytic streptococci. A subculture from a single colony of the latter proved only moderately virulent, and in all the guinea-pigs staphylococci only were isolated from the lesions in the lung as recovery seemed assured. The staphylococcus culture from a single colony was extremely virulent. The hemorrhagic lung and pleural fluid yielded, in addition to the staphylococcus, a few colonies of green-producing streptococci. A culture from a single colony of the latter, which showed no staphylococci when injected, yielded staphylococci in both of 2 guinea-pigs as well as in the culture tube after prolonged cultivation. The green-producing strain in the next animal passage produced marked leukopenia, increased respiration for a time, and then was lost as recovery ensued.

In case 2608 the sputum was injected directly intraperitoneally into a guinea-pig. It died from peritonitis. The blood showed the green-producing streptococcus in pure culture; the peritoneal fluid showed this organism and Staphylococcus aureus in moderate number. A well isolated single colony of the former was inoculated into glucose-brain broth. The twenty-four-hour culture was injected intraperitoneally into a guinea-pig. The blood-agar plate of this culture yielded only green-producing streptococci. The guinea-pig died in three days of hemorrhagic fibrinous peritonitis, pericarditis and pancreatitis. The leukocyte count dropped from 6,000 before injection to 4,480 in twenty-four hours, and to 3,600 in forty-eight hours. The cultures from the blood showed a pure growth of green-producing streptococci, whereas the pericardial and peritoneal fluid showed these together with a moderate number of the Staphylococcus aureus. In order to test whether or not the staphylococci found in the pericardial exudate possessed virulency, a culture in dextrose-brain broth from a single colony was injected intraperitoneally into a guinea-pig in the usual dosage (0.5 c c per 100 gm. weight). It died in three days from hemorrhagic peritonitis, with localized areas of hemorrhage and edema in the lungs. The leukocyte counts were 9,200 before injection, 3,200, 6,000, and 3,240, respectively, twenty-four and forty-eight hours later, and after death. Cultures from the peritoneal fluid and blood yielded a pure growth of Staphylococcus aureus.

A summary of a large number of experiments in animals injected with cultures proved to be pure by plate cultures, reveals that apparent mutations occurred in 11 of 75 injected intraperitoneally and intravenously, and in 14 of 73 injected intratracheally.

It is realized that the finding in these animals of bacteria that were not introduced might be interpreted as secondary invasion, if it were not for the fact that these mutation forms develop in the test tube under controlled conditions. Indeed until the pure line requirement and the remote possibility of contamination from the air in the test-tube experiments are met, conclusions with regard to the mutation of streptococci into staphylococci and mutation of influenza bacilli cannot be drawn. However, from a consideration of the precautions which have been taken to exclude accidental contamination, the regularity of its occurrence under certain conditions, and the high virulency of the staphylococci which at times displace the streptococcal flora in fulminating cases of influenzal pneumonia and the high and peculiar virulency of the mutants, the observations are believed worthy of record.

MORTALITY FROM INFLUENZAL INFECTION IN RELATION TO THE RISE AND FALL OF EPIDEMIC WAVES

It has been noted by physicians who have seen many cases of influenza that the attacks were more severe during the height of the epidemic and milder as the epidemic subsided. The mortality statistics of infectious diseases now available are based almost wholly on the number of patients who develop the disease and the number of deaths within a certain number of days, weeks or months. No records of epidemic diseases have come to my notice in which the mortality rate is studied strictly in relation to the time in the epidemic at which the disease was contracted. Owing to the changes noted on successive intratracheal application in the invasive power of streptococci from influenza it was thought worth while to determine the mortality in the patients with influenza admitted to the hospitals according to the period in the epidemic the disease was contracted. In chart 3 each black column represents the number of patients who developed influenza on that day. These columns show that there were four distinct waves and two lesser recrudescences between September, 1918, and April, 1919, and that each wave spent its force in about six weeks. Each wave was divided into three two-week periods, namely, two weeks before and including the day of the crest of the wave, the first two weeks following the crest, and the second two weeks following the crest of the wave. The first row of figures at the bottom of the chart indicates the number of persons with influenza admitted to the hospital in each of these periods. The second row indicates the percentage of deaths from influenzal infection, not during the two weeks, respectively, but during that time or later. In other words, 16 per cent. of the 43 persons contracting influenza during the first two weeks of the first wave ultimately died, 20 per cent. of the 112 persons contracting influenza during the second two weeks died, and 13 per cent. of the 54 persons contracting influenza during the third two weeks died, and so on. By a study of the mortality according to the time the disease was contracted, it was discovered that the highest mortality rate occurred in each of the three main waves in the second two weeks, the time when the largest number of cases developed. It was lower during the first two weeks as the epidemic was on the increase, and in each instance lowest the third two weeks as the wave subsided. The number of cases during the third wave was small and the mortality low; accordingly, the marked rise and fall in mortality did not occur. The slight recrudescence in November also carried with it a low mortality (15 per cent.). The mortality during the recrudescence in April was highest (26 per cent.) when the number of cases was largest (36), and much lower (12 per cent.) as the epidemic disappeared. The curve to the extreme right in the chart represents the average mortality percentage of the four waves, during the three periods of two weeks each, 14, 21 and 12 per cent., respectively.

Besides the change in mortality rate, there was a noticeable difference in the type of the disease during the early part, or the height of each wave, and that found as the wave subsided. The incidence and degree of exudation into the lung was more marked during the middle part of the epidemic. Thus, during the first two weeks of the first wave 24 per cent. of the patients admitted developed pneumonia, during the second two weeks, 30 per cent., and during the third two weeks, 27 per cent. The average percentage incidence of influenzal pneumonia during the four waves for the three biweekly periods was 30 per cent., 37 per cent., and 41 per cent., respectively. The lesions in the lung found at necropsy in our cases as in those of other observers were distinctly different early and late in the waves.

Voluminous lungs with marked hemorrhagic edema and relatively slight true consolidation were the rule at the height of the waves, while exudative pneumonia of the bronchopneumonic type with relatively slight hemorrhage and edema dominated the picture as the waves subsided.

In a previous paper [4] I have shown that the tendency to a persistence of leukopenia in patients contracting the disease late in epidemic waves is less marked than at the height of the waves. In the light of the animal experiments might not this difference as well as the greater tendency to true consolidation of the lung late in the waves be an expression of a diminished virulence on the part of the infecting microorganisms?

In another paper [4] I have shown also that as patients recover from influenza and especially influenzal pneumonia the leukocyte count goes up. Exceptionally this is true also in protracted cases in which the patient dies. This is generally considered to be due to secondary invasion or to a winning fight by the defensive mechanism of the host. The possibility that this is due to changes in the parasite must, in the light of the experiments on successive intratracheal injection, be taken into consideration. Leukocytosis following an initial leukopenia was noted commonly in guinea-pigs injected with sublethal doses of the green-producing streptococcus, and prolonged contact with the body fluids and cells was found to rob these strains of the power to produce leukopenia. The mortality curves in the epidemics studied represent in a general way those noted by others and indicate a rise and a fall of virulency of the infecting micro-organism. The severity of influenza as it passes through smaller groups, such as large families, often shows the same rise and fall.

The difficulties, however, in studying the severity of influenza in sequence in individual families in which quarantine is not strictly observed are obvious. Authentic information regarding the severity of attacks has been obtained, however, in the case of a number of families living in the country. The findings in a family of eleven living in isolation 15 miles from a railroad station are especially instructive in this connection. The date of onset, date of death in the fatal cases, the age of the patients, and the attacks according to severity are arranged chronologically in Chart 4. It will be noted that fifty-three days elapsed from the time the first became ill (September 27) until the last one contracted the disease (November 19). The interval between the groups of cases was about four, twelve, ten, twelve and fifteen days, respectively. The epidemic spent its force in the surrounding community during the same time. The first person to contract the disease had a mild attack, but because he persisted in working, he developed severe symptoms, was in bed with fever for six days, and then recovered. The 3 persons who came down last had mild attacks, and all recovered without developing pneumonia or other complications. The 7 who contracted the disease during the interval between the first and the last cases all had severe attacks; 3 died from influenzal pneumonia; 2 of those who recovered developed pneumonia, and 1 phlebitis of the leg; the fourth had a severe attack, but did not develop outspoken signs of pneumonia. The source of the infection was not known. From the dates of onset of symptoms in these cases, it seems that the

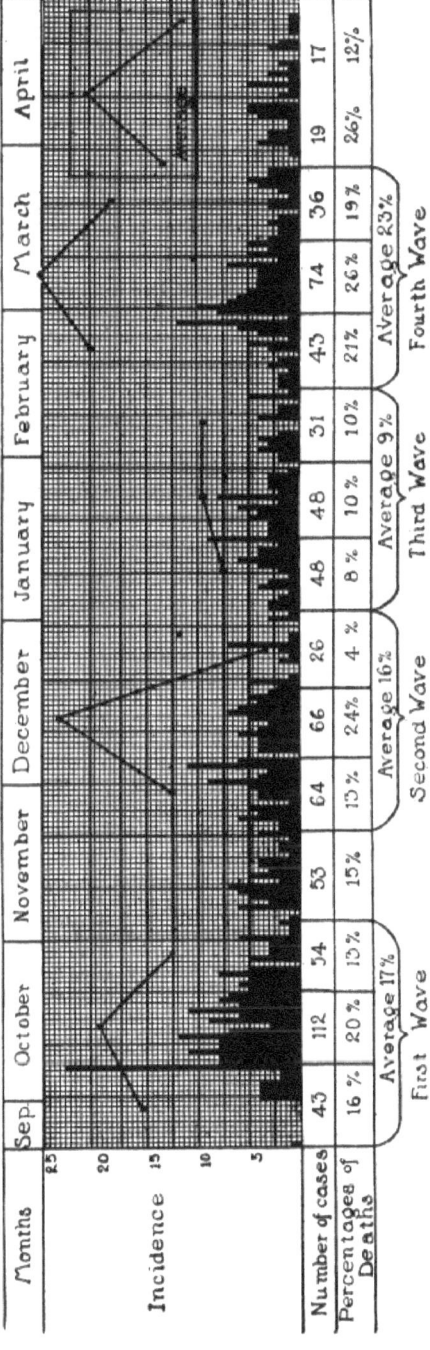

Chart 3.—Mortality from influenza in relation to the rise and fall of epidemic waves of the disease. The black columns show the number of cases of influenza. The curves show the percentage of deaths in persons who developed influenza during two weeks prior to the crest, first two weeks following the crest and second two weeks following the crest of the waves.

organism passed through five persons, and as this occurred the virulency, just as on successive animal passage on tracheal application increased during the earlier passages and then decreased, and was lost in the sixth passage.

CHART 4

THE RISE AND FALL IN VIRULENCY OF INFLUENZAL INFECTION AS IT PASSED THROUGH A LARGE FAMILY

William K., aged 31, farmer. Influenza Sept. 27, 1918; mild attack at first; would not give up work; then had severe attack. Recovered.

Mrs. K., aged 60. Influenza October 1. Severe attack with influenzal pneumonia, but recovered.

Walter K., aged 30. Influenza October 1. Death from influenzal pneumonia, October 13.

Laura K., aged 29. Influenza October 15. Death from influenzal pneumonia October 23.

Edwin K., aged 21. Severe influenza October 13, but no pneumonia. Recovered.

Meda K., aged 17. Influenza October 23. Severe attack with pneumonia, but recovered.

Selma K., aged 26. Influenza October 23; extremely ill; developed phlebitis of leg, but recovered.

Freda K., aged 21. Influenza November 4. Extremely ill and died November 17 of pneumonia.

Hired Girl, aged 22. Influenza November 17. Mild attack.

Ben K., aged 25. Influenza November 19. Mild attack.

Ezra K., aged 16. Influenza November 17. Mild attack.

SUMMARY

The results reported elsewhere following the intratracheal injection of the green-producing streptococcus from influenza have been verified and extended in this study.

The virulency and mortality in animals increased for one or two successive intratracheal injections of this organism, and on further animal passage progressively diminished. At the peak of virulency the symptoms of respiratory embarrassment are frequently violent and often resemble those of anaphylaxis. Cyanosis and leukopenia are marked, and death from hugely dilated lungs filled with hemorrhagic edema fluid with relatively slight exudative pneumonia frequently occurs. Microscopically, necrosis of alveolar epithelium and endothelium of the capillaries of all grades with marked hemorrhagic edema and little leukocytic infiltration are the chief findings. In subsequent intratracheal injection respiratory embarrassment becomes less marked, reduction in leukocytes less pronounced or wholly absent, and as this occurs the dilatation of the lung becomes less, exudation of leukocytes in the lung more pronounced, and extensive pneumonia with little hemorrhage and edema is the dominant picture.

TABLE 1
EFFECT OF SUCCESSIVE INTRATRACHEAL INJECTION OF STREPTOCOCCI FROM INFLUENZA, THE LEUKOCYTE COUNT AND MORTALITY

Animal Passage	Strains	Animals Injected	Average			Percentage Showing			Mortality per Cent.
			Before Injection	After Injection (24 hours)	Reduction, %	Leukopenia	Leukocytosis	No Change	
First	5	14	14,800	7,200	51	92	4	4	57
Second	5	8	12,300	4,200	66	88	0	12	100
Third	3	7	17,100	8,500	50	70	15	15	57
Fourth	3	13	14,700	13,300	9.5	47	25	25	38

From a study of the four epidemic waves as they occurred in Rochester, it has been found that a similar rise and fall in severity of symptoms, mortality and character of lung lesions occurred as the epidemic waves appeared and disappeared. The symptoms, cyanosis and leukopenia were most pronounced, and the mortality was the highest at the peak of the waves when the lungs were of huge size, and at necropsy hemorrhagic edema with relatively slight exudative pneumonia was the striking picture. Later as the symptoms became milder, leukopenia less persistent, and the mortality rate lower, exudative pneumonia became more common. Experimental evidence has thus been obtained to show that (1) the change in the type of the disease early and late in epidemics, (2) the rise and fall in mortality rate in the same epidemic and the virulency of different epidemics, and (3) the lesser tendency to leukopenia late in epidemic waves may be due, in the main, to changes in virulency and other properties of the green-producing streptococci isolated so constantly in influenzal infection.

These facts do not exclude the possibility that the influenza bacillus may play a rôle in the production of symptoms and lesions in influenza. In some cases they rather suggest the possibility that this organism may undergo similar changes, and that it may acquire peculiar and high infecting powers. Indeed the recent work of Blake and Cecil, in which symptoms and lesions simulating influenza have been produced experimentally in the monkey with the influenza bacillus made highly virulent by repeated monkey passages, supports this view.

Throughout the work the well marked examples in which green-producing streptococci suddenly acquired hemolytic power and hemolytic streptococci suddenly became green-producing streptococci, both in vitro and in vivo, suggest strongly that the complete or partial displacement of one type of streptococcal flora by another throughout, especially late in the epidemic waves, may be due to the development of mutation forms rather than the result of superimposed infection from the upper respiratory tract.

Since the mutants have been found to possess the power of producing the characteristic lesions in the lung and a sharp leukopenia on intratracheal application, might not the green-producing streptococcus isolated so constantly early in influenza and influenzal pneumonia, since it has high and peculiar invasive and other properties, be a mutation form of the pneumococcus-streptococcus group which humans normally harbor? Moreover, might not the sudden appearance and rapid "spread" of influenza among isolated groups and often almost simultaneously over wide areas be in part due to this cause?

1. Blake, F. G., and Cecil, R. L.: The Production of an Acute Respiratory Disease in Monkeys by Inoculation with Bacillus Influenzae. A Preliminary Report, Jour. Am. Med. Assn., 1920, lxxiv, 170-172.
2. Hirsch, E. F., and McKinney, M.: An Epidemic of Pneumococcus Bronchopneumonia, Jour. Infect. Dis., 1919, xxiv, 594-617.
3. Rosenow, E. C.: Studies in Influenza and Pneumonia. II. The Experimental Production of Symptoms and Lesions Simulating Those of Influenza with Streptococci Isolated During the Present Pandemic, Jour. Am. Med. Assn., 1919, lxxii, 1604-1609.
4. Rosenow, E. C.: Studies in Influenza and Pneumonia. VI. The Leukocytic Reaction in Influenza and Influenzal Pneumonia. (In press.)

STUDIES IN INFLUENZA AND PNEUMONIA

STUDY X. THE IMMUNOLOGIC PROPERTIES OF THE GREEN-PRODUCING STREPTOCOCCI FROM INFLUENZA

E. C. ROSENOW

Division of Experimental Bacteriology, The Mayo Foundation, Rochester, Minnesota.

In a previous report it was shown that most of the green-producing streptococci isolated so constantly in influenza were agglutinated specifically by a monovalent immune horse serum; that highly agglutinable strains absorb the agglutinins for the other strains; and that during convalescence in influenza the serum of patients acquires the power to agglutinate many of the freshly isolated green-producing streptococci. Attention was directed also to the fact that these organisms possess well marked antigenic properties, the serum of persons developing specific agglutinating power after injections of a mixed vaccine.

In this study I shall detail further results obtained by subjecting numerous strains of the green-producing streptococcus from influenza to the action of various immune serums, especially to the monovalent serum prepared with one of the strains of the green-producing streptococcus. The monovalent serum was prepared by injecting a large horse (horse 15) with increasing doses of one strain of green-producing streptococcus isolated from the blood after death in a case of influenza and influenzal pneumonia. The symptoms and findings in this case, reported elsewhere, were typical. The thorax was expanded and immobile, the patient expectorated a large amount of bloody, frothy fluid. The lung after death was voluminous, extremely wet with a dark colored bloody fluid and the seat of numerous coalescing areas of lobular pneumonia.

The strain as isolated from a single colony from the blood and after one animal passage was put aside on blood-agar slants and in deep tubes of dextrose-brain broth. Both of these produced typical, rather moist, spreading, greenish colonies on blood-agar plates, both fermented inulin, but they were not bile soluble. Cultures for immunization of the horse were made from the stock cultures in bottles of glucose broth containing 150 c c each. These were incubated over night, or until heavy growth had occurred, centrifuged and the sediment suspended in salt solution so that 1 c c of the sediment represented the growth from 15 c c of the broth. Control blood-agar plate cultures were made of the material inoculated in the bottle as well as of the growth injected into the horse. The dense bacterial suspension was used for intravenous immunizations. The first injection, made Jan. 9, 1919, consisted of 6 c c of the suspension or the growth from 90 c c of broth. The injections were given on three successive days in each week. The first six injections consisted of the heat killed bacteria (60 centigrade for thirty minutes). After that live cultures were injected. The dose by March 3, when 3 liters of blood were withdrawn, had been increased to 50 c c of the suspension or the growth from 750 c c of the glucose broth culture. The injections were continued and the dose gradually increased until April 4, when 14 liters of blood were withdrawn. The horse was given a rest for ten days, and the injections were resumed, but owing to marked reactions and loss of weight the dose had to be diminished and finally was discontinued, April 16. In spite of the fact that no more injections were given the horse continued to lose in weight and strength, and June 4 it was unable to get up, and was bled to death under ether.

The serums obtained before the injections were begun, and on March 3, April 4 and June 4 after immunization, were titrated against freshly isolated strains of the green-producing streptococcus. It was found that the upper limit of agglutinating power of the serum obtained before the injections were begun was about 1 to 10; the serum obtained March 3, about 1 to 500; April 4, 1 to 1,000 to 1 to 10,000; and June 4, 1 to 500 or 1 to 1,000. The serum of the highest titer obtained April 4 was mostly used in the agglutination experiments herein reported.

The antihemolytic streptococcus serum (horse 9) was prepared by repeated injections with four strains of highly virulent hemolytic streptococci from cases of severe ascending infections and cases of cellulitis. The injections were given between December 18, 1917, and July 1, 1918. The serum during this time had acquired marked agglutinating power over the strains injected. It should be emphasized that all of these strains were isolated before the epidemic of influenza occurred.

The pneumococcus immune serums were obtained from Dr. Rufus I. Cole, of the Hospital of the Rockefeller Institute for Medical Research, and from Dr. Augustus B. Wadsworth, of the New York State Department of Health. These were titrated against known strains of type pneumococci and were found to possess marked and specific agglutinating power.

METHODS

The freshly obtained sputum was sent to the laboratory for cultures throughout the four epidemic waves of influenza in 1918 and 1919. The cultures and agglutination experiments were made and recorded without knowledge of the history of the patients. The diagnosis, days of onset and other data were ascertained later from the records. A series of preliminary experiments in which various dilutions of serums were used (from 1 to 10 to 1 to 10,000), showed that a final dilution of these serums of 1 to 20 had the widest range of usefulness. Accordingly, for routine work the mixture in each tube consisted of 0.2 c c of the various serums diluted 1 to 10 with salt solution, and 0.2 c c of the antigen. The antigen consisted, for the most part, of the dextrose-blood broth or dextrose-acacia-broth culture, or of a salt solution suspension of bacteria grown in these after they had been preserved in 50 per cent. glycerol for a variable length of time. In some instances the peritoneal washings of mice and guinea-pigs which had succumbed to injections of sputum or primary culture from sputum, were also used as antigen. During the first two waves dense suspensions of the green-producing streptococci from primary cultures of sputum or blood of animals dead from injection of sputum were filed away in 50 per cent. glycerol, so that 1 c c equaled the growth from 15 c c of the dextrose-acacia-broth culture. These were kept in the ice chest and diluted with 15 parts of salt solution at the time the agglutination tests were performed. The mixtures of serum and antigen were thoroughly shaken and incubated at 37 C. for from one to one and one-half hours and placed in the ice chest over night, before readings were taken. The amount of agglutination, as indicated in the tables, was recorded by from 1 to 4 plus signs, 1 plus indicating slight but definite agglutination, 2 plus decided clumping but with little sedimentation, 3 plus marked agglutination and sedimentation but with supernatant fluid, not entirely clear, and 4 plus complete agglutination with the bacteria packed quite solidly at the bottom and the supernatant fluid completely cleared.

"Specific" agglutination is the term applied to the serum which agglutinated a particular strain to a greater degree than any of the other serums.

In most cases only one or two samples of sputum were cultivated and the agglutination tests made with the bacteria thus obtained. In some instances the agglutination experiments were done with strains isolated from the sputum daily or on alternate days throughout the illness and with the strains isolated after death. In selected cases cultures were made simultaneously of tonsil and of the throat or nasopharynx, and the strains isolated were subjected to the agglutinating action of the serums under identical conditions.

TABLE 1

AGGLUTINATION EXPERIMENTS WITH THE GREEN-PRODUCING STREPTOCOCCUS FROM INFLUENZA

Case or Strain	Date of Experiment	Date of Isolation	Source	Day of Disease	Antiserums					Controls	
					Pneumococcus			Streptococcus			
					I	II	III	Hemolytic Horse 9	Green Producing Horse 15	Normal Horse Serum	NaCl Solution
3218.2	3/ 9/19	3/ 7/19	Sputum	4	0	0	0	+	++	0	0
3218.2	3/ 9/19	3/ 7/19	Sputum	4	0	0	0	0	++	0	0
3225²	3/19/19	3/17/19	Sputum	3	0	0	0	++	+++	0	0
3225².5	6/17/19	3/17/19	Sputum	3	0	0	0	0	+	0	0
3266	3/25/19	3/24/19	Sputum	5	+	0	0	++	+++	+	0
3266².2	3/27/19	3/24/19	Sputum	5	0	0	0	0	0	0	0
3282	3/31/19	3/30/19	Sputum	2	0	+++	+++	+++	++++	0	0
3282	4/ 3/19	4/ 2/19	Sputum	5	0	++	+	++	+++	0	0
3332	4/ 7/19	4/ 6/19	Sputum	3	0	0	0	0	+++	0	0
3332.2	4/ 8/19	4/ 6/19	Sputum	3	0	0	0	0	++	0	0
3332	4/ 9/19	4/ 8/19	Tonsil	5	++	++	++	+++	+++	++	0
3332.2	4/10/19	4/ 8/19	Tonsil	5	0	++	0	0	+++	0	0
3332.6	11/18/19	4/ 8/19	Sputum	3	0	+	+	+	+	0	0
3334	4/ 7/19	4/ 6/19	Sputum	1	0	0	0	+++	++++	0	0
3334	4/ 8/19	4/ 7/19	Throat	2	0	0	++	+++	+++	0	0
3334.2	4/ 9/19	4/ 7/19	Throat	2	0	0	0	0	+++	0	0
3334.2	4/ 9/19	4/ 7/19	Throat	2	0	0	++	+	+++	+	0
3334.2	4/ 9/19	4/ 7/19	Throat	2	0	0	0	+++	++++	+	0
3334	4/10/19	4/ 9/19	Sputum	3	0	0	++	++	++	0	0
3334.6	11/11/19	4/ 9/19	Sputum	3	0	0	+	+++	+++	+	0
3365	4/14/19	4/13/19	Throat	3	0	0	++	0	+++	+	0
3365	4/14/19	4/13/19	Throat	3	0	0	0	0	++	0	0
3365.2	4/15/19	4/13/19	Throat	3	0	0	0	0	+++	+	0
3365	4/14/19	4/13/19	Sputum	3	0	0	0	0	+++	0	0
3365.2	4/14/19	4/13/19	Sputum	3	0	0	0	0	++	0	0
3365.3	4/16/19	4/13/19	Sputum	3	+	+	+	+	+++	0	0
3365.6	5/ 1/19	4/13/19	Sputum	3	0	0	0	0	++++	0	0
3365.6	5/ 1/19	4/13/19	Sputum	3	0	0	0	0	++++	0	0
3365.7	11/ 1/19	4/13/19	Sputum	3	0	0	0	+	+++	0	0
3366	4/14/19	4/10/19	Tonsil	2	0	0	0	0	0	0	0
3366	4/14/19	4/10/19	Throat	2	0	0	0	0	+	0	0
3366	4/14/19	4/10/19	Sputum	2	0	0	0	0	++	0	0
3366	4/14/19	4/12/19	Sputum	4	0	0	++	++	+++	+	0
3366.2	4/14/19	4/12/19	Sputum	4	+	+	+	+	+++	+	0
3366.3	6/17/19	4/12/19	Sputum	4	0	0	0	0	+++	0	0
3366.7	11/14/19	4/12/19	Sputum	4	0	0	0	0	++	0	0
3370	4/14/19	4/11/19	Sputum	2	0	0	0	0	++	0	0
3370.2	4/14/19	4/11/19	Sputum	2	0	0	0	0	++	0	0
3370.3	4/16/19	4/11/19	Sputum	2	0	0	0	+	++	0	0
3370.4	4/21/19	4/11/19	Sputum	2	0	0	0	0	++	0	0
3370.6	5/ 1/19	4/11/19	Sputum	2	0	0	0	0	+++	+	0
3370.7	11/22/19	4/11/19	Sputum	2	++	+	+	++	+++	++	0

RESULTS

In table 1 are summarized representative experiments indicating the results obtained with the green-producing streptococcus isolated from patients with influenza. In these and other experiments the following findings were noted:

1. The monovalent serum of horse 15 agglutinated specifically most of the strains isolated throughout short initial attacks of typical influenza (cases 3218, 3225 and 3332).

2. Specific agglutination occurred (often in duplicate) in the primary mass culture of sputum or throat swab and of material from animals dead from injection of sputum, and in the early subcultures of the green-producing streptococcus isolated from sputum, throat swab and animals injected with these strains (cases 3225, 3266, 3365 and 3366).

3. The immunologic condition of the green-producing streptococci, as manifested by their agglutinability in the various immune serums, varied between wide limits (cases 3282, 3332 and 3334).

4. Specific agglutinability of most of the strains was lost on prolonged cultivation (cases 3332 and 3370), but in some strains it was retained for a long time (cases 3334, 3365 and 3366).

In table 2 are summarized representative experiments with strains of the green-producing streptococcus isolated during life and after death in cases of influenzal pneumonia. The results with the strains isolated early in these cases were similar to those isolated in cases of influenza (cases 3206, 3207 and 3264), while late in the disease during life (cases 3265 and 3331), and after death (cases 3404, 3410, 3420 and 3436) the incidence of specific agglutination was decidedly lower, but even here the incidence was higher than that obtained with any of the other immune serums.

The agglutination experiments with the green-producing streptococcus isolated from the same patient throughout both the influenza attack and the influenzal pneumonia which followed showed that there was practically no difference in the immunologic condition of the strains isolated during influenza and during the early part of the influenzal pneumonia. Late in the pneumonic attack there was often a shifting of specific agglutination of these strains to one of the other serums, or agglutination to the same degree occurred in most of the immune serums; in other cases they might not be agglutinated by any of the serums. Thus in one case specific agglutination occurred in the serum of horse 15 of the primary culture from the sputum, and from the blood of a guinea-pig dead from an intraperitoneal injection of sputum, obtained on the third day of influenza. No agglutination occurred in any of the other serums. The colonies of the green-producing streptococci were quite moist and large, resembling type III pneumococci, but were not so mucoid in character, whereas on the

TABLE 2

Agglutination Experiments with the Green-Producing Streptococcus from Influenzal Pneumonia

Case or Strain	Date of Experiment	Date of Isolation	Source	Day of Disease	Antiserums					Controls	
					Pneumococcus			Streptococcus			
					I	II	III	Hemolytic Horse 9	Green Producing Horse 15	Normal Horse Serum	NaCl Solution
3097	3/12/19	3/11/19	Sputum	1	0	++	0	0	0	0	0
3175.2	3/14/19	3/11/19	Sputum	4	++	+++	++	++	++++	+	0
3175³.2	3/27/19	3/11/19	Sputum	4	0	0	0	0	++	0	0
3206	3/13/19	3/12/19	Sputum	2	0	0	0	0	+++	0	0
3207	3/13/19	3/12/19	Sputum	4	0	0	0	0	+++	0	0
3207².2	4/ 3/19	3/12/19	Sputum	4	0	++	0	0	+++	0	0
3264	3/25/19	3/24/19	Sputum	8	0	0	0	++	+++	0	0
3264	3/25/19	3/24/19	Sputum	8	0	0	0	++	+++	0	0
3264².2	3/28/19	3/24/19	Sputum	8	0	0	0	+	++	0	0
3265	3/25/19	3/24/19	Sputum	13	++	+	0	++	+++	+	0
3265.2	3/31/19	3/29/19	Sputum	18	0	0	++	0	0	0	0
3265.2	4/ 3/19	4/ 2/19	Sputum	21	0	0	0	0	0	0	0
3265².2	4/ 3/19	4/ 2/19	Sputum	21	0	0	0	0	0	0	0
3265.4	9/ 3/19	4/ 2/19	Sputum	21	+	++	+	++	+	+	0
3270	4/ 4/19	4/ 3/19	Sputum	12	0	0	0	+++	0	0	0
3270²	4/ 7/19	4/ 3/19	Sputum	12	0	0	0	++	0	0	0
3270.2	4/ 7/19	4/ 3/19	Sputum	12	0	0	0	++	0	0	0
3270².2	4/ 9/19	4/ 3/19	Sputum	12	0	0	0	++	++	0	0
3331	4/ 8/19	4/ 7/19	Sputum	2	0	0	++	++	+++	0	0
3331	4/ 8/19	4/ 7/19	Tonsil	2	0	0	0	0	++	0	0
3331	4/10/19	4/ 9/19	Sputum	4	0	0	0	0	0	0	0
3404	4/18/19	4/17/19	Throat	1	+	+	+	+	++	+	0
3404	4/21/19	4/20/19	Sputum	4	0	0	0	0	++	0	0
3404	4/21/19	4/20/19	Sputum	4	0	0		+	++	0	0
3404	4/25/19	4/24/19	Sputum	8	0	0	0	+++	0	0	0
3404	5/ 7/19	5/ 3/19	Lung after death	..	0	0	0	+	+	0	0
3404.2	5/ 8/19	5/ 6/19	Lung after death	..	0	0	0	++	++	0	0
2602.2	4/29/19	11/16/18	Lung after death	..	0	0	0	0	++	0	0
2630².2	4/29/19	11/30/18	Lung after death	..	+	+	+	+	+++	+	0
3228	3/19/19	3/18/19	Lung after death	..	0	0	0	++	+++	0	0
3287.3	4/ 8/19	3/31/19	Lung after death	..	0	0	0	0	+++	0	0
3287.3	4/ 8/19	3/31/19	Lung after death	..	0	0	0	0	+++	0	0
3410	4/21/19	4/19/19	Lung after death	..	0	0	0	0	0	0	0
3415	4/21/19	4/19/19	Lung after death	..	0	0	0	0	+++	0	0
3420	4/24/19	4/22/19	Lung after death	..	0	0	0	0	0	0	0
3433	4/25/19	4/24/19	Lung after death	..	++++	0	0	0	0	0	0
3436	4/26/19	4/25/19	Lung after death	..	0	0	0	+++	0	0	0

second and sixth days of the pneumonia which followed, specific agglutination occurred in type III pneumococcus serum of the primary culture from the sputum in four tests. Less agglutination occurred in the serum of horse 15 in three instances, and in two instances in each of the type II pneumococcus serum and hemolytic streptococcus serum of horse 9. In another case of typical influenza the green-producing streptococcus in the primary culture and in the first subculture from the sputum on the third day was agglutinated specifically by the serum of horse 9, while on the second day of the influenzal pneumonia which followed, and after death, it was not agglutinated by any of the serums. In still another case specific agglutination occurred in the serum of horse 15 during influenza and early in influenzal pneumonia, whereas

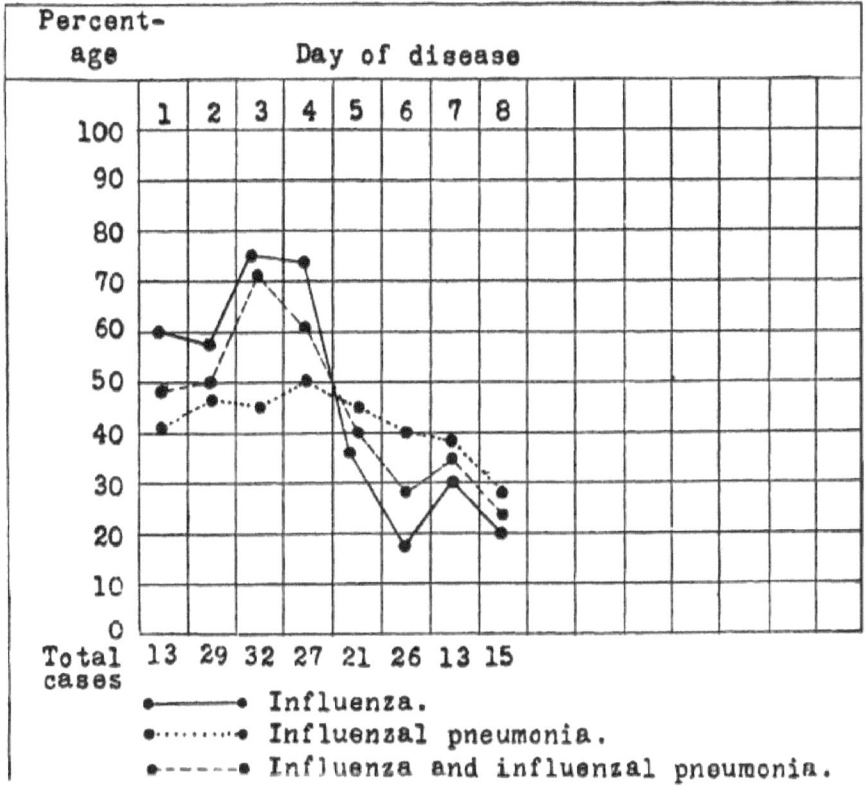

Chart 1.—Percentage of specific agglutination in the monovalent serum of the green-producing streptococcus from influenza and influenzal pneumonia according to the day of the disease.

later in the pneumonic attack specific and marked agglutination occurred in type II pneumococcus serum and lesser agglutination in the serum of horse 15.

In chart 1 is given graphically the average percentage incidence of specific agglutination by the monovalent serum of the green-producing streptococci from influenza and influenzal pneumonia, according to the days of the disease. The curves represent the results obtained on the days indicated. The antigen consisted throughout of the primary culture of the sputum in dextrose-blood broth or of animals injected with sputum irrespective of what the culture showed on plating, and with the early subcultures containing the green-producing streptococcus. The close parallelism between the strains isolated in influenza without frank signs of lung involvement and the cases of influenzal pneumonia is shown by the fact that the average incidence of specific agglutination, while somewhat lower in the latter, runs roughly parallel. The average incidence of specific agglutination for both influenza and influenzal pneumonia strains was highest during the first four days, when a gradual decline occurred up to and including the eighth day. A number of facts indicate that these strains of different agglutinability which appear late in the pneumonic attack are modifications of the strains which are agglutinated specifically by the monovalent serum early in the attacks, and that their appearance is not always the result of superimposed infections from without. The specific strains tend to lose this property on artificial cultivation. The various strains have been found to be unstable in their cultural character and fermentative reactions.

There was no parallelism between the occurrence of specific agglutination in the serum of horse 15 of the different strains and their power to ferment inulin, or their solubility in bile.

Moreover, marked changes in the immunologic condition as measured by agglutination tests have occurred in a number of strains following successive (intratracheal) animal passages.

Thus strain 2719 was agglutinated completely and specifically by the serum of horse 15, as isolated and after one animal passage. Less agglutination occurred in the serum of horse 9, but none in any of the other serums, whereas after the third and fourth animal passages agglutination in the serum of horse 15, while still specific, was less marked and some agglutination occurred in each of the other serums.

In strain 2749 a similar change in agglutinability occurred during the third and fourth animal passages.

In case 2800 the patient from whom the strain was isolated with which horse 15 was immunized, specific agglutination increased during the first and second animal passages over that noted before animal passage, and a marked diminution in agglutination occurred in the serum of horse 15 after the fourth animal passage.

In summarizing the agglutination tests which were made in a routine manner throughout the epidemic of 1918-1919 it was found that material from influenza and influenzal pneumonia, without regard to the time in the attack when the sputum or other material was obtained for culture, and without regard to the type of flora the cultures of the sputum or primary culture showed, was subjected to the agglutinating action of the monovalent immune serum in 567 experiments, representing 184 cases. Of these, 295 (52 per cent.) showed specific agglutination in the serum of horse 15. The primary culture of the sputum in many instances, especially late in the disease, and of the lung exudate after death, showed predominating numbers of hemolytic streptococci, less often staphylococci and rarely colon bacilli or bacillus mucosus.

Specific agglutination occurred in the serum of horse 15 in 29 instances (58 per cent.) of 50 experiments, representing 25 cases, and in 20 of the 25 cases in which the antigen consisted of a salt solution suspension of the primary culture of the sputum or blood of animals dead from injection of sputum, or of pure cultures of these after suspension in 50 per cent. glycerol for some months. All these were cultures from cases which occurred during the first two waves of the disease.

The relative significance of these figures becomes more apparent from a study of tables 1 and 2, in which it is shown that there is a relatively greater frequency and a greater degree of agglutination in the serum of horse 15 over those in the other immune serums; that the antihemolytic streptococcus serum (horse 9) ranks second, and that with few exceptions only a slight difference occurred between the type pneumococcus serums and normal horse serum. The exact figures of the total average incidence of agglutination from slight to marked agglutination in the different serums of the strains from influenza and influenzal pneumonia were found to be as follows: type I pneumococcus serum in 20 per cent. of 563 tests; type II pneumococcus serum in 22 per cent. of 525 tests; type III pneumococcus serum in 21 per cent. of 524 tests; horse 9 serum in 39 per cent. of 561 tests; horse 15 serum in 61 per cent. of 567 tests; normal horse serum in 23 per cent. of 556 tests; salt solution in 7 per cent. of 555 tests. It is certain that the high incidence of agglutination in horse 15 serum was not due to nonspecific effects, since its agglutinating power over 72 strains of green-producing streptococci or pneumococci from sources other than influenza was 25 per cent., or about that of normal horse serum. Moreover, the average amount of agglutination in the serum of horse 15 with the influenza strains was much higher than in the other serums. The control strains included, in addition to type pneumococci and hemolytic streptococci, green-producing streptococci from a wide range of sources, such as the nose and throat of normal persons, the nose of normal guinea-pigs, throats in simple nasopharyngitis, the central nervous system in poliomyelitis, ulcer of the stomach, and arthritis.

As I have pointed out, there was a tendency of the green-producing streptococci to become heterogeneous and to lose the property of specific agglutination after prolonged cultivation on artificial mediums. This varied greatly with different strains (tables 1 and 2). One hundred and fourteen strains after cultivation on artificial mediums (chiefly blood agar) for from 6 to 10 months were subjected to the agglutinating action of the monovalent and the other serums. In these only 26 strains, or 23 per cent., were agglutinated specifically by the monovalent serum. This low figure was no doubt due in part to the deterioration of the serum. It has been pointed out elsewhere (study III) that as these strains are cultivated on artificial mediums they tend to agglutinate spontaneously in liquid cultures, and many strains are unsuited for agglutination tests. This tendency was noted also in the strains which grew diffusely in that the incidence of nonspecific agglutination in the various serums was considerably higher than in the freshly isolated strains. Thus of the 114 experiments, nonspecific agglutination, usually slight, occurred in type I pneumococcus serum in 25 per cent.; type II, in 23 per cent.; type III, in 24 per cent.; antihemolytic streptococcus serum horse 9, in 54 per cent.; monovalent serum horse 15, in 78 per cent., and in normal horse serum, in 35 per cent.

The close relationship between the green-producing streptococcus and hemolytic streptococcus in influenza is shown by the fact that 18 per cent. of 44 strains of hemolytic streptococci isolated during life and after death in influenza were agglutinated specifically by the serum of horse 15.

Beside the time in the attack in which the cultures were made (chart 1) and the predominating flora at hand, the instability of the strains of green-producing streptococci had to be taken into consideration in properly interpreting the results of the agglutination experiments, for by plating the culture actually agglutinated it was found that nonspecific agglutination by the serum of horse 15 was often due either to the fact that green-producing streptococci were not inoculated, or marked changes had occurred in the culture. After these discrepancies, and the earlier experiments in which plates were not made of the cultures actually agglutinated are eliminated, there are in all 252 tests in which the culture subjected to the agglutinating action of the serum was proved to contain green-producing streptococci. Of the 252 tests, 120, representing 92 different cases, were made with the green-producing streptococci in the primary culture of dextrose-blood or acacia broth from sputum and throat exudate during life and lung exudate after death. In 72 (60 per cent.) specific agglutination occurred in the serum of horse 15. Of 27 tests, representing 16 cases, 19 (70 per cent.) showed specific agglutination in this serum in the primary culture of blood or peritoneal exudate of animals dead from injection of sputum, or primary culture of sputum. In the remaining 105 tests in which pure cultures of the green-producing streptococci in from the first to the sixth subcultures were used as antigen, representing 90 cases of influenza or influenzal pneumonia, 85 (81 per cent.) showed specific agglutination in the monovalent serum. Thus specific agglutination of the green-producing streptococci, which was proved to be contained in the antigen used, occurred in the monovalent serum in 176 of 252 agglutination experiments, an average of 70 per cent. Hence this figure may be taken to express roughly the percentage of the strains of green-producing streptococci which were immunologically identical and found throughout influenza and influenzal pneumonia.

Through the kindness of Major Fennell, of the Army Medical School, I have had an opportunity to test the behavior of strains of green-producing streptococci and type IV pneumococci, which he obtained from widely separated localities, toward the monovalent serum of horse 15. The source of these strains and their immunologic condition as measured by the various immune serums are given in table 3. Specific agglutination was obtained in 12 of 16 strains, or in 75 per cent. of the strains isolated from influenzal pneumonia, and in no instance in four other strains, one isolated from the normal mouth in Washington during the epidemic and three strains of pneumococci which Major Fennel isolated from spontaneous pneumonia in the monkey. A study of the results obtained with these strains in relation to their solubility in bile and their ability to ferment inulin shows that in these strains, as in those isolated in Rochester, specific agglutination does not depend either on whether they are or are not bile soluble, or whether they do or do not ferment inulin. Some of the negative agglutinations may be due to the fact that the strains had been cultivated for some time before the agglutination tests were made, all being in at least the eighth subculture. The incidence of agglutination of these strains by the other serums is about that of the strains isolated by us.

TABLE 3

AGGLUTINATION EXPERIMENTS WITH STRAINS OF GREEN-PRODUCING STREPTOCOCCI FROM WIDELY DISTANT LOCALITIES

Strain	Source	Antiserums					Controls		Solubility in Bile	Acid in Inulin
		Pneumococcus			Streptococcus		Normal Horse Serum	NaCl Solution		
		I	II	III	Hemolytic Horse 9	Green Producing Horse 15				
S 1	Influenzal pneumonia, Camp Wheeler	0	0	+	+	++++	0	0	0	+
S 3	Influenzal pneumonia, Camp Wheeler	0	0	0	0	++++	0	0	0	0
S 3	Influenzal pneumonia, Camp Wheeler	0	0	0	0	++++	0	0	0	0
S 5	Influenzal pneumonia, Camp Wheeler	0	+++	0	++	++++	0	0	0	0
S 6	Influenzal pneumonia, Camp Wheeler	0	0	0	0	++	0	0	0	0
55	Influenzal pneumonia, Camp Wheeler	0	0	0	0	+	0	0	+	+
S 14	Influenzal pneumonia, Chicago	0	0	0	0	+++	0	0	0	0
S 24	Influenzal pneumonia, Chicago	0	0	0	++	+++	0	0	0	0
S 17	Influenzal pneumonia, Walter Reed Hospital	0	0	0	0	0	0	0	0	0
24	Influenzal pneumonia, Walter Reed Hospital	0	0	0	++	+++	0	0	+	+
15	Influenzal pneumonia, Camp Sherman	0	0	0	0	++	0	0	+	+
S 19	Influenzal pneumonia, Camp Sherman	0	0	0	+++	++++	+	0	0	+
S 25	Influenzal pneumonia, Camp Sherman	0	0	0	0	0	0	0	0	0
S 27	Influenzal pneumonia, Johns Hopkins	0	0	0	0	0	0	0	0	0
113	Influenzal pneumonia, Camp Greene	0	0	0	0	+++	0	0	+	+
152	Influenzal pneumonia, Camp Greene	0	0	0	0	0	0	0	+	+
149	Normal mouth, Washington during epidemic	0	0	0	0	0	0	0	+	+
194	Spontaneous pneumonia, monkey	0	0	0	0	0	0	0	+	+
212	Spontaneous pneumonia, monkey	0	0	0	0	0	0	0	+	+
225	Spontaneous pneumonia, monkey	0	0	0	0	0	0	0	+	+
225	Spontaneous pneumonia, monkey	0	0	0	0	0	0	0	+	+

Owing to the instability of the green-producing streptococci from influenza, and the tendency to the development of mutation forms, it was found necessary to inoculate a blood-agar plate with the culture subjected to the agglutinating action of the different serums in order to interpret properly the results obtained.

Striking examples of the development of mutation forms as measured by changes in morphology in cultural characteristics and in immunologic conditions were noted in many instances. The source of the micro-organism, the culture medium inoculated and the effect of the various serums in some of the cultures which yielded mutation forms on plating are summarized in table 4. It will be noted that in the first nine experiments, hemolytic streptococci were obtained on the blood-agar plate in pure culture in eight and together with staphylococci in two when single colonies or groups of well isolated colonies of green-producing streptococci were inoculated, and that specific agglutination by the serum of horse 9 occurred in three, and in the serum of horse 15 in one instance. The rest were not agglutinated by any of the serums.

In experiments 10 to 13, inclusive, pure cultures of green-producing streptococci were obtained from the dextrose-blood or dextrose-acacia broth when single colonies of hemolytic streptococci were inoculated. One of these was agglutinated specifically by the hemolytic streptococcus, the other by the green-producing streptococcus antiserums. In these experiments it is assumed that the culture actually agglutinated contained the type of streptococcus homologous to the serum which agglutinated specifically. Proof that this was actually the case could not be obtained, because it is conceivable that mutation forms might develop not in the broth culture, but as growth occurred on the blood-agar plate, and the morphology of the two types of streptococci were so similar that differentiation in this way was not possible.

In experiments 14 to 24, inclusive, in which the mutant was a streptococcus, the morphology and immunologic condition were sufficiently different from that of the organisms inoculated to make it possible to determine where the mutation occurred. Specific or marked agglutination in the monovalent serum occurred in the dextrose-blood or acacia broth cultures in all but one of these strains. Smears of the cultures agglutinated in these showed no staphylococci, but typical elongated diplococci singly or in chains of variable length.

Smears of those in which agglutination did not occur (experiment 24) showed staphylococci, and agglutination experiments with streptococci from the sputum in influenza were not agglutinated by this or other serums (experiments 29 to 34). The number of staphylococcus colonies on the plates was often very large. Their number and distribution on the plates were such as to exclude the possibility of contamination from the air. Hence it is certain that mutation must have occurred on the blood-agar plates, and that many of the organisms in

TABLE 4

The Relation of the Agglutinability of Bacteria from Influenza to the Development of Mutation Forms

Number	Strain	Micro-organism Inoculated	Culture Used in Agglutination Test	Pneumococcus I	Pneumococcus II	Pneumococcus III	Streptococcus Hemolytic Horse 9	Streptococcus Green Producing Horse 15	Controls Normal Horse Serum	Controls NaCl Solution	Growth on Blood-Agar Plate of Culture Agglutinated
1	2666ª	Green-producing streptococcus from pleural fluid of guinea-pig injected with sputum	Dextrose-blood broth	0	0	0	+++	++	0	0	Hemolytic streptococci and staphylococci
2	3083.4	Single colony of green-producing streptococcus from sputum	Dextrose-blood broth	0	0	0	0	0	0	0	Slightly hemolytic streptococci
3	3270.2	Single colony of green-producing streptococcus from sputum	Dextrose-blood broth	0	0	•	0	0	0	0	Hemolytic streptococci and staphylococci
4	3296ª	Green-producing streptococcus from blood of mouse injected with sputum	Dextrose-blood broth	0	0	0	0	0	0	0	Hemolytic streptococci
5	3297.2	Single colony of green-producing streptococcus from sputum	Dextrose-blood broth	0	0	0	0	0	0	0	Hemolytic streptococci
6	3300.2	Group of green-producing streptococcus colonies from throat	Dextrose-blood broth	0	0	0	+++	0	0	0	Hemolytic streptococci
7	3358	Green-producing streptococcus from sputum	Dextrose-acacia broth	0	0	0	++	0	0	0	Hemolytic streptococci
8	3394².2	Single colony of green-producing streptococcus from blood of mouse injected with sputum	Dextrose-acacia broth	0	0	0	0	++	0	0	Hemolytic streptococci
9	3396.5	Single colony of green-producing streptococcus from sputum	Dextrose-blood broth	0	0	0	++	0	+	0	Hemolytic streptococci
10	2966².10	Single colony of slightly hemolytic streptococcus	Dextrose-blood broth	0	0	0	0	0	0	0	Green-producing streptococci
11	3048.3	Single colony of green-producing streptococcus from hemolytic streptococcus	Dextrose-acacia broth	0	0	0	++	+	0	0	Green-producing streptococci
12	3387².5	Slightly hemolytic streptococcus	Dextrose-blood broth	0	0	0	0	0	0	0	Green-producing streptococci
13	2666².2	Single colony of hemolytic streptococcus	Dextrose-blood broth	0	0	0	0	+++	0	0	Green-producing streptococci
14	2719	Green-producing streptococcus from pleural fluid of guinea-pig injected with sputum	Dextrose-blood broth	0	0	0	++	+++	0	0	Staphylococci
15	27194.4	Single colony of green-producing streptococcus	Dextrose-blood broth	+	++	+	+	++	0	0	Staphylococci
16	2757².4	Green-producing streptococcus from blood of guinea-pig injected with sputum	Dextrose-blood broth	0	0	0	++	+++	+	0	Staphylococci
17	2800ª	Green-producing streptococcus from blood of guinea-pig injected with sputum	Dextrose-blood broth	0	0	0	++	+++	+	0	Staphylococci
18	3225².3	Green-producing streptococcus from blood of mouse injected with sputum	Dextrose-blood broth	0	0	0	0	+	0	0	Staphylococci
19	3241ª	Green-producing streptococcus from blood of guinea-pig injected with sputum	Dextrose-acacia broth	++	0	0	0	++++	0	0	Staphylococci

INFLUENZA/PNEUMONIA 1918-1919

#	ID	Description	Medium							Result
20	3941².²	Single colony of green-producing streptococcus from blood of guinea-pig injected with sputum	Dextrose-acacia broth	0	0	0	++	++	0	Staphylococci
21	3270².²	Green-producing streptococcus from blood of guinea-pig injected with sputum	Dextrose-acacia broth	0	0	0	++	+++	0	Staphylococci
22	3296².²	Green-producing streptococcus from blood of mouse injected with sputum	Dextrose-acacia broth	0	0	0	++	++	0	Staphylococci
23	3334.2	Single colony of green-producing streptococcus from sputum	Dextrose-acacia broth	0	0	+++	0	+++	0	Staphylococci
24	3434²	Green-producing streptococcus from blood of mouse injected with sputum	Dextrose-blood broth	0	0	+++	0	0	0	Staphylococci
25	2917.3	Single colony of hemolytic streptococcus	Dextrose-acacia broth	0	0	0	0	0	0	Staphylococci
26	3211.2	Single colony of hemolytic streptococcus	Dextrose-acacia broth	0	0	0	0	0	0	Staphylococci
27	3296²	Single colony of hemolytic streptococcus	Dextrose-acacia broth	0	0	0	++	++	0	Staphylococci
28	3334.2	Single colony of slightly hemolytic streptococcus	Dextrose-acacia broth	0	0	0	++	0	0	Staphylococci
29	2606³.²	Single colony of staphylococcus from sputum	Dextrose-blood broth	0	0	0	0	0	0	Staphylococci
30	3175.4	Single colony of staphylococcus from sputum	Dextrose-blood broth	0	0	0	0	0	0	Staphylococci
31	3208.2	Single colony of staphylococcus from sputum	Dextrose-blood broth	0	0	0	0	0	0	Staphylococci
32	3302.2	Staphylococcus from sputum	Dextrose-blood broth	0	0	0	0	0	0	Staphylococci
33	3357.2	Single colony of staphylococcus from sputum	Dextrose-acacia broth	0	0	0	0	0	0	Staphylococci
34	3434.2	Staphylococcus from sputum	Dextrose-blood broth	0	0	0	0	0	0	Staphylococci
35	3334.2	Single colony of influenza bacillus from sputum	Dextrose-blood broth	0	0	+	0	++	0	Green-producing streptococci
36	3334.2	Single colony of influenza bacillus from sputum	Dextrose-blood broth	0	0	0	+++	+++	0	Green-producing streptococci
37	3341.2	Single colony of influenza bacillus from sputum	Dextrose-blood broth	0	0	0	0	0	0	Green-producing streptococci
38	3332.2	Single colony of influenza bacillus from sputum	Dextrose-blood broth	0	0	•	0	+	0	Slightly hemolytic streptococcus
39	3332.2	Single colony of influenza bacillus from sputum	Dextrose-blood broth	0	0		0	0	0	Hemolytic streptococcus
40	3248.2	Single colony of influenza bacillus from sputum	Dextrose-blood broth	0	0	0	0	0	0	Moist hemolytic streptococci
41	3283.8	Single colony of influenza bacillus from evaporated oil suspension	Dextrose-blood broth	0	+++	0	0	++	0	Green-producing streptococci and staphylococci
42	3201.3	Single colony (twice) of influenza bacillus from sputum	Dextrose-blood broth	0	+++	0	0	++	0	Staphylococci
43	3178.8	Group of colonies of influenza bacillus from sputum	Dextrose-blood broth	0	0	0	0	0	0	Bacillus influenza
44	3353²	Influenza bacilli from blood of mouse	Dextrose-blood broth	0	0	0	0	0	0	Bacillus influenza

the tall cultures of dextrose-blood or acacia broth took part in this process. The lack of specific agglutination when the cultures of hemolytic streptococci yielded staphylococci is also in harmony with this idea.

Similar results were obtained in many instances in which influenza bacilli were inoculated into the dextrose-blood broth (experiments 35 to 44). In most of these the culture of influenza bacillus was derived from a single colony on blood-agar plates inoculated with sputum, and in these it is conceivable, but not probable, that what appeared as a mutation might merely be the growth of this organism in the broth when inhibited on the blood-agar plate, the contact on the blood-agar plate inoculated with the sputum not being sufficiently intimate to allow growth of one or a few organisms.

Control inoculations from the colony fished in these as well as in the streptococcus experiments made in the immediate neighborhood of the colony or on another blood-agar plate showed only the growth characteristic of the colony from which inoculated. Moreover, similar results were obtained with some strains after many subcultures and after repeated platings from single colonies (experiments 41 and 42). The mode of occurrence, the immunologic condition, the control cultures of the blood used in the broth, and finally, the fact that the mutants were often highly virulent, rule out all reasonable possibility that we were dealing with contaminations, but, as pointed out elsewhere, final conclusions cannot be drawn until the pure line requirement has been fulfilled.

The suddenness and degree of the changes noted throughout these studies were similar to those I noted in a study on the transmutation of pneumococci and streptococci, and to those described by Clough in a study of pneumococci reacting with all of the three antipneumococcus type serums and in which a striking example of mutation occurred.

By the use of various immune serums, including the monovalent serum, it may be concluded that the somewhat peculiar green-producing streptococci noted at the outset of the epidemic and isolated so constantly since, both in influenza and influenzal pneumonia, are immunologically quite homogeneous. A high percentage of the strains, especially those isolated early in the attacks, are agglutinated specifically in the serum prepared with one of these strains. Highly agglutinable strains, as has been shown, absorb the agglutinins for other strains. The serum of patients recovering from influenza acquires agglutinating power over homologous and other strains. This finding is in accord with those of Tunnicliff and of Howell and Anderson, who also find immunologic evidence of the identity of green-producing streptococci from influenza. Specific agglutination occurred in the monovalent serum irrespective of whether or not they fermented inulin or of whether they were bile soluble or insoluble. After cultivation on artificial mediums, and after repeated animal passages, as well as late in influenza and influenzal pneumonia, the strains tend to become more heterogeneous.

The findings of immunologically dissimilar green-producing streptococci late in influenza is in harmony with the results obtained by Mathers in a study of pneumococci in reinfection in lobar pneumonia in which the type was also found to change. Evidence has been obtained to show that the mutation forms which develop in vitro and in vivo in animals are in general similar immunologically to the organisms commonly isolated in influenza. It has been shown elsewhere that they resemble these also in infecting power. Hence, it would seem that mutation may play an important rôle in the pathogenesis of influenza.

BIBLIOGRAPHY

Clough, Mildred C.: A Study of Pneumococci Reacting with Antipneumococcus, Sera of Types I, II and III, Jour. Exper. Med., 1919, xxx, 123-146.

Howell, Katherine, and Anderson, Ruth: Complement Fixation in Influenza, Jour. Infect. Dis., 1919, xxv, 1-5.

Mathers, G.: The Varieties of Pneumococci Causing Lobar Pneumonia, with Especial Reference to Their Biologic Differences, Jour. Infect. Dis., 1915, xvii, 514-521.

Rosenow, E. C.: Transmutations Within the Streptococcus-Pneumococcus Group, Jour. Infect. Dis., 1914, xiv, 1-32.

Rosenow, E. C.: Studies in Influenza and Pneumonia III. The Occurrence of a Pandemic, Strain of Streptococcus During the Pandemic of Influenza, Jour. Am. Med. Assn., 1919, lxxii, 1608-1609.

Tunnicliff, Ruth: Phagocytic Experiments in Influenza, Jour. Am. Med. Assn., 1918, lxxi, 1733-1734.

STUDIES IN INFLUENZA AND PNEUMONIA

XI. THERAPEUTIC EFFECTS OF A MONOVALENT ANTISTREPTOCOCCUS SERUM IN INFLUENZA AND INFLUENZAL PNEUMONIA

E. C. Rosenow

Division of Experimental Bacteriology, The Mayo Foundation, Rochester, Minnesota.

In this study I shall record the results obtained in the treatment of influenza and influenzal pneumonia with the serum prepared with one strain of the green-producing streptococcus, and a study of the immunologic condition of the streptococcal flora of the sputum made at the same time in the patients receiving the serum injections.

The serum was used in undoubted and, with one exception, in severe cases only. All injections were made slowly intravenously. The amount injected at one time varied from 25 c c to 100 c c of the undiluted serum. In some instances a desensitizing dose of 1 c c was given one hour previously. Twelve patients were given the serum. These may be conveniently divided into three groups according to the agglutination tests and therapeutic results.

Group 1 (*Four Patients*).—The sputum of all contained predominating numbers of green-producing streptococci which were agglutinated specifically by the monovalent serum. All four patients showed marked improvement and recovered promptly following the serum treatment. Three of the patients were experiencing the initial influenzal attack, and one had a recrudescence at the time of the serum treatment. The lung findings remained limited; none of the patients developed outspoken signs of extensive consolidation. In at least two, the improvement seems definitely attributable to the serum since the lung findings and symptoms were on the increase at the time of the serum treatment (cases 1, 2 and 3, and chart 1).

Case 1 (3283).—Mrs. H. C. L. came to the Clinic March 11, 1919, on account of nervousness, general weakness, fluttering of the heart and profuse menstruation. The symptoms followed a severe attack of influenza in October, 1918. Examination revealed a pelvic tumor for which a hysterectomy was advised.

March 28 the patient was admitted to the isolation hospital, with symptoms of influenza. She had been taken ill five days before with moderate headache, aching in the arms and back, sore throat, cough and slight nausea. These symptoms grew gradually less severe until the day before admission to the hospital, when she became worse with general aching, chilly sensations in the back, but no distinct chill or fever. The patient's throat was diffusely red, her tongue coated, she was cyanotic, and crackling râles were elicited over the bases of both lungs, especially on the right side. Findings of the heart, blood and urine were normal. On the day of admission the sputum was slightly blood streaked. No evidence of consolidation was noted at any time. A culture of the sputum showed predominating numbers of green-producing streptococci and a few staphylococci, and the primary culture in dextrose-blood broth was agglutinated specifically by the serum from horse 15 (table 1). March 29 the patient was given 50 c c of this serum; the aching disappeared during the course of the day, the cough lessened, and the following day the temperature dropped perceptibly and became normal (chart 1). The leukocyte count was 7,300 the day after admission and rose to 13,500 March 31 and April 1. The patient made an uneventful recovery.

Case 2 (3208).— A farmer of middle age, entered the hospital March 11, 1919. He complained of severe backache, headache, inability to sleep, sore throat and cough. The illness had begun the previous day with chilly

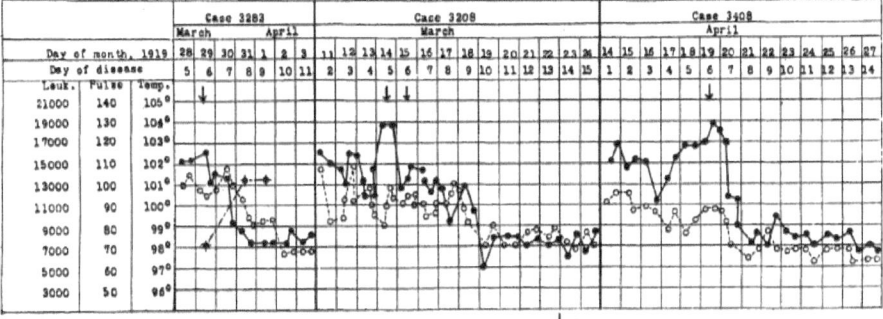

Chart 1.—Temperature, pulse and leukocyte curves in three patients in whom specific agglutination of the green-producing streptococcus from the sputum was obtained, and in whom marked improvement followed injection of the monovalent serum. In this and the following charts temperature is indicated by a solid line; leukocytes by a long and short dash line; pulse by a short dash line, and serum injections by arrows.

sensations but there had been no distinct chill. The patient's lips and fingernails were moderately cyanotic, he was mentally apathetic, although he complained of inability to sleep. His throat was diffusely red. The tonsils were also congested and the tongue was heavily coated. In the night of March 13 severe hemorrhage from the nose occurred and continued at intervals the following day. The lung findings were negative until March 17 when a small area of dulness was found at the inferior angle of the left scapula with slightly increased vocal fremitus and a suggestion of bronchial breathing. Later in the day dulness at the left base of the lung, fine crepitant râles in showers, and distinct bronchial breathing, especially at the inferior angle of the scapula near the spine, were noted. The sputum at first was mucopurulent, but March 13 it became serous in character and streaked with blood. Leukopenia was marked (chart 1). Blood-agar-plate cultures of the sputum obtained March 13, 15, and 17, showed countless numbers of green-producing streptococci, a

TABLE 1

Agglutination Experiments with Cultures from the Sputum in Cases of Influenza and Influenzal Pneumonia in which Immune Serum was Used

Case	Date on Which Sputum Culture Was Made	Condition of Culture at Time of Agglutination Test Dextrose-Blood-Broth Inoculated with	Antiserums							Controls	
			Pneumococcus			Streptococcus				
			I	II	III	Hemolytic of Horse 9	Green-producing of Horse 15	Normal Horse Serum	NaCl Solution
3208	3/13/19	Single green colony streptococcus............	0	0	0	0	+++	0	0
		Green-producing streptococcus after one animal passage............	0	0	0	++	++++	0	0
		Green-producing streptococcus in third generation after one animal passage...	+	+	+	+	+++	0	0
3276	3/28/19	Washed sputum............	0	0	0	0	+++	0	0
		Blood of mouse dead from intraperitoneal injection of sputum. Pure green streptococcus............	++	++	++	++	++++	++	0
	3/30/19	Washed sputum............	0	+	+++	+	++	+	0
		Blood of guinea-pigs injected intratracheally with moist, spreading greenish colony of streptococcus from sputum............	0	0	+++	0	0	0	0
	4/2/19	Washed sputum............	0	0	++	++	0	0	0
3282	3/30/19	Washed sputum............	0	+++	+++	+++	++++	0	0
	4/2/19	Washed sputum............	0	++	+	++	+++	0	0
3283	3/30/19	Washed sputum............	0	0	0	0	+	0	0
		Single colony moist, green streptococcus............	0	+	0	+	++	0	0
3338	4/7/19	Washed sputum............	0	0	0	++	++++	+	0
	4/8/19	Swab from throat............	0	0	0	0	+	0	0
	4/9/19	Washed sputum............	0	0	0	+	++	0	0
	4/11/19	Washed sputum............	0	++	0	++	0	0	0
	4/13/19	Washed sputum............	+	+	+	+	+	+	+
		Single colony green-producing streptococcus from sputum............	+	0	+	++	++	+	0
	4/16/19	Washed sputum............	0	0	0	0	0	0	0
	4/17/19	Washed sputum............	0	0	0	++	++	0	0
	4/25/19	Exudate right lung (hemolytic streptococci)............	0	++	0	+++	0	++	0
		Exudate right lung (hemolytic streptococci)............	+	+	+	+++	+	+	0
3341	4/8/19	Tonsil swab............	0	0	0	0	0	0	0
	4/9/19	Washed sputum............	0	+++	0	0	++	0	0
	4/11/19	Washed sputum............	0	+++	++	++	++	0	0
	4/12/19	Single colony green streptococcus............	0	+++	0	+++	++	0	0
3402	4/17/19	Throat swab............	0	0	0	0	0	0	0
		Washed sputum............	+	+	+	+	+	+	+
3408	4/18/19	Washed sputum............	0	0	0	0	++	0	0

few staphylococci, but no hemolytic streptococci nor influenza bacilli. A blood culture made March 12 was negative. Dextrose-blood-broth cultures of the green-producing streptococcus isolated directly from the sputum March 13 and from the lung of a guinea-pig injected intratracheally with the sputum were agglutinated specifically by the serum of horse 15 (table 1). March 14 the patient's condition was very serious. Cyanosis was increasing, the sputum became more bloody and frothy, the mental apathy was worse, and prostration and epistaxis were marked. In the afternoon the patient was given 60 c c of the serum intravenously. The hemorrhage from the nose stopped, the patient's general condition became much better, and he was brighter mentally soon after the injection. The following day the injection of serum was repeated. The temperature dropped gradually to normal, and uneventful recovery followed (chart 1). The effect of the serum in this case appeared strikingly favorable, and probably was not coincident, since the symptoms and lung findings were on the increase at the time the serum was given. A slight urticarial rash developed ten· days later. This patient was one of a group of five from the same locality who had severe attacks of influenza within a few days of each other after their arrival in Rochester; two of the patients died.

Case 3 (3408).—A middle aged man, entered the hospital April 14, 1919. He complained of severe aching, headache, malaise, weakness, sore throat, and slight cough. A general examination revealed moderate cyanosis, without manifest dyspnea, mental apathy, a diffusely red throat, and coated tongue. The chest findings were negative on the day of admission, but bubbling râles over both chests were elicited posteriorly April 15, 16, 17 and 18. The sputum obtained April 18 was mucopurulent. The cultures showed countless numbers of staphylococci and a moderate number of rather moist, spreading, green-producing and hemolytic streptococci. The leukocyte count on the fifteenth was 4,700. A blood culture made on the nineteenth proved negative. The primary culture of the washed sputum in dextrose-blood broth was agglutinated specifically by the serum of horse 15 (table 1). April 19, 25 c c of the serum were injected intravenously; the temperature and pulse rate dropped rapidly, and the general improvement was marked. The patient recovered promptly.

Group 2.—The three patients in this group were treated with the serum, and all showed marked improvement following injections during the initial attack of influenza when the green-producing streptococci from the sputum were agglutinated specifically by the monovalent serum. Later the patients developed bronchopneumonia due to green-producing streptococci that were not specifically agglutinated by this serum or by any of the immune serums tested (table 1, cases 4 and 5, and chart 2).

Case 4 (3282).—A woman, aged 48, came to the Clinic because of the recurrence of an abdominal tumor which had been operated on two years before. She was admitted to the isolation hospital March 28, 1919, stating that she had become ill the day before with a severe chill, sore throat, headache, and severe general aching. Her lips and fingernails were cyanotic, she was short of breath, even when lying quietly in bed, and abundant crepitant râles were found posteriorly at the left base of the lung and on the right side. A culture of the sputum obtained on the day of admission showed a large number of staphylococci and green-producing streptococci, and duplicate cultures in dextrose-blood broth were agglutinated specifically by the serum of horse 15 (table 1). March 29 and 30, 80 c c and 60 c c, respectively, of the serum of horse 15 were given intravenously. The patient's general condition improved following both injections, and her temperature and pulse rate dropped to normal (chart 2). The temperature remained normal for four days, and the abnormal lung findings almost disappeared. On the fifth day the temperature again rose and remained high for nine days, the pulse was rapid, and a sharp rise in the leukocyte count occurred. On the day following the rise of temperature an urticarial rash covered the entire body. With the increase in the temperature, dulness, bronchovesicular breathing and crepitant râles developed over the right side below the angle of the scapula. A culture of the sputum on the first day of normal temperature which followed the injection of the serum showed countless numbers of green-producing streptococci and staphylococci. The primary culture in dextrose-blood broth was

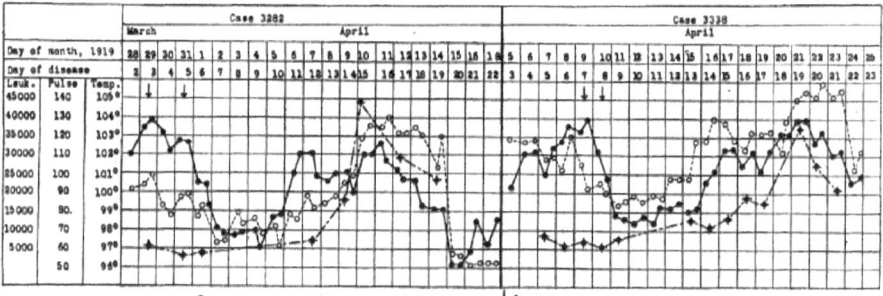

Chart 2.—Temperature, pulse and leukocyte curves in two patients in whom specific agglutination of the streptococcus was obtained during the initial attack, in whom there was marked improvement following injection of the monovalent serum, and in whom immunologically different green-producing streptococci were found during a reinfection.

again agglutinated specifically by the serum of horse 15. No cultures of the sputum were made subsequently. During the latter part of the attack of pneumonia, as the pulse rate crossed the temperature line (chart 2), the patient's condition was extremely critical for a number of days, but she finally made a complete, although slow, recovery.

Case 5 (3338).—A woman, aged 39, housekeeper, entered the isolation hospital April 5, 1919. Three days before the patient had felt chilly and could not get warm; she complained of moderate aching and was stiff in the joints and muscles. Two days afterward she developed a cough with a slight sore throat, and a moderately severe headache. If quiet in bed, she appeared well, but her lips and fingernails were decidedly blue. The examination of the chest was negative. On the morning of April 7 appeared a small area of slightly decreased resonance, bronchovesicular breathing, and a few râles below the angle of the left scapula near the posterior axillary line. The evening of April 8, crackling râles were heard on both sides in the lower axillae and posteriorly. On the morning of April 9 there were impaired resonance and crackling râles over the left base behind and at the side, and crackling râles on the right base posteriorly. The sputum was blood tinged and serous. By evening there was dulness over both lower lobes, but no definite bronchial breathing; crackling râles were heard over the entire chest. A culture of the sputum April 7 showed countless numbers of staphylococci and green-producing streptococci, a few hemolytic streptococci, and a moderate number of influenza bacilli. The primary culture in dextrose-blood broth of the washed sputum obtained April 7 and 9, and of a throat swab, showed almost pure cultures of green-producing streptococci which were agglutinated specifically by the serum of horse 15. Accordingly the patient was given intravenously 100 c c of serum April 9 and 10, respectively. The patient's general condition improved following both injections, the cyanosis became less marked, the expectoration diminished, and a drop in temperature and pulse rate occurred, the temperature reaching normal the day after the second injection (chart 2). The temperature remained normal for two days and then began to rise again, as evidence of a new involvement of the lung developed. The pulse rate remained high and continued unusually high throughout the fatal recurrence. Cultures of the sputum obtained on April 11, 13, 17 and 18 showed countless numbers of staphylococci, green-producing streptococci, an increasing number of hemolytic streptococci, and a few influenza bacilli. The green-producing streptococci, however, were no longer agglutinated specifically by the serum of horse 15 (table 1). The leukocyte count was persistently low throughout the first attack of fever, and at the onset of the recurrence, but then it rose to a high point, the maximum (43,000) being reached on the sixth day. On the two subsequent days the leukocytes diminished markedly and the patient died on the following day from what appeared to be cardiac failure from an overwhelming toxemia. After death the lung showed green-producing streptococci, hemolytic streptococci, and staphylococci, but no influenza bacilli. Duplicate cultures in dextrose-blood broth of the lung exudate showed hemolytic streptococci which were agglutinated by the antihemolytic streptococcus serum from horse 9. The reinfection in this case was clearly due to streptococci which were culturally identical, but immunologically were unlike those found during the initial attack. The anatomic diagnosis made at necropsy was: "Unresolved influenzal bronchopneumonia; marked enlargement of the tracheobronchial lymph nodes; purulent hemocatarrhal tracheal bronchitis; bilateral serofibrinous pleuritis; marked engorgement of the venous trunks of the body; petechial hemorrhages in the lining of the stomach and duodenum; hemorrhagic cystitis and marked hyperplasia of the spleen."

Group 3.—This group consisted of five cases in which no improvement followed the injection of the serum. In none of these was specific agglutination obtained at the time of the serum treatment, and all the patients died. In one case (case 3276) the agglutination of the streptococcus isolated from the sputum shifted from the serum of horse 15 to type III pneumococcus serum. In another case (case 3341) agglutination occurred in type II pneumococcus and hemolytic streptococcus serums. In the third case (case 3402) the sputum showed hemolytic streptococci which were not agglutinated by any of the serums (table 1). In two cases in this group countless numbers of green-producing streptococci were found in the sputum which were not agglutinated by any of the serums, and the patients were moribund at the time of the serum treatment. Cases 6, 7 and 8 illustrate the conditions found in this group of cases.

Case 6 (3276).—A farmer, aged 36, was admitted to the isolation hospital March 27, 1919. He had developed fever, backache, general aching, headache, dry throat, cough, and marked weakness the day before. On March 28 the throat was congested; the chest was negative except for a few scattered crackling râles. March 29 crackling râles and decreased resonance were found at the base of the left lung. The sputum was moderately bloody. On the afternoon of March 29 the patient was given 50 c c of serum from horse 15; the injection had no effect. April 1 there were definite signs of pneumonia on the left side, especially below the angle of the left scapula. The sputum was very frothy and bloody. The patient's condition grew rapidly worse, cyanosis and dyspnea increased, and he died from typical hemorrhagic pulmonary edema April 2. The leukocyte count was low at first, but it rose

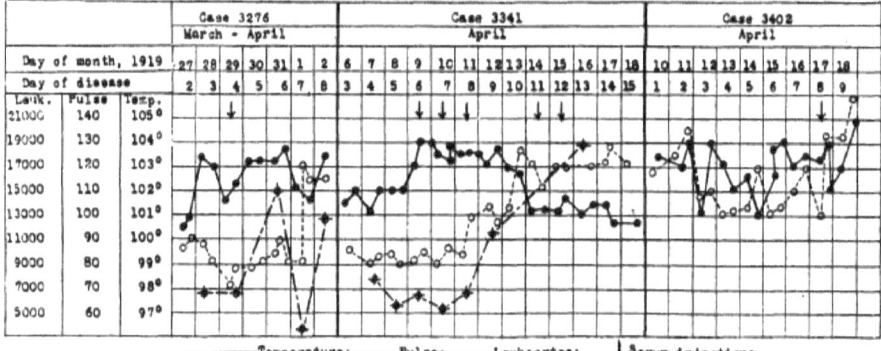

Chart 3.—Temperature, pulse and leukocyte curves in three patients in whom specific agglutination of streptococci from the sputum was not obtained and in whom the injection of the monovalent serum was without effect.

to 15,000 on March 31, and with the overwhelming toxemia showed a marked drop to 3,500 April 1, with another slight increase on the day of death (chart 3). Cultures from the sputum obtained March 28 showed countless numbers of moist, spreading, green-producing streptococci, a few staphylococci, but no hemolytic streptococci nor influenza bacilli. The primary culture in dextrose-blood broth of the washed sputum obtained on the twenty-eighth, and of the blood of a mouse, dead from intraperitoneal injection of sputum, were agglutinated specifically by the serum of horse 15. In contradistinction to this, March 30, the primary dextrose-blood-broth culture of the washed sputum, and of the moist, spreading, greenish colony of streptococci from the sputum was agglutinated specifically by type III pneumococcus serum. The primary culture of the sputum obtained April 2 was agglutinated slightly but equally by type III pneumococcus serum and antihemolytic streptococcus serum from horse 9 (table 1). The colonies on blood-agar from the dextrose-blood broth on all the days showed no change and resembled closely type III pneumococci, but they were not so elevated, and not so mucoid in character as pneumococcus mucosus.

Case 7 (3341).—A man, aged 38, undertaker, was admitted to the isolation hospital April 6, 1919. His illness had begun two nights before with a severe chill, vomiting, fever, backache, aching in the knees, general aching, slight nose bleed, and sore throat. The patient coughed and expectorated mucopurulent sputum. He was definitely short of breath and cyanotic. An examination of the chest was negative except for a few scattered râles. April 7 there were decreased resonance, and decreased breath sounds below the angle of the left scapula; April 8 decreased resonance and breath sounds and a few crackling râles were noted at the right base behind. On April 9 very definite signs of pneumonia were found on both sides. The sputum became bloody and serous. Cultures of the sputum and throat swab obtained April 7 and April 9 showed countless numbers of green-producing streptococci and staphylococci. On April 12 cultures showed countless numbers of staphylococci, a moderate number of green-producing streptococci, and larger, more moist spreading colonies resembling type III pneumococci. April 8, the primary cultures in dextrose-blood broth of the tonsil swab, and April 9, 11 and 13, of the sputum, were not agglutinated specifically by the serum of horse 15. Fermentative reactions showed that the green-producing streptococci from the sputum fermented inulin. The cultures of the sputum obtained on April 9 and 11 were agglutinated specifically by type II pneumococcus serum; those on April 13 by type II, and hemolytic streptococcus serum (table 1). The afternoons of April 9 and 10, 100 c c of serum from horse 15 were injected intravenously without effect. On April 11 and 14 injections of polyvalent antipneumococcus serums were given without effect. April 13 the urine showed a large amount of albumin and some red blood corpuscles. April 15 the patient was growing worse. He was bled 250 c c and was then given intravenously 250 c c of blood of a convalescent influenza patient, likewise without effect. The leukocyte count ranged from 5,500 in the earlier part of the attack to 19,200 in the latter (chart 3). The patient died April 18. The anatomic diagnosis was: "Bronchopneumonia, chronic cystitis with exacerbation, chronic parenchymatous nephritis, and old tuberculosis abscesses of the left lower lobe."

Case 8 (3402).—Woman, entered the hospital April 11, 1919; she complained of severe aching, fever, sore throat, and cough; she was toxic, cyanosed, and expectorated a small amount of mucopurulent sputum. The lung findings were negative. The heart showed mitral endocarditis with stenosis. April 14 and 15 crackling râles were elicited over both sides of the chest posteriorly, together with auricular fibrillation. April 16 the findings were definite for pneumonia of the left base. April 17 the expectorations became bloody, and profuse; the cyanosis and dyspnea increased. An injection of the serum of horse 15 had no apparent effect (chart 3), and the patient died April 18 with signs of acute hemorrhagic pulmonary edema. The sputum obtained April 17 showed countless numbers of hemolytic streptococci, staphylococci, and a few green-producing streptococci, but no influenza bacilli. The primary cultures in dextrose-blood broth of a throat swab and washed sputum were not agglutinated by any of the serums (table 1).

DISCUSSION

Of the twelve patients treated, all but one were critically ill at the time of serum treatment. Five recovered and seven died. Three of the patients who died were practically moribund at the time of the serum treatment and good effects could scarcely be expected. The two others that died showed green-producing streptococci immunologically different from the strain with which the serum was prepared, and in two, hemolytic streptococci caused death. In these cases also improvement could not be expected. In all cases in which specific agglutination was obtained, marked improvement followed the injection of the serum, and in no case were good effects noted at a time when agglutination tests were negative.

The influenza bacilli found in the sputum in two cases might be regarded as unimportant since both patients showed marked improvement following injections of the serum. The patients treated are of course too few to permit sweeping conclusions, but since the results were controlled by immunologic studies it would seem that diplostreptococci, closely related to pneumococci on the one hand and hemolytic streptococci on the other, bear important etiologic relationship to influenza and to influenzal pneumonia, especially early in the attack. The injection of properly prepared hyperimmune serums may prove curative in cases due to organisms immunologically identical to those used in the preparation of the serum, quite as has been found in the case of type pneumococcus infections in lobar pneumonia.

The changes which occurred in bacterial flora as measured by cultural and immunologic tests during the course of the disease, emphasize the complexity of the problem and the need for their consideration in the developement of specific methods of prevention and treatment of influenza and its complications.

APPENDIX A: *Minnesota Medicine* 12, June 1929, 366-368
Observations on the Cause and Prevention of Influenza and Influenzal Pneumnoia*
E. C. ROSENOW, M.D.
Rochester, Minnesota

In the pandemic of influenza of 1918 and 1919 extremely important experimental results bearing on the etiology of influenza were obtained with Bacillus influenza by Blake and Cecil, Duval, Parker and others, with green-producing and hemolytic streptococci by Rosenow and with staphylococci by several workers. On the basis of this work I suggest the following hypotheses: Peculiar strains of these organisms occurring individually or symbiotically should be considered the cause of the varied manifestations of influenza. Mutation or "dissociation" in the pneumococcus-streptococcus group normally present in the upper respiratory tract in human beings, sudden acquirement of exalted and peculiar virulence, especially of the streptococcus group, and hypersensitiveness or allergy to the bacterial proteins should be considered as important factors in the production of the peculiar manifestations of this disease.

To quote from one of my published reports: "The freshly isolated strains from influenza and its accompanying lesions have been found to produce relatively large amounts of 'anaphylatoxin' both in vitro and in vivo. The idea that the virulence of these bacteria may depend in part on their ability to produce 'anaphylatoxin' is in accord with my previous finding that virulent pneumococci and their filtrates produce a larger amount of this toxic substance than avirulent pneumococci. The picture in animals is clearly that of an anaphylactic intoxication, and suggests that the symptoms and lesions in man as recorded by numerous observers may likewise be due to this cause in which sensitization of the host to the bacterial proteins may or may not play a part. Findings as follows indicate this mechanism: (1) the delay in the coagulation time of the blood, leukopenia and cyanosis; (2) the marked tendency to develop acute pulmonary edema with a distended lung and relatively immobile expanded chest and extreme respiratory effort; (3) the voluminous lung as found at necropsy; (4) the occurrence of the rupture of alveoli and consequent subcutaneous emphysema (bronchial spasm); (5) the frequency of abortion (contraction of unstriped muscle) and other uterine disturbances."

The small anaerobic organism isolated from filtrates by Olitsky and Gates in the early stages of influenza should be regarded as being related to the streptococcus-pneumococcus group. They have shown that after long cultivation the organism becomes less anaerobic, of larger size, and of fairly typical streptococcal morphology.

The time, it seems to me, has fully arrived when epidemiologists and boards of health should acknowledge that while common-sense measures of quarantine are indicated the disease cannot be adequately controlled in this way. However important contact infection may seem to be, it is not the fundamental factor that causes epidemic and pandemic waves of this disease to appear and disappear so suddenly and so mysteriously at varying intervals of time.

I have found that the bacterial flora of the present epidemic in Rochester and in Minneapolis, Minnesota, and in Miami, Florida, is the same. Furthermore, it is like that of the pandemic of 1918 and 1919. The disease fortunately is milder and correspondingly the virulence of the streptococci is less marked. The green-producing streptococcus has been found constantly present in pure culture or in predominating numbers in the early stages of the disease, and the hemolytic streptococcus alone, or in mixture with the green-producing streptococcus, has been found later, especially in the secondary attack. Bacillus influenza and staphylococci have been found in goodly numbers in about one-fourth of the cases.
Instability and a marked tendency to the development of mutational forms have been noticed in the respective strains isolated in this epidemic. Similar features were noticed in the pandemic of 1918 and 1919. A summary of the results of the use of the vaccine during the pandemic of 1918 and 1919 is given in the tabulation.

The incidence of influenza and pneumonia, and the mortality rate, were consistently higher among the unvaccinated than among the vaccinated persons in each of the different groups studied.

The incidence of influenza was from three to six times as great and on the average was four times as great in the unvaccinated control groups as in the vaccinated groups. This observation was not anticipated since the vaccine was used only in the hope that the complicating pneumonia and the death rate might be lowered. Pneumonia occurred from three to twelve times as often in the unvaccinated as in the vaccinated groups. Deaths were from four and a half to nine and a half times as frequent in the unvaccinated as in the vaccinated groups. These differences are believed to be too great to be explained on the basis of statistical or other error in compiling the results, and therefore seem attributable to the vaccine. The largely negative results of Jordan and Sharp obtained in 1920 should not be interpreted as nullifying the positive results which I have obtained. In their work no particular care was exercised to incorporate freshly isolated strains, especially of the green-producing and hemolytic streptococci, which were so predominatingly present. I used freshly isolated strains.

TABULATION
RESULTS IN PERSONS VACCINATED THREE TIMES IN THE PANDEMIC OF INFLUENZA OF 1918 AND 1919

			Incidence in Each 1,000 Persons		
	Groups	Persons	Influenza	Pneumonia	Deaths
Nineteen counties in Minnesota	Vaccinated	17,532	102.8	4.2	0.8
	Unvaccinated	36,100	373.5	20.4	6.35
Olmsted County, Minnesota	Vaccinated	9,300	41.0	3.0	0.64
	Unvaccinated	8,700	248.0	13.1	4.00
Institutions	Vaccinated	8,306	31.0	1.0	0.5
	Unvaccinated	9,388	200.0	12.0	5.9
Hospitals	Vaccinated	57		21.0	5.0
	Unvaccinated	609		57.0	22.0
Results from questionnaires	Vaccinated	93,476	87.0	4.4	1.43
	Unvaccinated	345,133	281.0	21.0	8.55
Influenza complicating pregnancy	Vaccinated	997	109.0	27.0	14.0
	Unvaccinated	3,656	294.0	80.0	59.9

They worked at a time when the bacteria found, as well as the clinical manifestations, were far more heterogeneous and the disease less virulent. The amount of streptococcus viridans, the peculiar green-producing streptococcus in their vaccine, was approximately a half of the amount which was present in my vaccine. A sixth of their vaccine consisted of Bacillus influenza, against which, as is well known, it is more difficult to immunize than against pneumococci or streptococci. My vaccine contained at first a smaller proportion of influenza bacilli than theirs and later no influenza bacilli, but staphylococci instead. Their organisms were killed by heat; mine were killed by cresol. Moreover, in their series, as in mine, most of the patients declared that they had received definite protection against colds. Differences in epidemics and in the vaccines used may readily explain the discrepancies in the results obtained.

The bacterial flora of the present epidemic seems to be much like that of 1918 and 1919; at that time seemingly unmistakable good results were obtained from a mixed vaccine made to contain a high proportion of fleshly isolated strains.

I would recommend, therefore, that a concerted effort on a large scale be made against this disease by means of vaccines prepared from freshly isolated strains in proportions approximating the bacterial flora at hand in different localities. This work has already begun in Rochester.

The bacteria are grown in gallon bottles of broth; this is clarified, and the bacteria then are stored in dense suspension in glycerin and sodium chloride solution. The vaccine is made by diluting these dense suspensions with sufficient sterile sodium chloride solution. These dilutions are heated at 70° C. for one hour and 0.3 per cent phenol is added as a preservative. One cubic centimeter is made to contain 5,000,000,000 killed bacteria. Three subcutaneous injections of 0.3, 0.5 and 1.0 c.c., respectively, are given at weekly intervals and then a monthly injection of 1.0 c.c. for as long a time as needed. The dosage for children should be about half and for infants about a fourth that for adults.

The vaccine is sent gratis to physicians by The Mayo Foundation in the hope that information of value as regards the good that may be accomplished in this way will be forthcoming. In order to estimate the value of the vaccinations, physicians are requested to be sure to record the name, sex, age, occupation, the degree of reaction, the date and number of vaccinations and the date, duration and severity of attacks of respiratory infections in those vaccinated. So far as possible they are requested to give similar data concerning unvaccinated persons living under similar circumstances or who live or work in the same household, shop or office.

BIBLIOGRAPHY

1. Jordan, E. O., and Sharp, W. B.: Influenza studies ; effect of vaccination against influenza and some other respiratory infections. Jour. Infect. Dis., 1921, xxviii, 357-366.
2. Olitsky, P. K., and Gates, F. L.: Experimental studies of the nasopharyngeal secretions from influenza patients. VIII. Further observations on the cultural and morphological characters of *Bacterium pneumosintes*. Jour. Exper. Med., 1922, xxxv, 813-821.
3. Rosenow, E. C.: Studies in influenza and pneumonia. II. The experimental production of symptoms and lesions simulating those of influenza with streptococci isolated during the present pandemic. Jour. Am. Med. Assn., 1919, lxxii, 1604-1609.

*From the Division of Experimental Bacteriology, The Mayo Foundation, Rochester, Minn., presented at the National Conference on Influenza, Washington, D. C., January 10, 1929.

APPENDIX B: *A.M.A. Arch. Otolaryng.* 58: 609-622, Nov. 1953

DIAGNOSTIC CUTANEOUS REACTIONS, SPECIFIC PREVENTION AND TREATMENT IN EPIDEMIC RESPIRATORY INFECTIONS

EDWARD C. ROSENOW, M.D.
CINCINNATI

THE IMPORTANCE of cultivatable micro-organisms currently considered as secondary invaders and of the different strains of virus currently considered as primary in the causation of influenza and other epidemic respiratory infections is still a largely unsolved problem. The investigations on influenza virus have yielded information of the greatest importance as regards its presence and nature. The results of virus neutralization tests with convalescent serum for the identification of different strains in epidemics are reminiscent of the early studies on identification of different types of pneumococci by serologic means. At first there was but one type of the Pneumococcus and one strain of influenza virus and then two, three, and so on. The uncertainty as to presence of virus and the type at hand in current epidemic outbreaks, the changes that occur in influenza virus during epidemics, the difficulty and delay entailed in the identification of virus strains, the toxicity and sensitizing properties of virus vaccine made from chick embryo cultures, and the short duration of immunity that follows prophylactic immunization with virus vaccine have proved serious handicaps for the solution of this important problem. Studies from the purely virus standpoint have yielded little of practical value for treatment. The results from the use of antibiotics in the treatment of influenza, as of other epidemic disease due to or associated with virus infections and nonhemolytic streptococci, have also proved disappointing. The need for further information is therefore clearly indicated.

It is the purpose of this communication to review in some detail the existing evidence which bears on this problem and to report the results obtained by the use of new methods—especially those for the detection of specific circulating streptococcal antigen and antibody by the immediate reactions which follow intradermal injection of specific streptococcal antibody and antigen—on the etiology, diagnosis, and specific treatment of epidemic respiratory infections, including influenza.

REVIEW OF PUBLISHED STUDIES

Of the so-called secondary invaders, pneumococci,[1] staphylococci,[2] Bacillus influenzae,[3] and green-producing or nonhemolytic and hemolytic streptococci are by far

---

From the Department of Bacteriological Research, Longview Hospital.

1. Hirsch, E. F., and McKinney, M.: An Epidemic of Pneumococcus Bronchopneumonia, J. Infect. Dis. **24**:594-617, 1919.

2. Chickering, H. T., and Park, J. H., Jr.: Staphylococcus Aureus Pneumonia, J. A. M. A. **72**:617-626, 1919.

3. Huntoon, F. M., and Hannum, S.: The Rôle of Bacillus Influenzae in Clinical Influenza, J. Immunol. **4**:167-187, 1919.

the most important. Streptococci (including a pandemic strain [4] during the pandemic of influenza of 1918), especially of the alpha type, have been isolated consistently by various investigators [5] and by me from persons stricken,[6] from indoor and outdoor air,[7] from milk supplies,[8] from casual water and water supplies [9] during epidemics which have occurred chiefly in winter months since 1918 and by myself [10] and others [11] in studies of primary atypical or so-called "virus" pneumonia. The nonhemolytic streptococci isolated by the special methods used from persons ill during epidemics of respiratory infections and from air, milk, and water were shown to possess pneumotropic virulence which was roughly proportional to the severity of epidemics. The nonhemolytic streptococci isolated during the pandemic of 1918 were extremely virulent. Intratracheal insufflation in guinea pigs caused death in high incidence from widely disseminated areas of extreme emphysema, atelectasis, hemorrhagic edema, tracheitis, bronchitis, bronchopneumonia, and necrosis of alveolar epithelium and capillaries. These findings simulated the extraordinarily severe clinical, pathological, and histological picture of the naturally occurring disease in human beings during the pandemic.[12]

The nonhemolytic streptococci were isolated consistently, since in studies of milder epidemics of respiratory infections, including the common cold and "virus" pneumonia, they had a similar predilection for the respiratory tract on cerebral, nasal, and intraperitoneal inoculation in mice, guinea pigs, and rabbits, respectively. The symptoms and lesions were less pronounced and the mortality far lower than during

4. Rosenow, E. C.: Studies in Influenza and Pneumonia: III. The Occurrence of a Pandemic Strain of Streptococcus During the Pandemic of Influenza, J. A. M. A. **72**:1608-1609, 1919.

5. Blanton, W. B., and Irons, E. E.: A Recent Epidemic of Acute Respiratory Infection at Camp Custer, Mich.: Preliminary Laboratory Report, J. A. M. A. **71**:1988-1991, 1918. Falk, I. S.; Harrison, R. W.; McKinney, R. A., and Stuppy, G. W.: Experiments on the Etiology of Influenza: Preliminary Report, ibid. **93**:2030-2031, 1929. Weisner, R. R.: Streptococcus Pleomorphus und die sogenannte spanische Grippe, Wien. Klin. Wchnschr. **31**:1101-1104, 1918. Rosenow, E. C.: Studies in Influenza and Pneumonia: II. The Experimental Production of Symptoms and Lesions Simulating Those of Influenza with Streptococci Isolated During the Present Pandemic, J. A. M. A. **72**:1604-1608, 1919. Mathers, G.: The Bacteriology of Acute Epidemic Respiratory Infections Commonly Called Influenza, J. Infect. Dis. **21**:1-8, 1917.

6. Rosenow, E. C.: Studies on the Etiologic Relation of Streptococci to Acute Epidemic Respiratory Infections, Am. J. Clin. Path. **15**:319-333, 1945.

7. Rosenow, E. C.: Isolation from the Air of Streptococci and Streptococcal Antigens Resembling Those Associated with Certain Epidemic Diseases, J. Bact. **39**:73-74, 1940.

8. Rosenow, E. C.: Isolation from Milk Supplies of Specific Types of Green-Producing (Alpha) Streptococci and Their Thermal Death Point in Milk, Minnesota Med. **27**:550-556, 1944.

9. Rosenow, E. C.: Specific Types of Alpha Streptococci and Streptococcal Antigen in Unpotable Water and Water Supplies, Am. J. Clin. Path. **15**:513-528, 1945.

10. Rosenow, E. C.: Diagnostic Cutaneous Reactions to Intradermal Injection of Natural and Artificial Antibody and of Antigen Prepared from Streptococci Isolated in Studies of Diverse Diseases, Ann. Allergy **6**:485-496, 1948.

11. Thomas, L.; Mirick, G. S.; Curren, E. C.; Ziegler, J. E., Jr., and Horsfall, F. L., Jr.: Serological Reactions with an Indifferent Streptococcus in Primary Atypical Pneumonia, Science **98**:566-568, 1943.

12. LeCount, E. R.: The Pathological Anatomy of Influenzal Bronchopneumonia, J. A. M. A. **72**:650-652, 1919; Disseminated Necrosis of Pulmonary Capillaries in Influenzal Pneumonia, ibid. **72**:1519-1520, 1919. Bell, E. T.: The Pathology of the Lungs in Pneumonia Following Influenza, Journal Lancet **39**:3, 1919.

the pandemic, paralleling the severity of the disease of the epidemics in question. Moreover, the nonhemolytic streptococci on isolation in dextrose-brain broth from sputum and nasopharyngeal swabbings in studies of the different epidemics were found to have characteristic distribution curves of cataphoretic velocity or electrical potential.[13] Intradermal injection of solutions of the euglobulin fraction of the serum of horses that had been immunized with the nonhemolytic Streptococcus from influenza caused an immediate erythematous reaction indicating specific streptococcal antigen in skin or blood and hence a corresponding streptococcal infection in influenza and in influenzal and "virus" pneumonia.[6] The agglutinative titer of the serum of persons with influenza and influenzal and "virus" bronchopneumonia for the respective streptococci increased as recovery occurred.[14] Antistreptococcus serums were prepared in horses with the streptococci in which the antigenic specificity was preserved at 10 C. throughout the long period of immunization by partial dehydration of the freshly isolated strains in dense suspension (1,000,000,000,000 organisms per cubic centimeter) of glycerin (2 parts) and saturated NaCl solution (1 part). Such antiserums agglutinated the streptococci and precipitated specifically the antigen in NaCl solution washings of nasopharyngeal swabbings and in cleared suspensions of the streptococci whose specificity had been preserved in the glycerin-NaCl solution menstruum in interface precipitation tests. [15]

The high degree of protection afforded by prophylactic immunization in advance of anticipated epidemics or abreast with epidemics with vaccines containing a high percentage of the nonhemolytic Streptococcus whose specificity had been preserved in the glycerin NaCl solution menstruum further indicates the importance of bacterial infection in influenza. The protection afforded by three weekly subcutaneous injections of the vaccine and then one injection at three- or four-week intervals during epidemics was most striking. The incidence of influenzal attacks, the dreaded hemorrhagic edema and bronchopneumonia, miscarriages in pregnancy, and deaths from hemorrhagic edema and bronchopneumonia during the pandemic were from three- to eightfold lower in the vaccinated groups than in the control unvaccinated groups.[16] Persons having chronic bronchitis, sinusitis, myositis, or infectious arthritis

---

13. Rosenow, E. C.: (a) Cataphoretic Velocity and Virulence of Streptococci Isolated from Throats of Human Beings, from Raw Milk, Flies, Water, Sewage and Air During Epidemics of the Common Autumnal Cold, Am. J. Hyg. **19**:1-21, 1934; (b) Cataphoretic Time and Velocity of Streptococci and Pneumococci: Studies on Organisms Isolated in Cases of the Common Cold, Influenza, Bronchopneumonia and Lobar Pneumonia, J. Infect. Dis. **54**:91-122, 1934; (c) Cataphoresis as a Control of the Specificity of Streptococcal Vaccines: Influenzal Streptococcus Vaccine in the Prevention and Treatment of Infections of the Respiratory Tract, J. Immunol. **26**:401-433, 1934; (d) footnote 6.

14. Rosenow, E. C.: Studies in Influenza and Pneumonia: X. The Immunologic Properties of the Green-Producing Streptococci from Influenza, J. Infect. Dis. **26**:597-613, 1920.

15. Rosenow, E. C.: Demonstration of the Association of Specifically Different Alpha Streptococci with Various Diseases, and Methods for the Preparation and Use of Specific Antiserums and Vaccines in Diagnosis and Treatment, Am. J. Clin. Path. **12**:339-356, 1942.

16. (a) Rosenow, E. C., and Sturdivant, B. F.: Studies in Influenza and Pneumonia: IV. Further Results of Prophylactic Inoculations, J. A. M. A. **73**:396-401, 1919. (b) Rosenow, E. C.: Observations on the Cause and Prevention of Influenza and Influenzal Pneumonia, Minnesota Med. **12**:366-368, 1929. (c) Rosenow, E. C., and Osterberg, A. E.: A Method for the Preparation of Prophylactic and Autogenous Lipovaccines, J. A. M. A. **73**:87-91, 1919. (d) Rosenow, E. C., and Heilman, F. R.: Streptococcal Vaccines in the Prevention and Treatment of Respiratory Infections: A Clinical and Experimental Study, Am. J. Clin. Path. **8**:17-27, 1938.

to whom the vaccine was given also benefitted.[17] Others reported similar results.[18] Having found a method for preserving antigenic specificity and for reducing toxicity of the highly mutable nonhemolytic Streptococcus, an attempt was made to find a vaccine sufficiently nontoxic and broad in antigenicity that would afford protection not only for the common cold but also for the severer influenzal infections. Two vaccines were used, at first one prepared from the streptococci isolated in studies of the common cold and one containing the streptococci from patients with influenza. It was found that the former protected against the common cold but not against influenza. The latter afforded protection geographically against both the common cold and influenza.[19] Throughout these studies the vaccine was used also in treatment. Results obtained by us and by the large numbers of physicians to whom it was sent gratis for study were also uniformly favorable geographically.

Protective and curative action of the vaccine in animals was similar to that obtained in human beings,[20] and the monovalent antistreptococcal serum had curative action in persons having influenza due to serologically homologous nonhemolytic streptococci.

It should be emphasized that the results obtained in the studies reviewed are attributable to the special methods employed. The characteristic virulent and nonvirulent nonhemolytic streptococci, morphologically indistinguishable, were found in mixture in nasopharyngeal swabbings and in sputum. The former had a distinctive influenzal distribution curve; the latter had a normal distribution curve of cataphoretic velocity or electrical potential. The former was highly sensitive to oxygen and usually did not grow on blood agar in primary aerobic cultures; whereas the latter grew in large numbers in mediums affording a gradient or reduced oxygen tension and other conditions favorable for growth, such as 0.2% dextrose broth to which pieces of fresh calf brain (1 part to 6 or 7 parts of the broth) in tall columns were added before autoclaving. The virulent nonhemolytic streptococci in dextrose-brain broth outgrew the nonvirulent variants in young cultures. The use of this medium for primary isolations and for rapidly repeated subcultures for inoculation of animals and the preservation of antigenic specificity in the glycerin and sodium chloride solution menstruum for serologic studies and for the preparation of vaccines was found essential. The nonhemolytic Streptococcus having high pneumotropic virulence, as that isolated during the pandemic, commonly changed to hemolytic type in vivo and in vitro, and the hemolytic variant often reverted to nonhemolytic type. A rise and fall in severity of symptoms and mortality occurred in family groups and during successive epidemic waves during the pandemic and was shown to be due to changes in virulence of the Streptococcus. Similar changes in severity of the infection and mortality occurred on successive intratracheal guinea pig passage of the causative nonhemolytic Streptococcus.[21]

---

17. Rosenow.[13b] Rosenow and Sturdivant.[16a]

18. Fennel, E. A.: Prophylactic Inoculation Against Pneumonia: A Brief History and Present Status of Procedure, J. A. M. A. **71**:2115-2120, 1918. Cecil, R. L., and Vaughan, H.: Results of Prophylactic Vaccination Against Pneumonia at Camp Wheeler, J. Exper. Med. **29**:457-483, 1919. Moody, E., and Howard, W. M.: Control of Juvenile Asthma by Vaccine Therapy: Report of Small Series, Arch. Pediat. **58**:774-778, 1941.

19. Footnote 13c. Footnote 6. Footnote 16d.

20. Rosenow.[6] Footnote 13c.

21. Rosenow, E. C.: Studies in Influenza and Pneumonia: IX. Changes in the Green-Producing Streptococcus Induced by Successive Animal Passage and Their Significance in Epidemic Influenza, J. Infect. Dis. **26**:567-596, 1920.

The common occurrence of gastroenteritis during the course of epidemics of influenza and other respiratory infections is well known. Nonhemolytic streptococci having predilection for the gastrointestinal tract in animals have been consistently isolated from the nasopharynx and stools of persons so afflicted and often from the water supply.[22] Changes from pneumotropic to gastroenterotropic type of the Streptococcus have occurred on successive passage through animals,[22] and the occurrence of both the respective streptococci and the viruses in epidemics of influenza has been reported.[23] The occurrence of lethargic and other forms of encephalitis following epidemics of influenza is also well known. Most important, the strains of "neurotropic" nonhemolytic streptococci isolated in studies of encephalitis lost "neurotropic" virulence and acquired "pneumotropic" virulence, causing pneumonitis on successive cerebral passage through animals.[24] The results of these experiments indicate that the older classifications of influenza as "catarrhal," "brain," and "gastrointestinal" fever, respectively, were appropriately designated by these descriptive terms. Nonhemolytic streptococci having distinctive elective localizing properties were isolated respectively from these three disease entities, and in each of these—influenza and other epidemic respiratory infections, encephalitis, and gastroenteritis—characteristic viruses having respective specific disease-producing properties have been identified.

On the basis of facts such as these it was postulated that the respective streptococci and viruses may be related and that the respective specificities may be due to mutation or dissociation. A long series of experiments were made to determine the validity of such a hypothesis. The three respective filtrable agents resembling the natural viruses have been produced experimentally from the respective "neurotropic,"[25] "enterotropic,"[22a] and "pneumotropic"[26] green-producing or nonhemolytic streptococci. The strains of streptococci in each instance were so far removed from the original source as to eliminate the presence of the respective natural viruses.

The results of studies on the relation of pneumotropic streptococci to influenza virus were especially relevant. Pneumotropic nonhemolytic streptococci were isolated by the special methods employed from natural influenza virus and from the experimentally produced filtrable pneumotropic agents resembling virus. The nonhemolytic streptococci isolated from the nasopharynx of persons having influenza, from the experimentally produced virus, and from natural virus all produced pneumonitis on nasal inoculation in mice. Mice were immunized against the natural and the

22. Rosenow, E. C.: (a) Infectious Gastro-Enteritis: An Epidemiologic and Laboratory Study, Am. J. Digest. Dis. **11**:381-391, 1944; (b) Studies in Influenza and Pneumonia: VIII, Experiments on the Etiology of "Gastro-Intestinal" Influenza, J. Infect. Dis. **26**:557-566, 1920.

23. Rosenow, E. C.: Streptococci and Diplostreptococci and the Respective "Viruses" in the Etiology and Epidemiology of Epidemic Respiratory Infections and Infectious Gastroenteritis, Am. J. Digest. Dis. **17**:261-270, 1950.

24. Rosenow, E. C.: Changes in the Streptococcus from Encephalitis, Induced Experimentally, and Their Significance in the Pathogenesis of Epidemic Encephalitis and Influenza, J. Infect. Dis. **33**:531-556, 1923.

25. (a) Kendall, A. I.: Observations upon the Filterability of Bacteria, Including a Filterable Organism Obtained from Cases of Influenza: Studies in Bacterial Metabolism, Science **74**:129-139, 1931. (b) Rosenow, E. C.: Studies on the Virus Nature of an Infectious Agent Obtained from 4 Strains of "Neurotropic" Alpha Streptococci, J. Nerv. & Ment. Dis. **100**:229-262, 1944; (c) The Relation of Neurotropic Streptococci to Encephalitis and Encephalitic Virus, Proc. Staff Meet., Mayo Clin. **17**:551-560, 1942.

26. Rosenow, E. C.: Studies on the Relation of Pneumotropic Streptococci to Influenza Virus, Am. J. Clin. Path. **15**:362-380, 1945.

experimental virus with the influenzal streptococcic vaccine. Natural and experimental viruses were neutralized in parallel by influenzal antistreptococcic serum and by convalescent serum.[22a] In support of the results of these studies, it has since been shown with the electron microscope that the virus of influenza consists of small spheres, ovoids singly and doubly and in short and long filaments or in chain formation,[27] suggesting further that the Streptococcus and virus are related and antigenically similar.

Having reviewed the studies which bear so directly on the problem involved, I shall next report the results of further studies by new methods which further indicate the importance of nonhemolytic streptococci in influenza.

TABLE 1.—*Results in Mice After Cerebral and Nasal Inoculation of the Streptococcus Isolated from Nasopharynx of Persons Having Epidemic Respiratory Infection, from Outdoor Air During Epidemic Prevalence of Such Infection, and as Controls from Poliomyelitis and Persons Not Having Respiratory Infections*

Source and Type of Material Inoculated			Strains	Inoculated	Mice Percentage			Streptococci from			
						In which Developed		Lungs		Brain	
					That Died	Polio-encephalitis	Pneumonitis	Cultured	% Plus	Cultured	% Plus
Streptococci from	Nasopharynx of persons having epidemic respiratory infection		70	131	31	10	48	40	80	38	53
	Poliomyelitis	Nasopharynx of persons stricken	18	81	39	54	16	9	22	33	69
		Virus from monkey and mouse	8	88	27	47	9	11	27	37	70
	Well persons or persons ill not with respiratory infection		69	156	17	12	14	10	30	18	15
Outdoor air during general prevalence of epidemic respiratory infection	Streptococci*		1	33	24	24	64	19	78	17	18
	Filtrates*		1	18	0	0	39	12	50	17	18

RESULTS OF FURTHER STUDIES BY NEW METHODS

The results in control material and in mice, following inoculation of nonhemolytic streptococci isolated in dextrose-brain broth and obtained from the nasopharynx of well persons and of persons having respiratory infection and from the NaCl solution washings of absorbent material exposed to outdoor air on an automobile during a drive of 1,850 miles in November, 1950, through regions where respiratory infections were generally prevalent, are summarized in Table 1. While under ether anesthesia, the mice were inoculated cerebrally with 0.03 ml. and nasally with 0.06 ml. of 10:1 suspension in sodium chloride solution of pure cultures of the nonhemolytic streptococci from the end-point of growth of serial dilution cultures in dextrose-brain broth. Mice that died were examined as soon after death as possible. Those that survived

27. (*a*) Taylor, A. R.; Sharp, D. G.; Beard, D.; Dingle, D. H., and Feller, A. E.: The Isolation and Characterization of Influenza A Virus (PR8 Strain), J. Immunol. **47**:261-282, 1943. (*b*) Murphy, J. S.; Karzon, A. T., and Bang, F. G.: Studies of Influenza (PR8) Infected Tissue Cultures by Electronmicroscopy, Dept. Med., The Johns Hopkins Univ. School of Med., Baltimore, Md.

were killed with ether three to five days following inoculation. A high degree of specificity of the respective strains is shown by the incidence of lesions and isolations of streptococci from the lesions produced.

In order to determine further the epidemiologic importance of the Streptococcus isolated from the sampling of outdoor air and as a control, NaCl solution and a Seitz filtrate of NaCl solution washing of the exposed material were nebulized into sterilized gallon jars, into each of which five mice were placed. Into each of two of these jars was nebulized 5 ml. of a dextrose-brain broth culture isolated from the filtrate of sodium chloride solution washings of the exposed material. Into each of two other jars was nebulized the Seitz filtrate of such washings and, as a control, 5 ml. of sterile sodium chloride solution was nebulized into each of two jars. The mice were killed with ether on the third day after the nebulization. Four of the 10 that were made to respire the Streptococcus revealed slight to severe pneumonitis, and the Streptococcus was isolated from affected lungs. Five of the 10 that respired the filtrate of NaCl solution washings of material which had been exposed to outdoor air revealed pneumonitis, and the Streptococcus was isolated. The lungs of the 10 control mice were normal, and cultures for streptococci were negative.

Through studies on the in vitro production of antibodies, new materials suitable for diagnosis and specific treatment have become available.[28] When suspensions in sodium chloride solution containing 20,000,000,000 streptococci per milliliter prepared from dilutions of the dense glycerin-sodium chloride solution suspension are autoclaved at 17-lb. (7.7 kg.) of pressure for 96 hours, the organisms disintegrate; the remnants become sharply agglutinated and brownish in color, and substances resembling the natural antibody suitable for diagnostic cutaneous tests and treatment appear in the supernatant sodium chloride solution.

Erythematous reactions to intradermal injection of 0.03 ml. of the supernatant diluted with equal parts of NaCl solution containing 0.4% phenol have been found to serve as a measure of specific antigen in skin or blood and hence of a corresponding streptococcal infection. Erythematous reactions to the bacteria-free supernatant of streptococci containing 10,000,000,000 streptococci per milliliter after heating at 70 C. for one hour and similarly injected intradermally serve as a measure of antibody in skin or blood. Antibody produced by autoclaving suspensions containing 10,000,000,000 streptococci per milliliter for three hours after adding 1.5% hydrogen peroxide has been found to have high specific agglutinative titers and on subcutaneous therapeutic injection, after bringing the pH to 6.5, has been found to cause a sharp drop in antigen and rise in antibody on repeat intradermal tests and often a corresponding improvement in symptoms. Therapeutic response and diminution of cutaneous reaction occur also following injection of the supernatant of suspensions autoclaved for 96 hours without hydrogen peroxide.

The results of cutaneous tests in groups of persons having respiratory infections and in well control persons according to season for four consecutive years and in persons having acute and chronic sinusitis, bronchial asthma, and hay fever are summarized in Table 2. The average reactions indicating "respiratory" streptococcic antigen and antibody to intradermal injection of antibody and antigen respectively were uniformly far greater in persons having respiratory infections than in persons

---

28. Rosenow, E. C.: Production in Vitro of Substances Resembling Antibodies from Bacteria, J. Infect. Dis. **76**:163-178, 1945; Studies on the Nature of Antibodies Produced in Vitro from Bacteria with Hydrogen Peroxide and Heat, J. Immunol. **55**:219-232, 1947.

TABLE 2.—*Intradermal Antibody-Antigen and Antigen-Antibody Reactions in Persons Having Acute Respiratory Infection and Well Persons According to Season and in Persons Having Sinusitis, Bronchial Asthma, and Hay Fever or Allergic Rhinitis, Respectively*

Year	Season	Acute epidemic respiratory infection + or 0	Cutaneous reactions (sq.cm.) to intradermal injection of thermal antibody and antigen prepared from streptococci isolated in studies of										
			Epidemic respiratory infections		Chronic Encephalitis		Arthritis		Well persons		Control - Pneumococci Types I, II, III	
			Indicating in skin or blood respective streptococcal									
			Persons Tested	Antigen	Antibody	Persons Tested	Antigen	Persons Tested	Antigen	Persons Tested	Antigen	Persons Tested	Antigen
1947	Summer & Autumn	+	77	12.03	7.02			77	2.66				
		0	121	3.77	2.92	104	2.44	45	3.11				
1948	Spring & Autumn	+	60	12.67	7.45	9	4.60	33	2.43	16	1.34		
		0	165	4.02	2.19	94	2.59	54	2.59	45	2.21		
1949	Autumn & Winter	+	96	13.97	9.17	55	4.25	20	3.96	16	2.42	10	5.52
		0	124	8.61	6.29	124	1.10	124	1.87	16	3.42	10	3.51
1950		+	67	13.48	7.95	11	3.64	21	2.41			25	3.22
		0	119	7.09	5.26	40	2.92	18	1.27	23	1.67	58	2.99
Sinusitis	Acute		7	16.81	6.02	6	3.88	6	3.45				
	Chronic		16	7.34	5.43	7	4.40	16	2.10				
Bronchial Asthma			11	11.08	8.40	4	3.68	10	2.63				
Hay Fever and Allergic Rhinitis			22	6.93	1.14	14	2.90						

TABLE 3.—*Intradermal Antibody-Antigen and Antigen-Antibody Reactions Indicating Antigen and Antibody, Respectively, in Skin or Blood in Well Persons and Persons Having Respiratory Infection in Relation to the Seasonal Incidence of Respiratory Infection and Poliomyelitis*

Persons studied according to disease and season			General incidence of		Groups	Persons Tested	Erythematous reactions (sq.cm.) indicating streptococcal antigen and antibody in skin or blood on intradermal injection respectively of thermal antibody and of antigen prepared from streptococci isolated in studies of					
			Resp. Infection	Polio-myelitis			Resp. Infection		Poliomyelitis		Controls	
							Antigen	Antibody	Antigen	Antibody	Antigen	Antigen
Persons Tested Twice While	Well	Sept. 1948	Mod.	Mod.	4	99	6.61	4.29	11.32	8.32	2.12	2.34
		Feb. 1949	High	0			11.21	7.54	4.55	4.30	4.18	3.08
	Having Resp. Infection	Sept. 1948	Mod.	Mod.	4	79	12.77	5.52	12.55	8.35	3.99	3.30
		Feb. 1949	High	0			13.53	7.79	5.80	4.14	4.42	2.46
Persons Tested Once While	Well	May 1948	Mod.	0	1	78	6.46	5.20	3.26	2.85	3.41	1.88
		Sept. 1948	0	Mod.	8	383	4.86	3.52	11.77	8.79	1.66	1.24
		Feb. 1949	High	0	5	103	10.46	7.70	5.94	3.62	4.29	4.98
	Having Resp. Infection	May 1948	Mod.	0	1	35	13.91	6.70	4.05	3.50	3.57	1.55
		Sept. 1948	Mod.	Mod.	7	101	12.14	5.80	12.14	8.55	3.47	2.30
		Feb. 1949	High	0	5	60	15.17	9.45	5.20	5.47	4.94	4.24

having encephalitis or arthritis and in well persons. Reactions indicating "respiratory" antigen and antibody both in ill persons and in well persons were uniformly significantly greater during autumn and winter in 1949 and 1950 than during summer and autumn in 1947 and during summer in 1948 (not shown in the Table), corresponding to the usual seasonal incidence and severity of respiratory infections. Reactions to control antibody indicating antigen were uniformly far less, and there were no significant seasonal changes. The reactions indicating infection by the "respiratory" type of Streptococcus in sinusitis, bronchial asthma, and hay fever parallel roughly the clinical and bacteriological findings in these conditions.

The results of similar tests made in a large number of well persons and persons having respiratory infections in relation to the seasonal incidence of respiratory infection and poliomyelitis, respectively, are summarized in Table 3. Cutaneous reactions indicating "respiratory" streptococcic antigen and antibody in well persons but especially in persons having respiratory infection were greatest during winter months, when epidemics of influenza and other respiratory infections were prevalent.

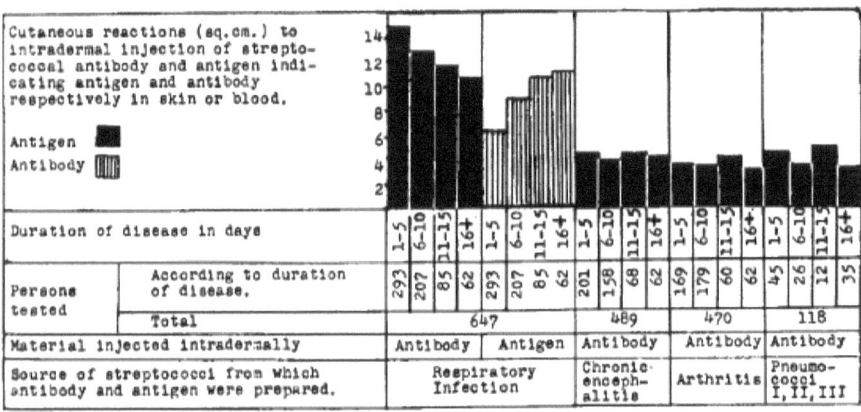

Chart 1.—Cutaneous reactions to intradermal injection of "respiratory" streptococcal antibody and antigen and in contrast to those of control antibody in persons having acute respiratory infection, according to the duration of the disease.

In sharp contrast, "respiratory" antigen and antibody were lowest and reactions indicating "poliomyelitis" streptococcic antigen and antibody were uniformly greatest in summer, when poliomyelitis occurs in highest incidence. Reactions to intradermal injection of the control antigen and antibody were uniformly far less and did not change according to season. The large number of persons tested and summarized in Tables 2 and 3 consisted of widely separated groups, chiefly nurses, college students, physicians, and personnel in hospitals in Ohio, Illinois, Wisconsin, and Minnesota.

The results of cutaneous reactions in a large number of controls and persons having respiratory infections, according to the duration of the disease, are shown graphically in Chart 1. Cutaneous reactions to the respiratory thermal antibody indicating streptococcal antigen in persons having respiratory infections were greatest at the onset of the disease and diminished with time as recovery ensued. Reactions to antigen indicating antibody were least pronounced at the onset and increased as recovery occurred. Reactions to the control antibody prepared respectively from streptococci isolated in studies of encephalitis and arthritis and pneumococci in pneumonia were minimal throughout.

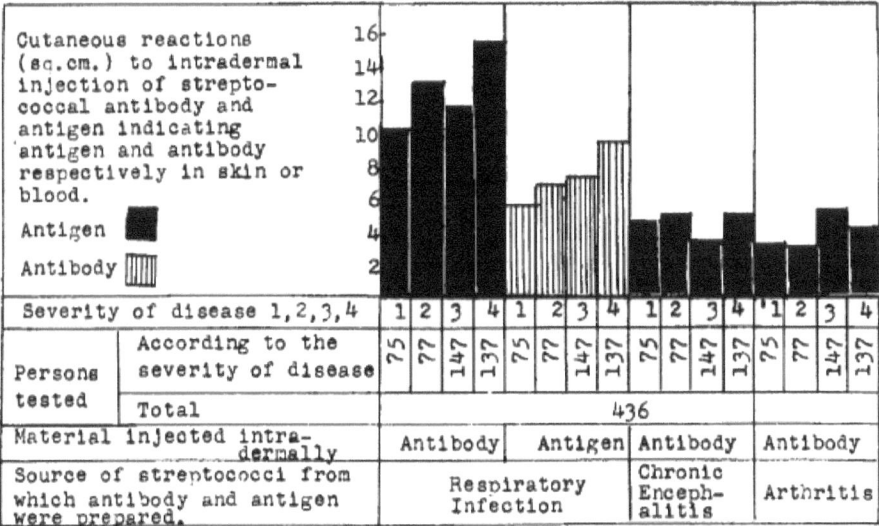

Chart 2.—Cutaneous reactions to intradermal injection of thermal "respiratory" streptococcal antibody and antigen and in contrast to those of control antibody in persons having acute respiratory infection, according to the severity of the disease.

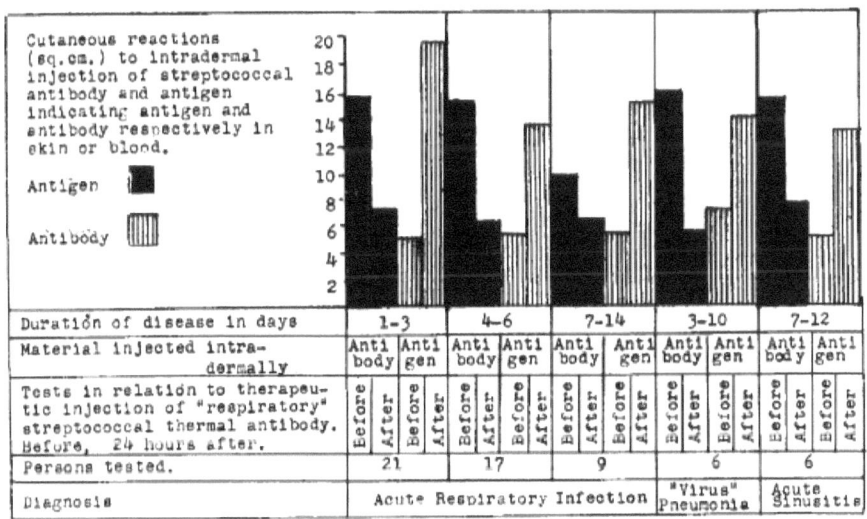

Chart 3.—Cutaneous reactions in relation to subcutaneous therapeutic injection of thermal antibody prepared from streptococci isolated in studies of respiratory infection in persons having acute respiratory infection, "virus" pneumonia, or acute sinusitis.

[AMA Arch Oto 58, 618]

The results of cutaneous reactions in persons having respiratory infection, according to severity of attacks, are summarized similarly in Chart 2. It will be noted that reactions indicating streptococcal antigen and antibody were directly proportional to the severity of the disease, but reactions indicating antibody were proportionately far less than those indicating antigen. Reactions to the control antibody were minimal.

The results of cutaneous reactions in response to subcutaneous therapeutic injection of "respiratory" streptococcal thermal antibody in three groups of persons having acute respiratory infection and one group each having "virus" pneumonia and acute sinusitis are shown graphically in Chart 3. It will be seen that a sharp drop in cutaneous reactions to repeat intradermal injection of thermal antibody, indicating circulating antigen, and a great increase in reactions to repeat intradermal injection of antigen, indicating antibody, often associated with a corresponding clinical improvement, occurred 24 hours after therapeutic injection of antibody. The diminution in antigen and increase in antibody were greatest during the early stages of the disease.

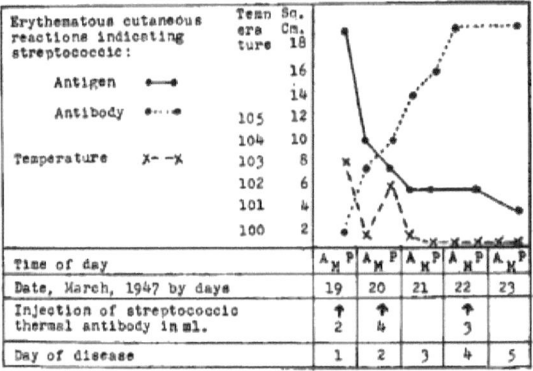

Chart 4.—Effects of therapeutic injection of influenzal streptococcic thermal antibody as indicated by cutaneous reactions to intradermal injection of thermal antibody and antigen, respectively, and temperature in a case of acute influenza.

The effect of therapeutic injection of thermal antibody prepared from streptococci isolated in studies of influenza and other respiratory infections is well illustrated in the following case.

The patient, a business man of robust health, 45 years of age, awoke March 19, 1947, with a sore throat but went to work as usual. The sore throat grew worse, as a dry cough, pain in the chest, and a chill developed during the afternoon. When seen at his home later that afternoon, he had a flushed face, ached severely, and felt exhausted. His temperature was 102.8 F. The blood leucocyte count was 6,500. The nasopharynx, uvula, and soft palate were congested and edematous. The chest was normal. The nasopharynx was swabbed. A pure culture of a greening streptococcus was isolated from the end-point of growth, 10^{-10} of serial dilution cultures in dextrose-brain broth, which on nasal inoculation produced pneumonitis in mice in high incidence. Two milliliters of the respiratory streptococcal antibody was injected subcutaneously. He felt quite well the next morning, went to work, and made a prompt and complete recovery without postinfluenzal exhaustion and was given two additional subcutaneous injections of thermal antibody. The erythematous reactions to intradermal injection of thermal antibody indicating "pneumotropic" streptococcal antigen and intradermal injection of streptococcal antigen indicating antibody in skin or blood, the concomitant drop in temperature, and the time and amounts of subcutaneous injection of thermal antibody are shown graphically in Chart 4.

During an institutional epidemic of influenza it was found that penicillin had little or no curative action in persons in whom the cutaneous test indicating antigen was high, and the reduction of antigen and increase in antibody to repeat tests were far less than in a control group not receiving penicillin, and improvement in symptoms for reasons still obscure was correspondingly delayed. The cutaneous tests have proved of great value in diagnosis of the type of infection at hand, and repeat tests have been of great value in determining the need for reinjection of antibody in treatment.[29]

SUMMARY AND CONCLUSIONS

The results of bacteriological and viral studies of influenza and other epidemic respiratory infections are reviewed, and results of further studies on etiology and treatment by new methods are reported.

The nonhemolytic or green-producing alpha Streptococcus was isolated consistently by special methods from the nasopharynx of persons stricken during life and from the pneumonic lungs after death during the pandemic of 1918-1919 and from the nasopharynx in recurring epidemics ever since. Culturally, morphologically, and antigenically the Streptococcus isolated throughout the years was identical or very similar, but pneumotropic virulence varied according to severity of the disease and epidemic. It was isolated in significant incidence from filtrates of nasopharyngeal washings, from natural influenza virus, from pneumonic lungs produced experimentally in mice with naturally and experimentally produced virus from which the Streptococcus had been isolated, from allantoic fluid of embryonated chicken eggs that had been inoculated with natural influenza virus, and from washings of absorbent material that had been exposed to outdoor air during epidemics of influenza and from filtrates of such washings. Realizing the importance of these experiments, special precautions in the making of these cultures were taken to prevent contamination from extraneous sources.

The importance of pneumotropic nonhemolytic streptococci is indicated furthermore by the formation of agglutinins specific for the Streptococcus during recovery from epidemic influenza, by the formation of specific agglutinin and precipitin and protective antibodies in the serum of horses immunized with the Streptococcus, by the high degree of protection afforded by prophylactic immunization of human beings with the heat-killed streptococcal vaccine containing the nonhemolytic Streptococcus freshly isolated in mediums, such as dextrose-brain broth, which furnish a gradient of oxygen tension and in which specificity was maintained on storage at 10 C. of the partially dehydrated streptococci in dense suspensions of glycerin (2 parts) and saturated NaCl solution (1 part).

Pneumotropic filtrable agents resembling influenza virus have been produced experimentally from the streptococcus isolated respectively from persons with influenza and from natural influenza virus.[30] Convalescent serum and antistreptococcal serums produced in horses, with the Streptococcus neutralized, parallel the natural and experimental influenza virus, and mice were successfully immunized against

---

29. (a) Rosenow, E. C.: Nonhemolytic Streptococci in Relation to an Epidemic of Influenza: Diagnostic Cutaneous Tests and Specific Treatment, A. M. A. Arch. Otolaryng. **54**:609-619, 1951; (b) Studies in Influenza and Pneumonia: Therapeutic Effects of a Monovalent Antistreptococcus Serum in Influenza and Influenzal Pneumonia, J. Infect. Dis. **26**:614-622, 1920.

30. Rosenow.[25b] Footnote 26.

inoculations of natural and experimental virus with composite streptococcic vaccines used successfully for prevention and treatment of influenza in human beings.

Relationship of the Streptococcus and the virus is indicated further (a) by the production in animals of pneumonitis with both the Streptococcus and the virus, (b) by specific agglutination of the pneumotropic Streptococcus and by neutralization of the virus by convalescent serum, (c) by the successful immunization of animals and human beings with the pneumotropic streptococcal vaccine and with the virus vaccine, and (d) by the demonstration in filtrates of the virus [27a] and in tissue cultures of the virus [27b] of spheres, ovoids, and pairs in short and long-chain formation with the electron microscope. The Streptococcus and virus are similar or alike in tropism and antigenicity but greatly different in size. The Streptococcus appears to be the toxicogenic, antigenic phase and the virus the relatively non-toxicogenic nonantigenic, but highly invasive phase.

Additional evidence indicating the importance of the pneumotropic Streptococcus in the epidemiology, etiology, prevention, and treatment of epidemic influenza and milder forms of respiratory infection has been obtained in these studies. The isolation, filtrability, and localizing properties of the Streptococcus isolated from the nasopharynx of persons having a respiratory infection or poliomyelitis and from poliomyelitis virus (Table 1) are in accord with previous studies. Most important, immediate cutaneous reactions to intradermal injection of the respiratory streptococcal thermal antibody in persons having epidemic influenza or related respiratory infections indicating specific circulating streptococcal antigen paralleled the severity of the disease and diminished slowly during natural recovery and abruptly following therapeutic injection of thermal antibody. Reactions indicating antibody as determined on intradermal injection of antigen increased slowly during natural recovery and abruptly after therapeutic subcutaneous injection of respiratory streptococcal antibody (Charts 1, 2, 3, and 4).

The demonstrated parallelism between cutaneous reactions indicating streptococcal antigen and antibody in skin or blood of persons having respiratory infection (Table 2) and to a less degree in well persons within epidemic zones and the isolation of the pneumotropic Streptococcus from outdoor air during such epidemics are considered of great epidemiological importance (Table 3).

The results reported were obtainable only if the underlying principles as regards methods for the isolation of the specific type of Streptococcus and maintenance of specificity were fulfilled. The usual bacteriological mediums and methods did not suffice. On the basis of the results of these combined studies of the Streptococcus and the virus in influenza, the admirable studies which have been made of viruses, especially of influenza virus, lack breadth of concept as regards their source and their relationship to the bacteria, resulting in inadequate bacteriological methods.

Prophylactic immunization against epidemic influenza, as should be expected, has been successful with both the streptococcal and the viral vaccines. Protection with the streptococcal vaccine was afforded in numerous annual outbreaks by many physicians throughout 34 years. Composite pneumotropic streptococcal vaccines made from the undenatured streptococci from a central source were found to protect geographically against influenza and milder respiratory infections. Under proper dosage such streptococcal vaccines proved harmless and nonsensitizing. Recurring respiratory infections in highly susceptible persons have been prevented by prophylactic immunization with composite pneumotropic streptococcal vaccines. Preliminary time-consuming and expensive studies to determine the presence and the type of virus at hand often prove fallacious, because new strains appear during the course of epidemics. These studies are not necessary to afford protection with the streptococcal vaccine. The streptococcal vaccines alone or in combination with the newly developed streptococcal thermal antibody prepared from composite suspensions have been found to be highly efficacious in treatment of epidemic influenza, of milder types of acute respiratory infection, of bronchitis, bronchial asthma, and sinusitis, that so often follow influenza and other types of respiratory infection due to or associated with the Streptococcus. Immunity to influenza induced with virus vaccines, while more enduring than with the streptococcal vaccine, has certain disadvantages. Protection should accrue, because by special methods both the specific type of Streptococcus and the filtrable "virus" phase have been demonstrated. The preparation and use of the virus vaccines are difficult and expensive. Untoward local and constitutional reactions due to primary toxicity of the vaccine prepared from chick embryo cultures of the "virus" or to sensitization to egg and chicken on repeat injections do occur. Antiviral serums suitable for treatment of influenza are nonexistent; whereas pneumotropic antistreptococcal serums and now the pneumotropic streptococcal thermal antibody have been shown to be effective in causing a prompt reduction of circulating antigen, an increase in circulating antibody, and a concomitant clinical improvement.[29b]

On the basis of long-continued studies, it is suggested that the nonhemolytic Streptococcus normally present in the nasopharynx of human beings and broadly in nature tends to acquire "pneumotropic" virulence of varying degree in temperate climates during winter months and sometimes otherwise, resulting in epidemics of influenza and milder types of respiratory infections. As such infections occur, a "virus" or filtrable phase of the "Streptococcus may develop and propagate in varying proportions during the course of the disease and epidemics. Cessation of epidemic outbreaks according to these studies would appear to be due mainly to two factors: (*a*) the acquisition of specific resistance from subclinical and clinical infection in the general population and (*b*) the seasonal loss of "pneumotropic" virulence of the Streptococcus and perhaps of the associated virus.

[*AMA Arch Oto* 58, 622]

[Reprinted per provision 17 USC 107; request in process.]

AFTERWORD: **INFLUENZA, ENCEPHALITIS, IMPLICATIONS**

On the Relation between Influenza and Post-Influenzal (Von Economo's) Encephalitis, and Implications for the Study of the Role of Infection in Epilepsy and Schizophrenia; A Review of the Historical Works and Perspective of E.C. Rosenow (1875-1966), longtime head of Experimental Bacteriology (1915-44) for the Mayo Foundation, Rochester, Minnesota.

By S. H. Shakman, Institute Of Science, *InstituteOfScience.com / I-o-S.org*
July 1, 2003*

Many of the component research pathways supporting and comprising the growing modern consensus that infection is involved in the cause of schizophrenia and related conditions find independent support in the historical record of the Mayo Foundation's former head of Experimental Bacteriology, the late E.C. Rosenow, MD (1875-1966). In particular, Rosenow's extensive, multi-decade experience while at the Mayo Foundation (1915-44) with influenza and encephalitis, respectively, and the relation between them, provided the requisite foundation for his later extension of studies, over the decade following his departure from Mayo in 1944, into epilepsy, schizophrenia and other associated conditions.

It may be noted at the outset that the scope of Rosenow's microbiology was far more comprehensive than that which might be strictly-defined by the term "bacteriology", incorporating as essential components transmutations among microbial species, as well as considerations of reversibly dissociative, filter-passing forms, and their toxins, and comparisons with natural filter-passing (viral) forms.

The backdrop for Rosenow's role at the Mayo Foundation in the 1918-9 influenza pandemic, and indeed for his monumental body of work spanning more than a half-century of publication in the medical literature, dates back more than a decade earlier to his works with pneumonia, wherein he presented evidence from blood cultures that lobar pneumonia may be a "secondary localization of a primary blood invasion and not a local disease ... " [1,2], and to 1912 studies of the relation of a peculiar streptococcus to epidemic sore throat [3,4]. Over the ensuing years he investigated the potential role of microbes, particularly pneumococci and streptococci, in these and other conditions.

Special studies of the streptococcus-pneumococcus group were reported in 1914 [5], based on prior works by himself and others since 1906, whereby variations in oxygen tensions and salt concentration, growth in symbiosis with other bacteria, and injections into cavities in animals were found to commonly call forth mutational forms in streptococci. Virulence and fermentative powers were found to be diminished in vitro, and increased in vivo. To assure that the claimed mutations were not the result of mixed cultures from the start, cultures of each main variety were initiated with single organisms obtained by the Barber method; and all tests available were incorporated to demonstrate that these were indeed complete transformations, including, morphology, presence of capsule, fermentative powers, solubility or insolubility in NaCl solution, and behavior toward the respective broth culture filtrates (Marmorek's test).

Table 1. Transmutations; Streptococci to/from Pneumococci [5]

Original strain	Mutation	(number of strains mutated)
S.hemolytic to	S.rheumatism	(1)
	S.viridans	(21)
	pneumococci	(3)
	S.mucosis	(1)
S viridans to	pneumococci	(17)
	S.mucosus	(2)
	S.hemolytic	(10)
pneumococci to	S.hemolytic	(11)
	S.rheumatism	(3)
	S.viridans	(7)
S.mucosis to	hemolytic S.	(5)
	S.viridans	(2)

Also in 1914 he published details of his evolving methodology for making cultures from excised tissues, blood and other fluids through the use of tall tubes affording an oxygen pressure gradiant, from aerobic at the top to anaerobic at the bottom, aided by a sterile piece of tissue at the bottom if strictly anaerobic conditions are required. [6] Rosenow would continue to use fundamentally the same methodology for the next four decades, using calf or beef brain tissue to assure anaerobism at the bottom of the tubes as early as 1919 [7]; and modifying the method of isolating streptococci through the use of serial dilution cultures as early as 1935, associated with the finding that growth at higher dilutions often occurred despite absence at lower dilutions presumably due to inhibiting substances rendered inactive by dilution. [8]

The finding that relatively avirulent strains might be made virulent by successive animal passage, and the reverse by cultivation, along with other studies suggested to Rosenow that diseases of widely different symptomatology might be associated with microbes of related species but with differing infecting powers. Accordingly he undertook associated studies of other conditions of uncertain etiology, including conditions of the nervous system. In 1916 he reported that intravenous injections of cultures from multiple sclerosis, neuralgia, and multiple neuritis resulted in production of characteristic lesions in the spinal cord, dorsal nerve roots, and peripheral nerves, respectively, of experimental animals. [9]

Table 2. Intravenous Injection of Bacteria (Mixed, Primarily Streptococci) [9]

Source of Bacteria	% of Animals with Lesions in:			
	Spinal Cord	Dorsal Roots	Nerve Trunks	Muscles
multiple sclerosis	58	0	0	29
neuralgia	6	83	28	33
multiple neuritis	5	0	79	27
"Myalgia"	3	0	7	93

These results were to be revisited five years later as the basis of detailed studies of post-influenzal encephalitis, this as a sequel to his major involvement on behalf of the Mayo Foundation with the 1918-9 influenza pandemic.

In Rosenow's words, "The epidemic was severe, and the need and the demand for vaccination were great; a large number of cases were available for bacteriologic study, and to supply the proper strains for the vaccine. ... Owing to the foresight of the founders of the Mayo Foundation, necessary funds to meet the emergency were available. A large amount of the vaccine has been prepared and sent gratis on request to numerous physicians on condition that reports of the results be returned." [10]

On the basis of responses involving nearly a half-million persons, it was reported that unvaccinated persons were more than three times as likely to contract influenza, and six times as likely to die, as compared to persons receiving three prophylactic inoculations.

Table 3. Results reported in questionnaires from all sources [10]

	Number of Persons	Incidence per thousand of:		
		Influenza	Pneumonia	Deaths
One inoculation	26,936	118.2	8.7	3.0
Two inoculations	23,348	97.0	3.04	2.62
Three inoculations	93,476	87.9	4.4	1.43
Not vaccinated	345,133	281.8	21	8.55
	488,893			

Whereas Rosenow's initial vaccine used in 1918 had contained a small portion of influenza bacilli, these were rarely found later in the epidemic and thus were omitted from the vaccines used in this report; for the most part these reported vaccines were comprised of mixed cultures of fixed types of pneumococci (30%), pneumococci group IV and allied green-producing diplostreptococci (40%), hemolytic streptococci (20%) and staphylococcus aureus (10%). Of these, Rosenow suggested "that of all the bacteria isolated, the somewhat peculiar green-producing streptococcus or diplostreptococcus is the most important. This organism is present in large numbers at the very outset of symptoms of influenza and of the accompanying pneumonia; it is commonly present after death." Further, intraperitoneal injections of sputum or mass cultures in animals resulted in death, usually from invasion of the green-producing streptococci or pneumococci; and intratracheal injections closely simulated influenzal pneumonia.

In 1924 Rosenow discussed the extreme specificity of the characteristic green-producing streptococci, particularly in the case of nervous system diseases. In addition to the 1916 results for nervous system diseases discussed above, he cited the reproduction of characteristic lesions in intervertebral ganglions in rabbits and dogs by IV injection of green-producing streptococci from herpes zoster; in the posterior or sensory roots of rabbits, in the case of intercostal neuralgia; in the sheaths of large nerve trunks, in the case of sciatica; and paralysis with hemorrhagic lesions in the cord, in a series of animals, from infectious transverse myelitis.

These results had prompted him to apply these same methods, over a four-year period from 1921 to 1924, to the study of epidemic encephalitis, and encephalitis contacts, epidemic hiccup, spasmodic torticollis and respiratory arrhythmia (plus normal controls). In these conditions, he noted a constant finding of a low grade pharyngitis, and, as in his earlier experiments with other nervous system diseases, was able to isolate a similar streptococcus using methods affording a gradient of oxygen pressure.

Whereas intravenous injections had been found to yield striking results in the case of some nervous system conditions such as MS, neuralgia and multiple neuritis, it was found that intracerebral injections of small amounts of suspensions (in NaCl solution) were more likely to produce characteristic symptoms in the case of encephalitis. This method enabled the production of "profound lethargy never before seen or described in rabbits" from a fatal case of epidemic encephalitis, and similar results from eighty-one additional cases of various forms of encephalitis. [11]

It was noted that in sharp contrast to the production of epidemic or other forms of encephalitis by intracerebral injection of a strain from epidemic encephalitis, intratracheal injection of this strain produced little or no effect. However, following a series of rapid animal passages the virulence increased whereby intracerebral injection produced acute encephalitis associated with meningitis, and intratracheal injection produced marked hemorrhagic edema of the lungs associated with leukopenia. Rosenow stated at the time that these were "experimental facts in accord with the observation that epidemics of encephalitis usually follow, or occur coincidental with, influenzal outbreaks." [12]

In 1928 Rosenow followed up on his earlier results, noting that they had been recently confirmed by Evans and Freeman [13].

At this time he reported results of further experiments involving encephalitis and other nervous system diseases. He noted as particularly striking, among rabbits injected with organisms from epidemic encephalitis, a high percentage exhibiting lethargic behavior, 54%, compared to much lower percentages of such behavior in rabbits injected with organisms from other strains. In those rabbits exhibiting lethargy, "It varied in intensity and duration from slight somnolence lasting for a day or two to deep sleep continuing for a number of days, from which the animal could be aroused only with difficulty." It was noted that certain symptoms such as ataxia, tremors, hyperpnea and paralysis are relatively common in most of the conditions in this study, particularly in fatal cases; and in the case of parkinsonian encephalitis, that ataxia and tremors were "often pronounced", despite a lack of particularly high incidence among symptoms listed.

Table 4. Symptoms in Rabbits from Intracerebral Injection of Streptococci [11]

Source of strains	Number Injected	% Spasms of Diaphragm	% Lethargic	% Ataxia
Epidemic Hiccup	15	33	7	33
Epidemic encephalitis	50	2	54	20
Myoclonic encephalitis	31	3	9	23
Parkinsonian encephalitis	128	2	2	38
Respiratory arrhythmia	20	0	5	45
Spasmodic torticollis	52	0	0	44
Chorea	52	0	0	57

Over the years numerous investigators were able to replicate Rosenow's results through strict adherence to his protocols. [14] The extreme specificity noted by Rosenow in the case of nervous system diseases was independently and dramatically characterized by others who witnessed his results. For example, Jarlov and Brinch described how "Rosenow ... demonstrated in his laboratory an experiment on a single rabbit which was infected with material from a patient who had died under violent encephalitic hiccoughs. Already 48 hours after the injection, the animal died in front of the visitors' eyes after having hiccoughed violently for several hours." [15]

And Rowntree had related how Rosenow was able to "repeatedly by intracerebral injections ... set off syndromes in rabbits the exact counterparts of the clinical manifestations observed in the patients - especially tics of one kind or another. When the patient and the rabbit were placed side by side the resemblance of syndromes [was] often unbelievable and at times almost ludicrous and suggestive of plagiarism. ... he prepared autogenous vaccines that worked miracles in innumerable patients." [16]

In 1929 Rosenow reported that viability and specific properties of streptococci could be preserved for long periods of time in dense suspensions in two parts glycerol to one part saturated NaCl solution. [17] Use of such suspensions was retained as a tool throughout the remainder of Rosenow's career. He would later report that heat-killed vaccines prepared from dilutions of these suspensions were much less toxic and more antigenic than vaccines prepared directly from cultures and elicited a more rapid and more favorable, response." [18]

In 1933 Rosenow recorded seasonal changes in cataphoretic measurements as well as similarities between organisms isolated during convalescence from influenza and those from remote cases of chronic encephalitis. He also noted a "striking parallelism" between measurements of streptococci from ill persons and those from the raw milk supply during epidemics, and the return to normal patterns of both after the epidemics. These results were cited as further evidence of a role for these organisms in both influenza and encephalitis. [19]

In 1935 he reported on a new medium for cultivation of the streptotoccus, autoclaved chick mash; intracerebral inoculation of streptococci cultured in this medium enabled the replication of typical lesions of encephalitis, both in type and distribution, as well as symptoms; whereas the streptococcus from encephalitis that had been derived from dextrose-brain broth had enabled replication of symptoms, but lesions induced had often been atypical both in type and distribution. Added attributes of this chick mash medium were that it was highly favorable for rapid growth and long-term maintenance of viability of streptococci, and it did not turn acid from growth of streptococci. [20]

But its two most remarkable attributes were that (a) on prolonged storage of streptococci in the chick mash medium, changes in agglutinative titer and virulence occurred seasonally in accord with current epidemics of encephalitis and respiratory infection, and (b) as cultures in the chick mash medium became old, very small and filtrable forms appeared, which were found to behave "quite like the 'natural' viruses of these diseases." [21] Thus, with this new medium Rosenow was able over the next two decades to more fully explore prospective relations of the streptococcus to seasonal epidemics; as well as the relation between the streptococcus and dissociative filtrable forms, and between these "artificial" filtrable forms and the natural virus.

Noting that changes in cataphoretic velocity and virulence of streptococci had been induced by exposure to the high frequency field, by Rosenow and others as early as 1933, and that mutations or dissociations in bacteria and viruses had been produced by others on exposure to x-rays, ultraviolet, and other radiation, Rosenow hypothesized that the responsible agent for the observed changes may be some form of radiant energy. [21] This hypothesis was tested in three long-lasting storage experiments, in which organisms derived from "neurotropic" (poliomyelitis) and "pneumotropic" (from influenza) sources were stored (in the chick mash medium) in a mine 5000 feet under limestone and compared with samples stored (in this same medium) at ground level where they would be exposed to solar radiation and also in a lead-lined safe where they would not be so exposed. Rosenow found that the samples exposed to radiation changed properties seasonally, as indicated by measurements of cataphoretic velocity, but that samples shielded from solar radiation did not change. [22] In contrast, organisms stored at ground level for up to 7 years in glycerol-NaCl (2:1) suspensions were found to retain their original specificity regardless of season or current epidemic.

In a subsequent series of experiments, Rosenow was able to demonstrate parallel altered infectivity in the case of both non-filtrable (streptococcal) and filtrable forms in accord with seasonal occurrence of neurotropic and pneumotropic epidemics respectively. [23] The concept of a phasal nature of the involved organisms, critical to an understanding of how Rosenow's well-documented and monumental studies of the role of streptococcal forms in a range of diseases might be integrated with bodies of work implicating filtrable (viral) forms, was by no means originated by or isolated to Rosenow's works.

As precedents he prominently cited the 1927 work of Phillip Hadley and his comprehensive discussions of the large body of earlier literature on dissociation, including numerous investigators from the 19th Century. These included Nägeli, who in 1877 advocated extreme variability, and Cohn, whose contrary views had become the accepted dogma after being adopted by Robert Koch and followers. Hadley had discussed in detail "an ever-increasing mass of evidence pointing to the instability of bacterial species [which] ... may have a more significant bearing on problems of virulence, infection and immunity than many have supposed." [24]

While results from preliminary studies of epilepsy and schizophrenia, conducted in association with studies of other conditions as early as 1935, were noted as "highly suggestive", it was not until 1943-4 that Rosenow was able to undertake a more concentrated study of cases of epilepsy and dementia precox at Rochester, Minnesota State Hospital from an infectious standpoint. Following his retirement from Mayo in 1944, he was able to resume full time studies in this area a year later at Longview Hospital in Cincinnati Ohio. Results of this work were published in a three-part series of articles in 1947-8 [25].

Part I of this series recorded (in 14 tables) results of agglutination, agglutinin absorption, and precipitation experiments between streptococci, streptococcal polysaccharides, and/or nasopharangeal swabbings from patients; and serum of patients, thermal [26] antibody, and/or serums of and antiserums prepared in horses and rabbits. [25(a)] For example, Table 5 below illustrates some results of his agglutination experiments:

Table 5. Agglutination of Alpha Streptococci Isolated in Studies of Epilepsy, Schizophrenia and Arthritis by Serums of Persons Suffering From these Respective Conditions [25(a)]

Source of Streptococci	Number of Strains	Percent of Total Possible Agglutination by Serum of Persons Suffering From:			
		Epilepsy	Schizophrenia	Arthritis	Control
Epilepsy	23	64	45	19	20
Schizophrenia	22	45	68	26	19
Arthritis	43	14	19	53	16

Part II of this three-part series reported on symptoms and signs in rabbits and mice following intracerebral inoculation of streptococci from persons with epilepsy and schizophrenia. [25(b)] Part III recorded cutaneous reactions in persons with schizophrenia and epilepsy to intradermal injection of antigen and natural and in vitro streptococcal antibody, comparisons of results on admission and recovery, and comparative results for relatives and married couples. Also incorporated were effects of electro-shock in relation to circulating antibody and antigen, as reflected in cutaneous reactions. He concluded that the data implicated "specific types of alpha streptococci of low general but high and specific 'neurotropic' virulence ... [which] produce neurotoxins which have predilection for certain structures in the brain and thus may play a role in pathogenesis ... " of epilepsy and schizophrenia. [25(c)] (Rosenow's antibody-antigen tests were based on and a new application of Foshay's classic 1936 work [27].)

Also in 1948, in an article recapping studies of multiple sclerosis, Rosenow provided details of animal experiments indicating a great degree of specificity as among nervous system diseases, including schizophrenia, epilepsy, poliomyelitis and MS:

Table 6. ANIMAL EXPERIMENTS Schizophrenia, Epilepsy, Polio, MS [28]

	(% Symptoms in rabbits; and % positive brain cultures)				
Organism from:	Normal Control	Schizophrenia	Epilepsy	Polio	MS
% Died	25	87	74	46	60
% Hyperactivity	2	87	25	26	36
% Tremors	4	79	75	33	70
% Spasms	2	21	75	35	23
% Convulsions	0	3	34	2	1
% Ataxia	16	10	13	23	66
% Nystagmus	7	0	5	2	29
% Paralysis	8	9	16	70	49
% Positive Brain Cultures	25	83	93	91	62

It may also be noted that histamine was reported to decrease antigen and increase antibody.

In a subsequent article Rosenow reported production of epilepsy in mice by intracerebral injection of streptococci, recording spasms in 93% and convulsions in 69% of 130 mice inoculated, versus spasms in 7% and convulsions in 2% of 44 control mice. In this article he discussed an apparent prenatal passage of epilepsy, this in the case of a pregnant mouse intracerebrally inoculated with a streptococcus cultured from a case of epilepsy; one of four offspring died in a grand mal seizure several weeks after birth. A pure culture of streptococcus was isolated from the brain, and produced spasms in 19 and convulsions in 16 of 22 mice that were repeatedly inoculated intranasally. Notwithstanding these results and modern documentation of a higher than normal incidence of epilepsy in association with autism, there seems to have been no mention of the latter by Dr. Rosenow in this or other discussions of epilepsy. [29]

One of the most unusual sets of experiments conducted by Rosenow followed from an unexpected occurrence in a study of a prison population. Nervous prisoners with intercurrent arthritis, myositis, stomach ulcer or respiratory infection reacted not only to specific respective "thermal" (artificial) antibody, but even more strongly to antibody from streptococci isolated in studies of chronic encephalitis. This led to study of violent criminality from a bacteriologic standpoint, where it was found that streptococci isolated from incorrigible prisoners in accord with Rosenow's methodology, on intracerebral inoculation, tended to produce behavior which in some respects simulated incorrigible behavior. This included "severe tremors and excitation, hyperirritability, dashing about wildly, jumping up at the wall of the cage at repeated intervals, burying the head in bedding on the floor or under other mice and dashing over the huddle of more normal mice. Others walked slowly about in a dazed manner." Cutaneous reactions and agglutinative titer tests substantiated specificity of infection associated with incorrigibility. [30]

In his last article specifically directed at schizophrenia and related disorders, Dr. Rosenow once again emphasized that "These highly specific results were obtained by the use of special methods. The usual methods did not suffice." Herein he reported results of numerous additional sets of tests involving cutaneous reactions and agglutinative titer, and indicating specificity of infection with organisms cultured exclusively from nasopharyngeal swabbings. These included cutaneous reactions to thermal antibody, to the implicated streptococcus before and after vaccine, and to antibody with and without chlorpromazine and before and after oral chlorpromazine.

Additional agglutinative titer tests reported involved pooled blood serum, blood and spinal fluid on admittance, A.M. urine specimens, serum by season, serum and urine in relation to chlorpromazine, serum with and without chlorpromazine, A.M. urine with and without chlorpromazine, and serum on admittance and later in relation to chlorpromazine. It may be noted that based on these tests chlorpromazine was contraindicated immunologically.

In this article Rosenow also reported positive correlations between schizophrenia and some psychoneurotic and psychophysiologic disorders in terms of agglutinative titer of blood serum, in sharp contrast to distinctly negative results for well controls and chronic brain syndromes due to syphillis. He also found surprisingly strong indications of specificity (for an infectious agent isolated from schizophrenia cases) in cases of "mental deficiency", implying that such a condition might be amenable to therapy, etc. Also noted were relatively higher agglutinative titers of patients on admission during Winter and Spring, as compared to lower levels in Summer and lowest in Autumn.

Rosenow's conclusion: "It is realized how contrary to current psychiatric tenets the concept that schizophrenia and related mental disorders can possibly be due to an infectious process, but the results of bacteriological studies by the special methods used indicate that such is nevertheless the case." [31]

1. Rosenow, E.C., The Blood in Lobar Pneumonia, with remarks concerning treatment, JAMA 44:871-873, (March 18) 1905, 871-3.

2. Rosenow, E.C., Virulent pneumococci, opsonin, and phagocytosis. Illinois Med. Jour. 13: '3-19. 1908.

3. Rosenow, E.C., An epidemic of sore throat due to a peculiar streptococcus. Jour. Am. Med. Assn. 58:773, 1912. (With D. J. Davis.)

4. Rosenow, E.C., A study of streptococci from milk and from epidemic sore throat, and the effect of milk on streptococci. Jour. Infect. Dis. 11:338-346 1912.

5. Rosenow, E.C., Transmutations within the streptococcus-pneumococcus group. Jour. Infect. Dis. 14:1-32, 1914.

6. Rosenow, E.C., The newer bacteriology of various infections as determined by special methods, JAMA LXIII (Sept. 12, 1914), 903-908.

7. Rosenow, E.C., Studies on elective localization. Focal infection with special reference to oral sepsis. Jour. Dental Res. 1:205-267, 1919.

8. Rosenow, E.C., The relation of streptococci to the viruses of poliomyelitis and encephalitis: preliminary report. Proc. Staff Meetings of Mayo Clinic 10:410-414 (June 26) 1935.

9. Rosenow, E.C., Elective localization of bacteria in diseases of the nervous system. Jour. Am. Med. Assn. 67:662-665, 1916.

10. Rosenow, E.C., Studies in influenza and pneumonia. IV. Further results of prophylactic inoculation. Jour. Am. Med. Assn. 73:396-401, 1919. (With B. F. Sturdivant.)

11. Rosenow, E.C., Localization in animals of streptococci from cases of epidemic hiccup, encephalitis, spasmodic torticollis, and chorea. Arch. Neurol. and Psychiat. 19:424-436, 1928; abstract J.A.M.A., April 28, 1928, 1407.

12. Rosenow, E.C., Specificity of streptococci in the etiology of diseases of the nervous system. Jour. Am. Med. Assn. 82:449-453, 1924.

13. Freeman, Walter, JAMA 87: 1601, Nov. 13, 1926); and Alice C. Evans, U.S. Public Health Rep. 41:1095, 1926; and Evans, Alice C., U.S. Public Health Rep. 42:171, 1927.

14. (a) Haden RL, Dent. Infect.& Systemic Diseases, Lea & Febiger, 1928.
    (b) Barnes AR & AS Giordano, J.Indiana Med.Ass. 15: 1-7, 1932.
    (c) Nickel AC, AR Hufford, Arch.Int.Med 41:210-30, 1928.
    (d) Nickel AC, Staff Meet.Mayo Clinic 3 Aug.8,1928,232-5.
    (e) Nickel AC and WW Sager, ibid Oct 10, 1928, 297-9.
    (f) Cooper ML, Tr.Am.Pediat.Soc. 43:32-33, 1931.
    (g) Jarlov, E. and Brinch, O., Hospitalstid 81:80-5, 1938.
    (h) Welsh AL, Arch.Derm.&Syph. 30:611-629, 1934.
    (i) Welsh A, J.Invest.Dermat. 7:7-42, 1946.
    (j) Meisser JG & BS Gardner, J.Nat.Dental Assn.19:578-592,1922.
    (k) Cook TJ, J.Amer.Dent.A. 18, 2290-2301, 1931.
    (l) Bernhardt H, Z.f.Klin.Med. 117:158-174, 1931.
    (m) Irons EE, etal, J.Inf.Dis. 18:315-334, 1916.

(n) Kelley TH, Ohio State MJ 14:221-223, 1918.
(o) Topley WWC, and HB Weir, J.Path.& Bact. 24:333-346, 1921.
(p) Wilkie DPD, Brit.J.J. 1:481-4, 1928.
(q) Jones NW & SJ Newsom, Arch.Path. 13:392-414, 1932.
(r) E.A. Bering, J Neurol., Neurosurg. & Psych 14:205-8, 1951.
(s) Stortebecker, J. Canad. Dent. Ass.33:301-311, 1967.

15. Jarlov E., Brinch O, Danish Section, Assoc.Internationale Pour les Recherches sur la Paradentose, Copenhagen: Lassen and Stiedl, 1938; abstr.- JAMA 111 (1938), 290.

16. Leonard G. Rowntree, Amid Masters of Twentieth Century Medicine, Charles C. Thomas, Springfield Ill. 1958.

17. Rosenow, E.C., Results in various diseases from elimination of foci of infection and use of vaccines prepared from streptococci having elective localizing power. Jour. Lab. and Clin. Med. 14:504-512, 1929.

18. Rosenow, E.C., Streptococcal vaccines in prevention and treatment of respiratory infections; clinical and experimental study, Am. J. Clin. Path. 8: 17-27, Jan. 1938 (with F. R. Heilman).

19. Rosenow, E.C., Seasonal changes in the cataphoretic velocity and virulence of streptococci as isolated from well persons, from persons having epidemic or other diseases, and from raw milk. Jour. Infect. Dis. 53: 1-11 (July-August) 1933.

20. Rosenow, E.C., Seasonal changes of streptococci isolated in studies of poliomyelitis, encephalitis and respiratory infection, Postgrad. Med. 7: 117-123, Feb. 1950.

21. Rosenow, E.C., The relation of streptococci to the viruses of poliomyelitis and encephalitis: preliminary report. Proc. Staff Meetings of Mayo Clinic 10:410-414 (June 26) 1935.

22. Rosenow, E.C., Radiant energy as probable cause of seasonal changes in specificity of nonhemolytic streptococci, Postgrad. Med. 8: 290-292, Oct. 1950.

23. Rosenow, E.C., Parallel production of altered infectivity of Streptococcus and related filtrable agents isolated from outdoor air, J. Aviation Med. 22: 225-243, June 1951.

24. Hadley, Phillip: Microbic dissociation; the instability of bacterial species with special reference to active dissociaton and transmissible autolysis. J. Infect. Dis. 40:1-312, 1927.

25. (a) Rosenow, E.C., Bacteriologic, etiologic, and serologic studies in epilepsy and schizophrenia, Postgrad. Med. 2: 346-357, Nov. 1947.
(b) Rosenow, E.C., Bacteriologic, etiologic, and serologic studies in epilepsy and schizophrenia; effects in animals following inoculation of alpha streptococci, Postgrad. Med. 124-136, Feb. 1948.
(c) Rosenow, E.C., Bacteriologic, etiologic, and serologic studies in epilepsy and schizophrenia; cutaneous reactions to intradermal injection of streptococcal antibody and antigen, Postgrad. Med. 3: 367-376, May 1948.

26. Rosenow, E.C., Production in vitro of substances resembling antibodies from bacteria. J. Infect. Dis. 76: 163-178, May-June 1945; Diagnostic cutaneous reactions to intradermal interjection of natural and artificial antibody and of antigen prepared from streptococci isolated in studies of diverse diseases, Ann.Allergy 6: 485-496, Sept.-Oct. 1948.

27. Foshay, Lee, J. Infectious Dis. 59 (1936) 330-339, "The Nature of the Bacterial-Specific Intradermal Antiserum Reaction".

28. E.C.Rosenow, Ann. Allergy 6, 1948, 271-92.

29. Rosenow, E.C., Bacteriological studies in idiopathic
epilepsy and schizophrenia, South Dakota J. Med. and Pharm. 5: 243-248; 262; 272, Sept. 1952.

30. Rosenow, E.C., Influence of streptococcal infections on compulsive behavior of criminals, Postgrad. Med. 10: 423-432, Nov. 1951 (with O. F. Rosenow).

31. E.C. Rosenow, J. Nerv. and Ment. Dis. 122, 321-331, October 1955

***

*© S. H. Shakman / Institute Of Science July 1, 2003 All Rights Reserved. (Solicited by SH Fatemi,MD for his proposed 2003 book, Infectious Etiologies of Neuropsychiatric Disorders, submitted as requested July 1, 2003; book cancelled Feb. 17, 2004 by Wiley.co.uk /Charlotte Brabant); Posted at InstituteOfScience.com on November 10, 2009.

www.ingramcontent.com/pod-product-compliance
Lightning Source LLC
Chambersburg PA
CBHW030917180526
45163CB00002B/371